Before You Dive into Your Bo[ok]

Scan this code to unlock additional bonus features!

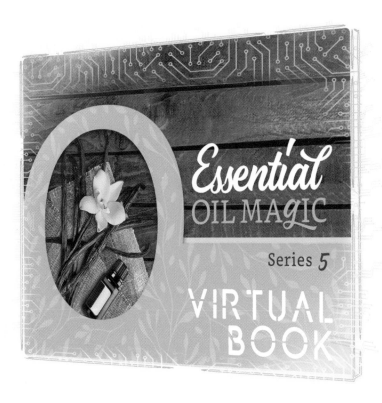

Scan here!

oilmagicbook.com/aeom

The QR Codes in this book unlock additional features in the Essential Oil Magic mini virtual book!

> *All your essentials available on-the-go*
> *Hundreds of common ailments*
> *Popular protocols*
> *All your favorite oils & blends*
> *Extra bonus content*

It's the original Oil Magic book, now in an amazing virtual format. It's interactive, accessible on any device, and makes using oils easier than ever...

...and we'd like you to enjoy it for free.

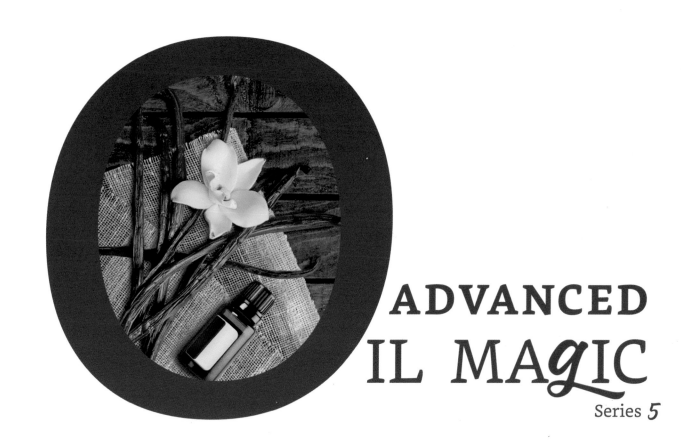

ADVANCED

OIL MAGIC

Series 5

Advanced Oil Magic
Essential Oil Guidebook, Usage & Protocols, and DIY & Diffuser Recipes

Series 5 - September 2021

ISBN: 978-0-9993689-8-5

Published by:

Oil Magic Book
Salt Lake City, UT
contact@oilmagicbook.com

"We do not need magic to transform our world. We carry all of the power we need inside ourselves already."

-J.K. Rowling

Get Your *Aromatherapy Bracelet,*
Support Empowering Women

Try the Custom LETS Aromatherapy Blend on Your Bracelet!

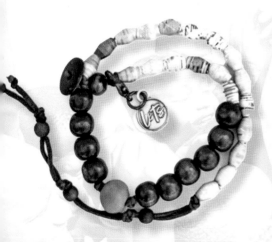

2 drops Myrrh

1 drop Black Spruce

1 drop Siberian Fir

2 drops Wild Orange

1 drop Ylang Ylang

1 drop Patchouli

2 drops Lime

Combine oils and drop a few drops onto your LETS bracelet to enjoy the aroma of liberation, courage, and hope.

LETS empowers women, men, and young people to make informed choices about their fertility, health and well-being through proven educational programs and tools.

The beautiful LETS aromatherapy bracelet helps women track their menstrual cycles, and is accompanied by critical fertility and health education in areas of the world where families are in need of this empowerment.

The positive benefits include preventing unplanned pregnancies, improving quality of life, and eliminating human trafficking, child poverty, and abuse before it begins.

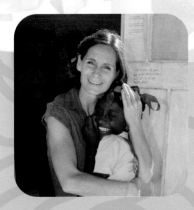

Order your aromatherapy bracelet or subscribe to the monthly *LETS Empowerment Club* to continue empowering women.

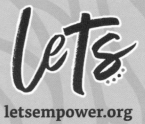

letsempower.org

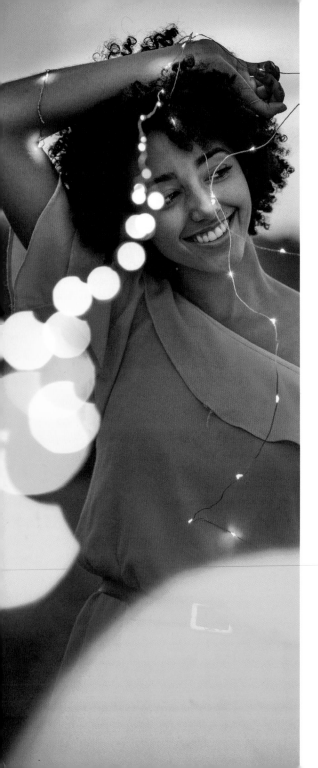

About this book

ADVANCED Oil Magic brings the balance of essential magic and science. The magic is in the protocols. The science backs it up.

The contents of this book have been compiled with influence from the best resources, researchers, doctors, naturopaths, and holistic specialists. While a true relationship with essential oils and natural remedies comes from discovering what works best for your body, following the recommendations in this book will get you off to a perfect start.

ADVANCED Oil Magic features gorgeous artwork from up-and-coming photographers featured on Unsplash. Visit www.oilmagicbook.com to learn more and find your favorite featured artists.

A most common complaint among essential oil users is that they want more specific instruction. Many people are used to explicit usage instructions from traditional healthcare providers. ADVANCED Oil Magic provides similar guidance for the natural world.

Use this guide as your first go-to. Turn to nature as your first resort, and remember that you also have the power of western medicine when needed.

Enjoy all the things your oils can do for you. Play the aromas and have fun blending oils to make your own experiences. Try creative DIY projects found on the individual oil pages. Discover how unlimited the possibilities are.

Most importantly, see what happens to your confidence as you learn to trust nature and yourself with your family's wellness.

Use the A-Z Quick Reference to find quick options for hundreds of ailments. Discover the top uses of popular essential oils in the Single Oils and Oil Blends sections. Use the Protocols section to get serious results. Once you've become accustomed to solving health challenges with natural solutions first, uplevel your experience with Emotions & Energy and Lifestyle Protocols!

Here's to all the magic you'll create.

Table of *Contents*

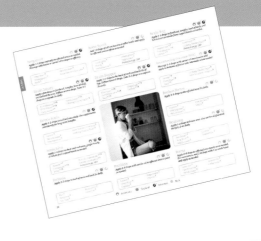

Start by looking up quick suggestions for your health challenges & needs.

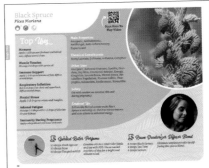

Then get to know your essential oils a bit more.

Commit to a Protocol or a Lifestyle Protocol to get big, long-term results.

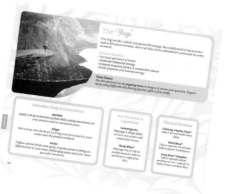

Explore more in this book!
Simply flash your smart phone's camera at the QR codes throughout this book to pull up videos and other amazing insights.

Oil Magic does not provide technical support for QR codes. Please refer to your smart phone manufacturer for help scanning codes.

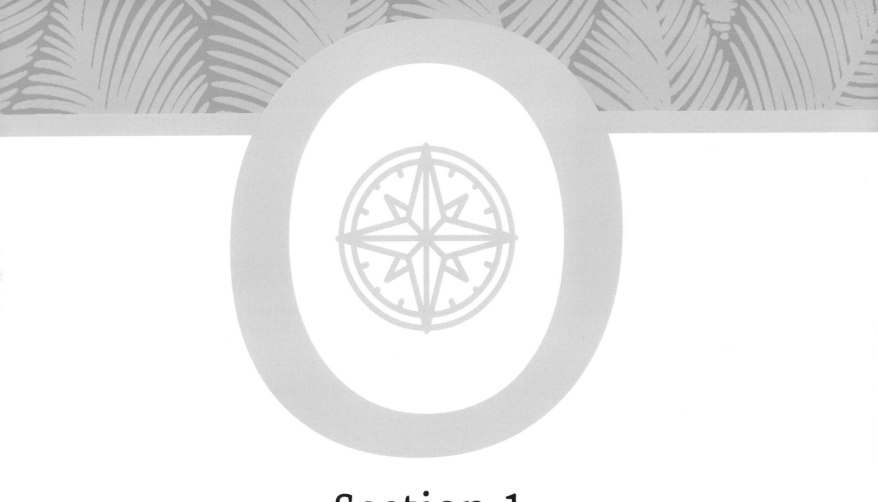

Section 1
Advanced Usage Guide

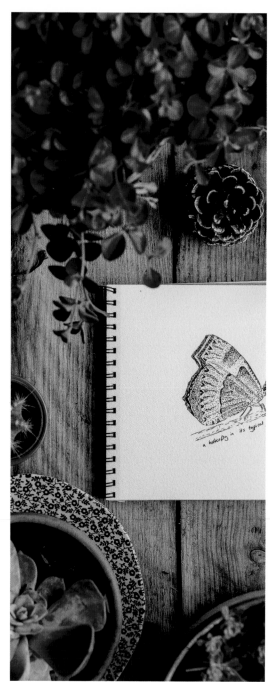

What is an Essential Oil?

Volatile Aromatic Compounds
Essential oils are volatile compounds naturally occurring in certain plants. They are extracted from seeds, flowers, bark, resins, leaves, rinds, and roots. The word "volatile" means they easily evaporate at normal temperatures.

Distillation
While many essential oils on the market are extracted using practices that render the oil impure and non-therapeutic, a true essential oil is carefully distilled using either steam distillation or cold pressing (citrus oils).

Benefits
Essential oils provide a number of benefits to plants, and many of those benefits are passed onto the human body with appropriate application:

- Anti-bacterial, anti-fungal, anti-viral, and anti-parasitic protection
- Restoration and regeneration from physical damage
- Communication via chemical signals

Misconceptions
Contrary to occasional misconception, essential oils do not contain vitamins or minerals. The health benefits they provide occur from the interactions of their naturally occurring chemical constituents with the human body in various ways.

Another misconception is that essential oils are the "lifeblood of the plant." Oils contribute significantly to a plant's well-being, but they do not keep the plant alive.

Original Medicine
While the term "alternative medicine" is a buzz word frequently used to describe remedies like herbs and essential oils, plant medicine is indeed *original* medicine.

Plants have been used for medicinal purposes for thousands of years in every culture. Modern science is quickly recognizing and validating the usefulness of plants as medicine (see the Science and Research section).

The Power of Aroma
Essential oils affect the body quickly and powerfully. When used aromatically, aromatic compounds interact with the olfactory system and limbic system to effectively instigate therapeutic chemical changes in the body. When used internally or topically, they interact directly with cells, organs, and entire body systems for health benefits.

Uses

It's hard to go wrong when using essential oils. This book suggests ways to use your oils for specific conditions, but you can try what feels best for your body.

Over time you'll discover your favorite ways to use your oils.

Aromatic

Diffuse

Put 4-8 drops in a diffuser to spread the oil throughout the room.

From Hands

Inhale a couple drops from cupped hands.

From Bottle

Enjoy the aroma directly from the bottle.

Not sure *what to do?*

Apply oils in ways that make sense for your needs. For example, use oils topically on location for a rash. If it's digestive upset, use them internally (though some people rub oils outside their tummy area!).

Again, you won't do it wrong. Discover and enjoy.

Topical

Neat

Apply certain oils directly to skin without dilution.

Diluted

Dilute with Fractionated Coconut Oil or other carrier oil/ lotion as needed.

Roller Bottle

Put 10-20 drops in a roller bottle. Fill the rest with Fractionated Coconut Oil.

Internal

Veggie Capsule

Put oils in an empty veggie cap, and take with water.

Drink with Water

Drink 1-2 drops with water (for oils with a friendly taste).

Sublingually

Place a drop under the tongue for rapid absorption.

*Most brands of oils are not safe for internal use. Be sure yours has undergone strict gas chromatography and mass spectrometry to ensure purity and chemical soundness.

11

Safety

Topical & Internal Use
True essential oils are safe to use topically and internally. The smaller the body, the less essential oil should be used. Be conservative and use your oils more frequently.

Age	Topical Dilution Ratio*	Internal Use
Birth - 12 months	1:30	not recommended
1-5 years	1:15	1 drop (1-6 drops in 24 hours)
6-12 years	1:5	1-2 drops (3-12 drops in 24 hours)
Adults	as needed	2-4 drops (12-24 drops in 24 hours)

*essential oil : carrier oil

Medication
Always consult with a physician if you have questions about using an essential oil with a medication. While certain foods may interact with medications, essential oils frequently require less restraint because of the chemical makeup of the oil vs. the food.

Pregnancy
Essential oils are wonderful for pregnancy support. Some women wish to use oils only aromatically during their first trimester.

Oils can be used in smaller doses, and certain oils should be avoided: Birch[ATI], Cassia[TI], Cinnamon[TI], Cypress[I], Eucalyptus[I], Rosemary[ATI], Thyme[ATI], Wintergreen[TI].

Sensitive Skin
Dilute as needed for sensitive skin. Apply to the bottoms of feet to avoid sensitivity.

A Few Precautions

If it Burns
If an oil causes burning or irritation to the skin, immediately dilute it with a carrier oil. You can also use soap to wash the oil off.

Mixing with Water
Oil and water don't mix, and water will usually make discomfort from an essential oil worse.

Avoid Sensitive Areas
Do not put essential oils in your eyes, nose, ears, or other sensitive areas.

If You Use Too Much
If too much oil comes out of the bottle, simply wipe up the excess with a napkin (or give it to someone near you!).

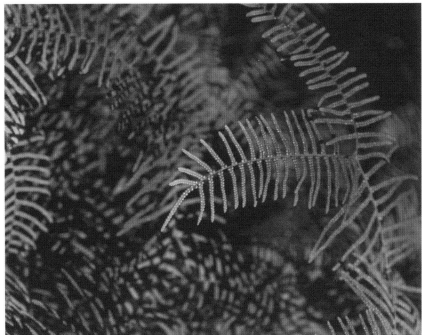

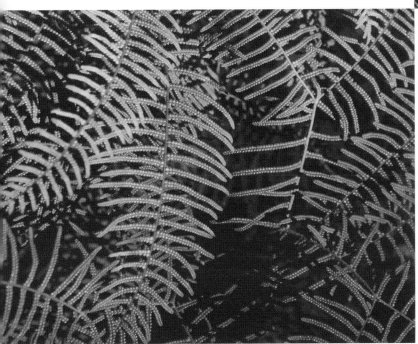

Photosensitivity
Certain oils, like citrus oils, can cause photosensitivity. This means that the skin can be more sensitive in sunlight, and that sunlight can even cause unsightly temporary hyper-pigmentation. Heed photosensitivity warnings in this book.

Lifestyle Habits
Keep your oils accessible. Have favorite ones in your bag, in high-traffic areas of the home, in the car, and at work. The easier they are to find, the more benefit you'll get from them.

How Much Should You Use?
Discover what works best for your body. Take heed of the safety warnings for each oil in this book.

Remember - small amounts more frequently tend to produce the best results.

Reflexology

Reflexology refers to contact points on the feet where nerve endings connect to other parts of the body. This is an ideal way to apply essential oils when the area of concern isn't accessible or when sensitivities limit application methods. It is also an ideal way to expose energy pathways such as those studied in Chinese medicine to the effects of essential oils.

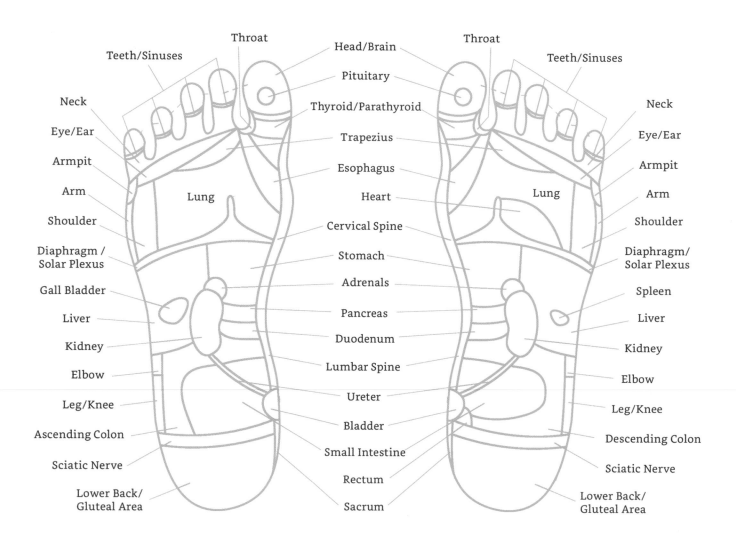

Preferences & Blending

Find the Right Solution for You

Remember that while essential oils have a most useful purpose, you should also enjoy what you use! Enjoying the use of oils makes it easier to create lifestyle habits with them.

If you love the smell of an essential oil, use away! If you don't love the smell, try an application method that limits exposure to the fragrance (like in a veggie cap or on the bottoms of feet), or look for a different oil that has similar properties.

Use oils you have on hand. Sometimes you'll find an oil in this book that you don't have, but that you do have in a blend. Sometimes you'll need to use an oil that has similar chemical properties to another oil you're missing. That's fine!

Blending

You won't break your oils. If you experiment with blending, but don't succeed, try again. You'll learn the smells that resonate best with you.

If you find yourself in need of an oil you may not love, try combining it with another oil to create a new fragrance.

Here are some blending tips:

• Pay attention to low, mid, and high notes in your oils for a well-rounded fragrance. (e.g. Vetiver is a low note, Lavender is a mid note, and Lemon is a high note.)

• Add FCO to your blends to help the fragrance last longer.

• When layering oils topically (using multiple oils one on top of the other), the oils on top will generally smell the strongest.

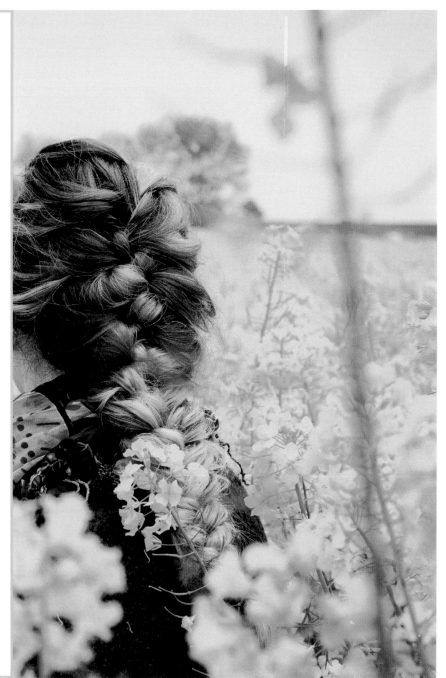

Purity & Potency

A properly sourced and produced essential oil is both pure and potent.

Purity means that the essential oil has *no contaminants or fillers.* It was cold-pressed or distilled using steam distillation.

Potency (or chemical accuracy) means that the essential oil has an *ideal chemical profile* for that particular plant in order to produce the intended therapeutic benefits. Plant chemistry develops differently based on where the plant is grown, climate, altitude, soil conditions, and growing practices.

You should verify that you are using oils that are scientifically shown to be both pure and potent. Don't take a company's word for it. A trustworthy company will make available the tests performed on every essential oil.

Know what you are putting in, on, and around your body.

Adulteration & Testing

The complexity of essential oils makes adulterating them too easy sometimes. Because some constituents appear in such small amounts, only sophisticated lab equipment with sufficiently comprehensive databases are able to detect skillful adulteration.

Unethical essential oil manufacturers use synthetic agents, fillers, and look-alike oils to produce inferior oils at cheaper costs.

Examples of Adulteration
(Tisserand, 2014)

Grapefruit   Orange terpenes, purified limonene

Jasmine Absolute   Indole, α-amyl cinnamic aldehyde, Ylang Ylang fractions

Lavender   Lavandin, Spike Lavender, Spanish Sage, White Camphor fractions, rectified Ho, acetylated Lavandin

Lemon   Synthetic citral or limonene

Peppermint   Cornmint

Rose   Ethanol, 2-phenylethanol, Geranium fractions, Rhodinol

Sandalwood   Australian Sandalwood, Sandalwood terpenes and fragrance chemicals

Ylang Ylang   Gurjun Balsam, Cananga oil, Benzyl Acetate, ρ-cresyl methyl ether

Standard Tests to Verify Purity & Potency

- Gas Chromatography
- Mass Spectrometry
- High Performance Liquid Chromatography
- Nuclear Magnetic Resonance Spectroscopy
- Fourier Transform Infrared Spectroscopy
- Chiral GC Testing
- Isotope Carbon 14
- Total Plate or Bacterial Count (TPC)/Microbial

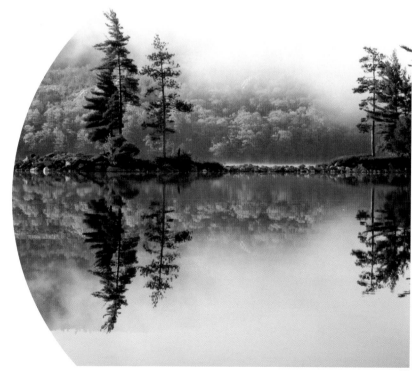

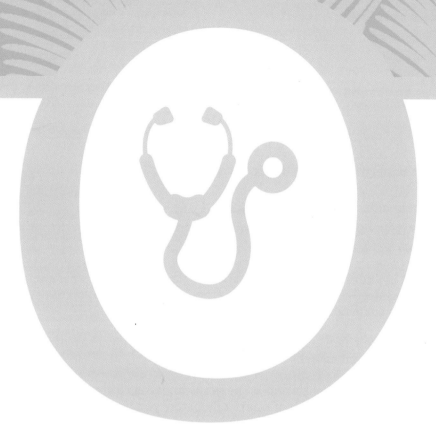

Section 2

A-Z Quick Reference

How to Use the *A-Z Quick Reference*

Using plant-based medicine is simple:

1. Look up your ailment or condition.
2. Try one or a few oils from the suggested list.
3. Decide what works best for your body.

Each ailment includes the primary oils and supplements that are beneficial for that ailment. You don't need to use all five products listed. Try the ones you have on hand, and consider trying some new ones in the near future.

Every solution listed here is only a recommendation. You may learn of other oils that help with your ailment as well!

Remember that trying essential oils is the same process as trying any remedy; you may go through a few oils, or combinations of oils, before you find what your body responds best to.

Many of the ailments listed reference a protocol found later in the book. While this section is intended to provide quick answers, the protocols give detailed instructions for serious results.

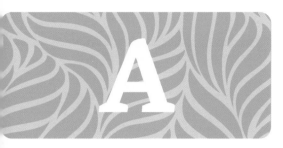

A

Abscess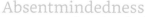

Apply 2-4 drops 3x daily over affected area.

Lavender T	Arborvitae T
Tea Tree T	Neroli T
Roman Chamomile T	

Absentmindedness

Massage 1-3 drops into forehead, temples, back of neck, and chest as needed; inhale from cupped hands.

Rosemary A T	Lavender A T
Peppermint A T	Frankincense A T
Bergamot A T	*Protocol on pg. 222*

Abuse Recovery

Apply 1-3 drops to top of head, forehead, and back of neck 3x daily.

Hope A T	Bergamot A T
ClaryCalm® A T	Lavender A T
Rose A T	*Protocol on pg. 237*

Aches

Massage 2-4 drops into affected muscles and joints as needed

Marjoram T	AromaTouch® T
Lemongrass T	Helichrysum T
Deep Blue® T	*Protocol on pg. 201*

Acid Reflux

Take 2-4 drops internally or rub over stomach as needed

Peppermint T I	Cardamom T I
DigestZen® T I	DigestTab® I
Ginger T I	*Protocol on pg. 184*

Acne/Blemishes

Apply a drop topically to affected areas 1-2x daily. Add 2-3 drops to facial lotion and apply after cleansing routine.

Tea Tree T	Neroli T
HD Clear® T	Lavender T
Juniper Berry T	*Protocol on pg. 184*

Actinic Keratosis

Apply 3-5 drops to affected area 4x daily.

Frankincense T	Neroli T
Lavender T	Myrrh T
Tea Tree T	

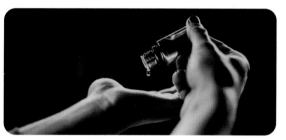

ADD/ADHD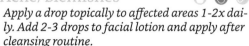

Apply a few drops on forehead and back of neck; inhale a few drops from cupped hands.

InTune® A T	Frankincense A T I
Vetiver A T I	Balance A T
Peace A T	*Protocol on pg. 183*

Addiction: Alcohol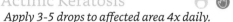

Apply a couple drops to back of neck, temples, ears, and below chest as often as needed.

Bergamot A T I	Black Pepper A T I
Hope A T	Lemon A T I
Motivate A T	*Protocol on pg. 214*

Addiction: Caffeine

Apply a couple drops to back of neck, temples, ears, and below chest as often as needed.

Peppermint A T I	Motivate A T
Wild Orange A T I	Lavender A T I
Jasmine A T	*Protocol on pg. 214*

Addiction: Drugs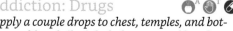

Apply a couple drops to chest, temples, and bottoms of feet daily; inhale from cupped hands as needed; use a drop under tongue.

Copaiba A T I	Black Pepper A T I
Zendocrine® A T I	Frankincense A T I
Purify A T	*Protocol on pg. 214*

Addiction: Food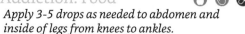

Apply 3-5 drops as needed to abdomen and inside of legs from knees to ankles.

Bergamot A T I	Ginger A T I
Lemon A T I	Coriander A T I
Cinnamon A T I	*Protocol on pg. 214*

Addiction: Internet/Video Games

Apply 3-5 drops to bottom of feet and outside of legs from knees to ankles

Lavender A T	Cedarwood A T
Wild Orange A T	Vetiver A T I
Bergamot A T	*Protocol on pg. 214*

 Aromatic   Topical   Internal   N/A

Addiction: Pain Medication

Apply a couple drops to back of neck, temples, and outside of ears as often as needed.

Lavender ᴬᵀ	Hope ᴬᵀ
Ylang Ylang ᴬᵀ	Eucalyptus ᴬᵀ
Cinnamon ᴬᵀ	*Protocol on pg. 214*

Addiction: Sex/ Pornography

Apply 3-5 drops to back of neck, forehead, and crown of head as often as needed.

Bergamot ᴬᵀ	Vetiver ᴬᵀ
Lavender ᴬᵀ	Siberian Fir ᴬᵀ
Cedarwood ᴬᵀ	*Protocol on pg. 214*

Addiction: Smoking

Ingest 2-4 drops daily; inhale from cupped hands as needed when experiencing cravings.

Black Pepper ᴬᵀᴵ	Bergamot ᴬᵀᴵ
Grapefruit ᴬᵀᴵ	Zendocrine® ᴬᵀᴵ
Basil ᴬᵀᴵ	*Protocol on pg. 214*

Addiction: Sugar

Apply 3-5 drops as needed to abdomen and inside of legs from knees to ankles. Also add a few drops to water throughout the day.

Slim & Sassy® ᴬᵀᴵ	Motivate ᴬᵀ
Ginger ᴬᵀᴵ	Elevation ᴬᵀ
Coriander ᴬᵀᴵ	*Protocol on pg. 214*

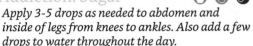

Addiction: Work

Apply 3-5 drops to bottoms of feet and outside of legs from knees to ankles.

Lavender ᴬᵀ	Cedarwood ᴬᵀ
Wild Orange ᴬᵀ	Vetiver ᴬᵀ
Bergamot ᴬᵀ	*Protocol on pg. 214*

Addison's Disease

Apply 3-5 drops 3x daily to lower back and front of legs near the shins and knees.

Whisper ᵀ	Cinnamon ᵀ
Ylang Ylang ᵀ	Bergamot ᵀ
Lavender ᵀ	

Adenitis

Apply 3-5 drops to the lower right quadrant of the abdomen and take internally.

On Guard ᴬᵀᴵ	Frankincense ᴬᵀᴵ
Oregano ᴬᵀᴵ	Lavender ᴬᵀᴵ
Tea Tree ᴬᵀᴵ	

Adrenal Fatigue

Massage 1-3 drops onto lower back over adrenals, or inhale from cupped hands. Ingest 1-3 drops as needed.

Basil ᴬᵀᴵ	Black Spruce ᴬᵀ
Juniper Berry ᴬᵀᴵ	Peppermint ᴬᵀᴵ
Rosemary ᴬᵀᴵ	*Protocol on pg. 185*

Age Spots

Apply 3-5 drops diluted to face at bed time.

Frankincense ᵀ	Immortelle ᵀ
Sandalwood ᵀ	Neroli ᵀ
Helichrysum ᵀ	*Protocol on pg. 215*

Aging

Apply 1-3 drops to target areas. Combine 2-8 drops with facial lotion or carrier oil and apply after cleansing.

Immortelle ᵀ	Sandalwood ᵀ
Frankincense ᵀ	Lifelong Vitality Pack® ᴵ
Cedarwood ᵀ	*Protocol on pg. 215*

Agitation

Apply 3-5 drops 3x daily over forehead, back of neck, and top of the head. Also use a drop under the tongue.

Bergamot ᴬᵀᴵ	Roman Chamomile ᴬᵀᴵ
Lavender ᴬᵀᴵ	Peace ᴬᵀ
Citrus Bloom® ᴬᵀ	*Protocol on pg. 206*

AIDS

Apply 3-5 drops to lower back, back of neck, and bottoms of feet. Also combine a few drops in a veggie cap 2-3x daily .

Oregano ᵀᴵ	Frankincense ᵀᴵ
Sandalwood ᵀᴵ	Tea Tree ᵀᴵ
Myrrh ᵀᴵ	*Protocol on pg. 185*

Air Pollution

Diffuse several drops or apply 3-5 drops over the lungs and nose as often as needed.

Air-X™ ᴬᵀ	Basil ᴬᵀ
Litsea ᴬᵀ	Lavender ᴬᵀ
Northern Escape ᴬᵀ	

Airborne Bacteria

Apply 3-5 drops 3x daily over chest and around the nose. Also diffuse several drops throughout the day.

On Guard ᴬᵀ	Eucalyptus ᴬᵀ
Breathe ᴬᵀ	Tea Tree ᴬᵀ
Pink Pepper ᴬᵀ	

 Aromatic   ᵀ Topical   Internal   N/A

Alertness

Apply 1-2 drops to forehead, temples, or base of skull as needed; inhale a few drops from cupped hands

Peppermint ^{A T}   Rosemary ^{A T}
Frankincense ^{A T}   InTune® ^{A T}
Basil ^{A T}

Alkalosis

Apply 3 drops of the oils on hand (preferably all 5 listed) over the chest and ribs.

Lavender ^T   Rose ^T
Vetiver ^T   Rosemary ^T
Roman Chamomile ^T

Allergies (Seasonal, Pet Dander)

Apply to back of neck, on bridge of nose, or chest as needed; use a drop under the tongue; diffuse several drops.

Lavender ^{A T I}   Peppermint ^{A T I}
Breathe ^{A T}   Zendocrine® ^{A T I}
Purify ^{A T}   *Protocol on pg. 186*

Alzheimer's/ Dementia

Massage 1-2 drops into scalp daily; ingest 2-4 drops 1-2x daily; supplement daily

Frankincense ^{A T I}   Rose ^{A T}
Rosemary ^{A T I}   Lifelong Vitality Pack® ^I
DDR Prime® ^{A T I}   *Protocol on pg. 186*

Amnesia

Diffuse several drops daily and apply 3 -5 drops 3x daily to forehead and top of head.

Rosemary ^{A T}   Wild Orange ^{A T}
Peppermint ^{A T}   Frankincense ^{A T}
Bergamot ^{A T}

Analgesic

Apply 3-5 drops as needed over the affected area. Also use a drop under the tongue.

Frankincense ^{T I}   Peppermint ^{T I}
Lavender ^{T I}   Rosemary ^{T I}
Marjoram ^{T I}

Anemia

Apply 1-3 drops to bottoms of feet and inside of wrists; take a few drops internally; inhale from cupped hands periodically

On Guard ^{A T I}   Lavender ^{A T I}
Basil ^{A T I}   Lifelong Vitality Pack® ^I
Lemon ^{A T I}

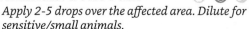

Aneurysm

Diffuse several drops and apply 3-5 drops 3x daily to forehead and top of head.

Frankincense ^{A T}   Vetiver ^{A T}
Rosemary ^{A T}   Myrrh ^{A T}
Helichrysum ^{A T}

Anger

Apply 1-3 drops to temples and chest; inhale a few drops from cupped hands as needed.

Balance ^{A T}   Melissa ^{A T}
Forgive ^{A T}   Magnolia ^{A T}
Peace ^{A T}   *Protocol on pg. 225*

Angina

Apply 3-5 drops over the chest as needed.

Rose ^T   Vetiver ^T
Lavender ^T   Siberian Fir ^T
Bergamot ^T

Anguish

Apply 3-5 drops 3x daily over forehead, back of neck, and top of the head.

Hope ^{A T}   Vetiver ^{A T}
Peace ^{A T}   Siberian Fir ^{A T}
Console ^{A T}   *Protocol on pg. 239*

Animals: Bleeding

Apply 1-2 drops to affected area every 15-30 minutes until bleeding stops. Dilute for sensitive/ small animals.

Helichrysum ^T   Lavender ^T
Geranium ^T   Tea Tree ^T
Rose ^T

Animals: Bone Pain

Apply 2-5 drops over the affected area. Dilute for sensitive/small animals.

Wintergreen ^T   Rosemary ^T
Eucalyptus ^T   Sandalwood ^T
Peppermint ^T

Animals: Cancer (skin)

Apply 2-5 drops to affected area 4-5x daily. Dilute for sensitive/small animals.

Frankincense ^T   Hope ^T
Lavender ^T   Geranium ^T
Sandalwood ^T

 Aromatic   **Topical**   **Internal**   **N/A**

Animals: Colds & Cough

Apply 2-5 drops over chest, and around ears and throat 3x daily. Dilute for sensitive/small animals.

On Guard ^AT Rosemary ^AT
Lime ^AT Oregano ^AT
Tea Tree ^AT

Animals: Stress & Anxiety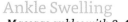

Apply 2-5 drops over the forehead, back of neck, and top of head as needed. Dilute for sensitive/ small animals.

Peace ^AT Serenity ^AT
Rose ^AT Neroli ^AT
Lavender ^AT

Ankle Swelling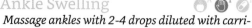

Massage ankles with 2-4 drops diluted with carrier oil if desired.

Juniper Berry ^T Deep Blue® ^T
Grapefruit ^T PastTense® ^T
Lemongrass ^T

Ankylosing Spondylitis

Apply 2 drops of each to spine, back of the neck, and other affected areas.

Ginger ^T Wintergreen ^T
Frankincense ^T Bergamot ^T
Myrrh ^T

Anorexia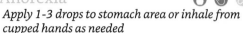

Apply 1-3 drops to stomach area or inhale from cupped hands as needed

Grapefruit ^AT Elevation ^AT
Ginger ^AT Cheer ^AT
Citrus Bliss® ^AT

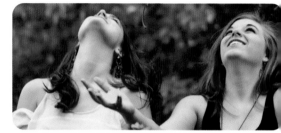

Antibacterial

Combine 3 drops of oils on hand into a capsule and take internally 4x daily; apply topically or diffuse as needed.

On Guard ^ATI Tea Tree ^ATI
Oregano ^ATI Melissa ^ATI
Cinnamon ^ATI

Anticoagulant

Add 2 drops of each to a capsule and take internally 2x daily; Apply 2 drops to bottoms of feet.

Basil ^TI Birch ^T
Oregano ^TI Cassia ^TI
Wintergreen ^T

Antidepressant

Apply 3-5 drops over the forehead, back of neck, and top of head 3x daily. Also diffuse several drops.

Elevation ^AT Frankincense ^ATI
Magnolia ^AT Tea Tree ^ATI
Rose ^AT *Protocol on pg. 193*

Antifungal

Combine 3 -5 drops of oils on hand with carrier oil and rub into affected area.

Tea Tree ^T Clove ^T
Oregano ^T Geranium ^T
Thyme ^T

Antioxidant

Apply 3-5 drops to outside of legs and feet. Use a few drops in a capsule.

Clove ^TI Rosemary ^TI
Blue Tansy ^T Oregano ^TI
Yarrow|Pom ^TI

Antisocial

Apply 3-5 drops over the forehead and back of neck. Also diffuse several drops.

Motivate ^AT Lime ^AT
Siberian Fir ^AT Ginger ^AT
Spearmint ^AT

Antiviral

Combine 3 drops of oils on hand into a capsule and take internally 4x daily. Rub 2-3 drops on bottoms of feet. Also diffuse several drops.

Melissa ^ATI Tea Tree ^ATI
Oregano ^ATI Green Mandarin ^ATI
On Guard ^ATI

Anxiety

Apply 1-3 drops to bottoms of feet, chest, or temples, or inhale from cupped hands as needed; use a drop under the tongue.

Adaptiv™ ^AT Balance ^AT
Vetiver ^ATI Lavender ^ATI
Peace ^ATI *Protocol on pg. 186*

Apathy

Apply 1-3 drops to bottoms of feet, chest, or temples, or inhale from cupped hands as needed. Also diffuse several drops.

Patchouli ^AT Ylang Ylang ^AT
Neroli ^AT Forgive ^AT
Peppermint ^AT

^A Aromatic ^T Topical ^I Internal ● N/A

Aphrodisiac

Apply 2-4 drops to wrists and neck. Also diffuse several drops.

Passion [AT]	Sandalwood [AT]
Jasmine [AT]	Rose [AT]
Cinnamon [AT]	*Protocol on pg. 231*

Appetite Stimulant

Apply 3-5 drops over the abdomen or drink a couple drops in water. Also diffuse several drops.

DigestZen® [ATI]	Coriander [ATI]
Ginger [ATI]	Fennel [ATI]
Bergamot [ATI]	

Appetite Suppressant

Apply 1-3 drops to stomach, chest, bottoms of feet, or inside of wrists or take 2-4 drops internally.

Slim & Sassy® [ATI]	Ginger [ATI]
Peppermint [ATI]	Wild Orange [ATI]
Grapefruit [ATI]	

Arrhythmia

Apply 3-5 drops to inside of arms and chest 3x daily.

Lemon [T]	Marjoram [T]
Lavender [T]	Cypress [T]
Ylang Ylang [T]	

Artery Issues

Apply 3-5 drops to inside of arms and chest 2x daily.

Basil [T]	Cassia [T]
Clary Sage [T]	Eucalyptus [T]
Cypress [T]	

Arteriosclerosis

Place 2 drops of oils on hand in a capsule and take internally 3x daily.

Frankincense [I]	Cinnamon [I]
Ginger [I]	Tea Tree [I]
Clary Sage [I]	

Arthritic Pain

Apply 1-3 drops and massage into affected areas with lotion or carrier oil as needed.

Deep Blue® [T]	AromaTouch® [T]
Copaiba [T]	DDR Prime® [T]
Wintergreen [T]	*Protocol on pg. 187*

Asthma

Apply 1-3 drops topically to chest, neck, under nose, and on bridge of nose, or inhale from cupped hands as needed.

Breathe [AT]	Roman Chamomile [AT]
Eucalyptus [AT]	Lavender [AT]
Peppermint [AT]	*Protocol on pg. 187*

Atherosclerosis

Place 2 drops of oils on hand in a capsule and take internally 3x daily.

Lemon [I]	Cinnamon [I]
Ginger [I]	Grapefruit [I]
Clary Sage [I]	

Athlete's Foot

Apply 1-3 drops to area between toes and around toenails 2-3x daily. Ingest 1-3 drops of Tea Tree or oregano once a day (no more than 10 days.)

Tea Tree [TI]	Geranium [TI]
Oregano [TI]	Lemon [TI]
HD Clear® [T]	

Autism/Asperger's

Apply 1-3 drops to bottoms of feet and back of neck. Ingest 1-3 drops of Cilantro or DDR Prime® 1-2x daily.

Frankincense [ATI]	Rose [AT]
InTune® [ATI]	DDR Prime® [ATI]
Cilantro [ATI]	*Protocol on pg. 187*

Autoimmune Disorders

Apply 1-3 drops to stomach, chest, bottoms of feet, or inside of wrists. Ingest 2-4 drops 3x daily.

DDR Prime® [TI]	Immortelle [T]
Zendocrine® [TI]	Lifelong Vitality Pack® [I]
Frankincense [TI]	*Protocol on pg. 188*

Autointoxication

Apply 1-3 drops to stomach, chest, bottoms of feet, or inside of wrists. Ingest 1-3 drops 2-3x daily for additional support.

Zendocrine® [ATI]	Grapefruit [ATI]
Cilantro [ATI]	Geranium [ATI]
Thyme [ATI]	

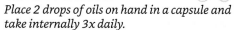

Back Pain

Apply 1-3 drops and massage into affected areas as needed. Use a carrier oil or lotion for increased efficacy.

Deep Blue® [AT]	Copaiba [ATI]
AromaTouch® [AT]	Deep Blue® Complex [I]
Turmeric [ATI]	*Protocol on pg. 188*

 Aromatic   Topical   Internal   N/A

Back Stiffness

Combine 3-5 drops of oils on hand and massage into affected area as often as needed.

Deep Blue®ᵀ	Peppermint ᵀ
Wintergreenm ᵀ	Cypress ᵀ
Ylang Ylang ᵀ	*Protocol on pg. 188*

Bacterial Infection

Apply 1-3 drops with a carrier oil to affected areas as needed. Ingest 1-3 drops every 2-3 hours for systemic/internal infections.

Oregano ᴬᵀᴵ	Tea Tree ᴬᵀᴵ
Thyme ᴬᵀᴵ	Pink Pepper ᴬᵀᴵ
On Guard ᴬᵀᴵ	

Bags Under Eyes

Combine 2 drops with carrier oil and gently rub under eyes at bedtime.

Rose ᵀ	Lavender ᵀ
Fennel ᵀ	Cypress ᵀ
Roman Chamomile ᵀ	

Balance Problems

Apply 1-3 drops topically to forehead, temples, back of neck, and behind the ears or inhale from cupped hands. Ingest 1-3 drops of Ginger as needed.

Balance ᴬᵀ	Basil ᴬᵀᴵ
Peppermint ᴬᵀᴵ	Cypress ᴬᵀ
Ginger ᴬᵀᴵ	

Balding

Dilute 5 drops in 20 drops of carrier oil. Massage into scalp every night. Supplement with DDR Prime® and Lifelong Vitality Pack® daily.

Rosemary ᵀ	DDR Prime® ᵀᴵ
Arborvitae ᵀ	Lifelong Vitality Pack® ᴵ
Spikenard ᵀ	

Basal Cell Carcinoma

Combine 3-5 drops of oils on hand and apply directly to affected area.

Frankincense ᵀ	Myrrh ᵀ
DDR Prime® ᵀ	Vetiver ᵀ
Sandalwood ᵀ	*Protocol on pg. 189*

Bed Bugs

Combine 10 drops of oils on hand (preferably all 5 listed oils) into 20 oz glass spray bottle of water and spray on bed or upholstery.

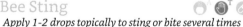

Tea Tree ᵀ	Sandalwood ᵀ
Lemon ᵀ	Cinnamon ᵀ
Lavender ᵀ	

Bed Sores

Apply 3-6 drops with carrier oil to affected area 3x daily.

Frankincense ᵀ	Neroli ᵀ
Tea Tree ᵀ	Helichrysum ᵀ
Lavender ᵀ	

Bed-wetting

Massage 2-4 drops over bladder and kidneys before bedtime.

Cypress ᵀ	Lemongrass ᵀ
Black Pepper ᵀ	Roman Chamomile ᵀ
Ylang Ylang ᵀ	

Bee Sting

Apply 1-2 drops topically to sting or bite several times daily until symptoms cease.

Lavender ᵀ	Basil ᵀ
Purify ᵀ	Magnolia ᵀ
Roman Chamomile ᵀ	

Bell's Palsy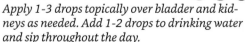

Massage 1-3 drops into spine and bottoms of feet or ingest 2-4 drops every 2-3 hours as needed.

Clove ᵀᴵ	Thyme ᵀᴵ
Melissa ᵀᴵ	Lifelong Vitality Pack® ᴵ
Frankincense ᵀᴵ	

Bipolar Disorder

Apply 1-3 drops to bottoms of feet, chest, or temples, or inhale from cupped hands as needed.

Frankincense ᴬᵀᴵ	Melissa ᴬᵀᴵ
Peace ᴬᵀ	Lifelong Vitality Pack® ᴵ
Vetiver ᴬᵀᴵ	*Protocol on pg. 188*

Bites

Apply 2-4 drops to affected area as often as needed.

Lavender ᵀ	Roman Chamomile ᵀ
Tea Tree ᵀ	Petitgrain ᵀ
Yarrow|Pom ᵀ	

Bladder Control

Apply 1-3 drops topically over bladder and kidneys as needed. Add 1-2 drops to drinking water and sip throughout the day.

Rosemary ᵀᴵ	Marjoram ᵀᴵ
Juniper Berry ᵀᴵ	Sandalwood ᵀᴵ
Cypress ᵀᴵ	

 Aromatic   Topical   Internal ⬤ N/A

Bladder Infection

Rub 3-4 drops over bladder. Take 3-5 drops in a capsule after food 3x daily.

Cypress ᵀ	Eucalyptus ᵀ
Oregano ᵀ ᴵ	Tea Tree ᵀ ᴵ
Clove ᵀ ᴵ	*Protocol on pg. 208*

Blocked Tear Ducts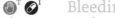

Apply 1-2 drops to bridge of nose; avoid getting in the eyes; dilute if using on an infant.

Lavender ᵀ
Clary Sage ᵀ
Tea Tree ᵀ

Blood Pressure (Low)

Apply 1-3 drops to stomach, chest, bottoms of feet, or inside of wrists, or ingest a few drops as needed.

Helichrysum ᴬ ᵀ ᴵ	Cedarwood ᴬ ᵀ
Frankincense ᴬ ᵀ ᴵ	Lifelong Vitality Pack® ᴵ
Jasmine ᴬ ᵀ	

Blurred Vision

Mix oils in a roller bottle with carrier oil and carefully apply around eyes 2-4x daily.

Clary Sage ᵀ	DDR Prime® ᵀ
Helichrysum ᵀ	Lavender ᵀ
Immortelle ᵀ	

Bleeding

Apply a drop topically to affected area as needed.

Helichrysum ᵀ	Lemon ᵀ
Geranium ᵀ	Tea Tree ᵀ
Myrrh ᵀ	

Blisters on Feet

Apply a few drops topically to affected area.

Lavender ᵀ	Tea Tree ᵀ
Frankincense ᵀ	Myrrh ᵀ
Patchouli ᵀ	

Blood Clotting

Apply 1-3 drops over affected area or ingest a few drops internally as needed.

Wintergreen ᵀ	Peppermint ᵀ ᴵ
Helichrysum ᵀ ᴵ	Ginger ᵀ ᴵ
Cypress ᵀ	

Blood Sugar (High)

Apply 2-4 drops over pancreas and bottoms of feet daily; take a few drops internally.

On Guard ᵀ ᴵ	Coriander ᵀ ᴵ
Slim & Sassy® ᵀ ᴵ	Ginger ᵀ ᴵ
Cinnamon ᵀ ᴵ	

Body Odor

Take 3-5 drops of Cilantro, Zendocrine®, or Dill at least once daily. Apply 1-3 drops on bottoms of feet.

Cilantro ᵀ ᴵ	Tea Tree ᵀ ᴵ
Zendocrine® ᵀ ᴵ	Petitgrain ᵀ
Citronella ᵀ	*Protocol on pg. 192*

Blisters from Sun

Apply a few drops liberally to affected area.

Frankincense ᵀ	Tea Tree ᵀ
Lavender ᵀ	Myrrh ᵀ
Patchouli ᵀ	*Protocol on pg. 207*

Bloating

Apply 1-3 drops to stomach, rubbing in a clockwise direction. Use 1-3 drops internally as needed.

Fennel ᵀ ᴵ	Juniper Berry ᵀ ᴵ
DigestZen® ᵀ ᴵ	Peppermint ᵀ ᴵ
Ginger ᵀ ᴵ	*Protocol on pg. 194*

Blood Pressure (High)

Apply 2-4 drops to stomach, chest, bottoms of feet, or inside of wrists; ingest 2-4 drops 2x daily.

Cypress ᴬ ᵀ	Ylang Ylang ᴬ ᵀ ᴵ
Marjoram ᴬ ᵀ ᴵ	Jasmine ᴬ ᵀ
Lemon ᴬ ᵀ ᴵ	

Blood Sugar (Low)

Apply 1-3 drops to stomach, chest, bottoms of feet, or inside of wrists, or ingest 1-3 drops as needed.

Cinnamon ᵀ ᴵ	Wild Orange ᵀ ᴵ
Melissa ᵀ ᴵ	Lifelong Vitality Pack® ᴵ
Cassia ᵀ ᴵ	

Boils

Apply 1-3 drops topically to affected areas several times daily.

Tea Tree ᵀ	Myrrh ᵀ
HD Clear® ᵀ	Bergamot ᵀ
Lavender ᵀ	

 Aromatic   Topical   Internal   N/A

Bone Pain/Break

Apply 3-5 drops topically to affected areas as needed. Massage with lotion or carrier oil to improve efficacy.

Deep Blue® T	Helichrysum T
Wintergreen T	Bone Nutrient Complex I
Bergamot T	

Bone Spurs

Massage 1-3 drops into affected area as often as needed.

Eucalyptus T	Wintergreen T
Myrrh T	Peppermint T
Frankincense T	*Protocol on pg. 189*

Brain Fog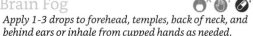

Apply 1-3 drops to forehead, temples, back of neck, and behind ears or inhale from cupped hands as needed.

Peppermint A T	Rosemary A T
Frankincense A T	Lifelong Vitality Pack® I
Lemon A T	*Protocol on pg. 195*

Brain Injury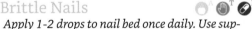

Apply a few drops to forehead, temples, base of skull, and behind the ears. Diffuse several drops. Take 3-5 drops in a capsule 3x daily.

Frankincense A T I	Sandalwood A T I
DDR Prime® A T I	Lifelong Vitality Pack® I
Cedarwood A T	

Brain Support

Apply 3-5 drops to the back of neck and backside of legs. Diffuse Several Drops. Take 3-5 drops in a capsule 3x daily.

Rosemary A T I	Grapefruit A T I
Frankincense A T I	Lemon A T I
Basil A T I	

Breastfeeding (Increase Milk)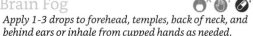

Massage 1-3 drops with carrier oil over breasts and apply to bottoms of feet or take internally when needed

Fennel T I	Lifelong Vitality Pack® I
Clary Sage T I	Bone Nutrient Complex I
Basil T I	

Brittle Nails

Apply 1-2 drops to nail bed once daily. Use supplements consistently for long-term benefits.

Lemon T	Bone Nutrient Complex I
Helichrysum T	Lifelong Vitality Pack® I
Frankincense T	

Broken Bones

Apply 3-5 drops to the affected area 5x daily.

Cypress T	Frankincense T
Wintergreen T	Vetiver T
Helichrysum T	

Bronchitis

Apply 2-4 drops to chest and neck area, gargle hourly, or inhale from cupped hands as needed.

Breathe A T	Roman Chamomile A T I
Cardamom A T I	Lemon Eucalyptus A T
Lime A T I	*Protocol on pg. 189*

Bruising

Apply 2-4 drops to bruise area. Use carrier oil if desired. Reapply 2-4x daily

PastTense® T	Cypress T
Deep Blue® T	Immortelle T
Helichrysum T	

Bulimia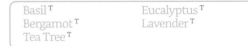

Apply 3-5 drops to back of neck and back 2x daily.

Basil T	Eucalyptus T
Bergamot T	Lavender T
Tea Tree T	

Bunions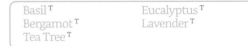

Apply 2-4 drops with carrier oil to affected area or joint as needed.

Lemon T	Peppermint T
Deep Blue® T	Cypress T
Copaiba T	

Burns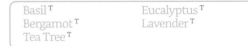

Apply 2-4 drops to affected area hourly or as needed. For more severe, mix 2-8 drops with 4 oz witch hazel and apply as needed.

Lavender T	Immortelle T
Frankincense T	Cedarwood T
Helichrysum T	

 Aromatic   Topical   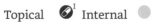 Internal   N/A

Burping
Apply 3-5 drops to upper abdomen as often as needed. Drink a couple drops in water if desired.

Coriander T I	Fennel T I
DigestZen® T I	Peppermint T I
Ginger T I	

Bursitis
Combine 5 drops of oils on hand to carrier oil and apply liberally to affected area as often as desired.

Wintergreen T	Helichrysum T
Deep Blue® T	Blue Tansy T
Ylang Ylang T	

C

Calluses
Rub 3-5 drops onto affected area, followed by a pumice stone to remove.

Rosemary T	Roman Chamomile T
Tea Tree T	Oregano T
Lemon T	

Cancer
Ingest 3-5 drops 3-5x daily. Apply topically if appropriate. Diffuse several drops. Supplement for added support.

DDR Prime® A T I	Geranium A T I
Frankincense A T I	Lifelong Vitality Pack® I
Sandalwood A T I	*Protocol on pg. 189, 190*

Candida
Apply 2-4 drops over abdomen and bottoms of feet. Take 3-5 drops in a capsule at least twice daily until symptoms subside.

Oregano T I	Tea Tree T
Thyme T I	GX Assist® I
Lemon Eucalyptus T	*Protocol on pg. 190*

Canker Sores
Apply a drop diluted with carrier oil directly to canker sore or gargle several times daily until sore is gone.

Tea Tree T I	Tulsi T
On Guard T I	Frankincense T I
Oregano T I	*Protocol on pg. 190*

Cardiovascular Disease
Apply 2-4 drops over chest 3x daily. Ingest 3-5 drops as needed.

DDR Prime® T I	Coriander T I
Geranium T I	Cypress T
Black Pepper T I	

Carpal Tunnel
Apply 2-4 drops to affected area several times daily. Massage with carrier oil or lotion for improved efficacy.

Deep Blue® T	Marjoram T
Wintergreen T	Oregano T
Lemongrass T	

Cartilage Injury
Apply 1-3 drops to affected area several times daily. Massage with carrier oil or lotion for improved efficacy.

Deep Blue® T	Helichrysum T
Lemongrass T	Copaiba T
Frankincense T	

Cataracts
Apply 1-3 drops under eyes, lower back and temples 3x daily.

Frankincense T	Lifelong Vitality Pack® I
Rosemary T	
Cypress T	

Cats (Anxiety, General Health)
Dilute 1 drop of oil to 2 Tbs FCO. Apply sparingly to back of coat.

Jasmine T	Turmeric T
Basil T	Frankincense T
Rose T	

Cavities
Apply 1-2 drops directly on tooth 2x daily. Dilute with carrier oil if necessary.

Clove T I	Bone Nutrient Complex I
On Guard T I	Lifelong Vitality Pack® I
Tea Tree T I	

Celiac Disease
Apply 2-4 drops to abdomen as often as needed. Also take 2-5 drops in a capsule.

Ginger T I	Coriander T I
Peppermint T I	DigestZen® T I
Fennel T I	*Protocol on pg. 190*

Cellulite
Massage 4-8 drops onto target areas daily, especially before exercising. Add to drinking water and consume throughout the day.

Slim & Sassy® T I	Juniper Berry T I
Grapefruit T I	Cinnamon T I
Lemon T I	*Protocol on pg. 209*

 Aromatic Topical Internal ● N/A

Cellulitis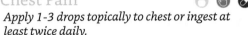

Apply 3-5 drops liberally to affected areas 3x daily. Dilute with carrier oil if needed.

Lavender ᵀ   Roman Chamomile ᵀ
Tea Tree ᵀ   Lemon ᵀ
Helichrysum ᵀ

Chapped Skin

Apply a drop or two to affected area as often as needed. Use a carrier oil to increase efficacy.

Myrrh ᵀ   Cedarwood ᵀ
Roman Chamomile ᵀ   Magnolia ᵀ
Yarrow|Pom ᵀ

Charley Horse

Massage 1-3 drops onto area of concern. Use a carrier oil or lotion for improved efficacy.

AromaTouch® ᵀ   Black Pepper ᵀ
Deep Blue® ᵀ   Bergamot ᵀ
Marjoram ᵀ

Chest Pain

Apply 1-3 drops topically to chest or ingest at least twice daily.

DDR Prime® ᵀ ᴵ   Wild Orange ᵀ ᴵ
On Guard ᵀ ᴵ   Marjoram ᵀ ᴵ
Lemon ᵀ ᴵ

Chicken Pox

Dilute 2-4 drops with a carrier oil and dab lightly on spots a couple times a day or ingest for immune support

Lavender ᵀ ᴵ   DDR Prime® ᵀ ᴵ
Thyme ᵀ ᴵ   Melissa ᵀ ᴵ
Tea Tree ᵀ ᴵ

Chiggers

Dilute 2-4 drops with a carrier oil and dab lightly on bites a couple times a day.

TerraShield® ᵀ   Zendocrine® ᵀ
Lemongrass ᵀ   Arborvitae ᵀ
Tea Tree ᵀ

Cholera

Apply 1-3 drops with a carrier oil to the affected areas as needed. Ingest 1-3 drops every 2-3 hours for systemic/internal infections.

Thyme ᵀ ᴵ   Tea Tree ᵀ ᴵ
Oregano ᵀ ᴵ   Arborvitae ᵀ ᴵ
On Guard ᵀ ᴵ

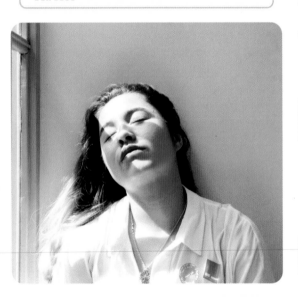

Cholesterol (High)

Apply 2-4 drops to chest area, bottoms of feet, or inside of wrists; ingest 2-4 drops once daily.

DDR Prime® ᵀ ᴵ   Zendocrine® ᵀ ᴵ
Lemon ᵀ ᴵ   Lifelong Vitality Pack® ᴵ
Rosemary ᵀ ᴵ   *Protocol on pg. 191*

Chronic Fatigue

Apply 2-4 drops to chest area, bottoms of feet, or inside of wrists; inhale 1-3 drops from cupped hands; supplement regularly for long-term benefits.

Lemon ᴬ ᵀ ᴵ   Mito2Max® ᴵ
Melissa ᴬ ᵀ ᴵ   Lifelong Vitality Pack® ᴵ
Basil ᴬ ᵀ ᴵ   *Protocol on pg. 195*

Chronic Pain

Apply 1-3 drops to affected areas as needed, using carrier oil for improved efficacy; supplement regularly for long-term care.

Deep Blue® ᴬ ᵀ   Turmeric ᴬ ᵀ ᴵ
Copaiba ᴬ ᵀ ᴵ   Lifelong Vitality Pack® ᴵ
DDR Prime® ᴬ ᵀ ᴵ

Circulation (Poor)

Apply 1-3 drops to bottoms of feet; ingest 1-3 drops twice daily or as needed.

Cypress ᵀ   DDR Prime® ᵀ ᴵ
Ginger ᵀ ᴵ   Mito2Max® ᴵ
Black Pepper ᵀ ᴵ

Cirrhosis of the Liver

Apply 3 drops of oils on hand (preferably all 5 listed) with carrier oil over the liver 3x daily.

Clove ᵀ   Rosemary ᵀ
Grapefruit ᵀ   Frankincense ᵀ
Geranium ᵀ

Cold (Common)

Ingest 2-4 drops 3-4x daily until symptoms subside. Diffuse several drops.

On Guard ᴬ ᵀ ᴵ   Melissa ᴬ ᵀ ᴵ
Breathe ᴬ ᵀ   Thyme ᴬ ᵀ ᴵ
Oregano ᴬ ᵀ ᴵ   *Protocol on pg. 191*

 ᴬ Aromatic   ᵀ Topical   ᴵ Internal   N/A

Cold Extremities

Apply 2-4 drops to bottoms of feet, chest area, and inside of wrists; ingest 2-4 drops daily as needed.

Cypress ^{ATI}	On Guard ^{ATI}
Black Pepper ^{ATI}	Mito2Max® ^I
Cinnamon ^{ATI}	

Cold Sores

Dilute with carrier oil and apply a drop to affected area as needed.

Melissa ^T	Clove ^T
On Guard ^T	Bergamot ^T
Tea Tree ^T	*Protocol on pg. 191*

Colic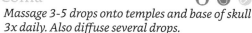

Dilute 1-2 drops with a carrier oil and apply topically to stomach and back before baby goes to sleep.

DigestZen® ^T	Neroli ^T
Peppermint ^T	Roman Chamomile ^T
Fennel ^T	

Colitis

Add 2 drops of oils on hand to capsule and take after eating 3x daily.

Lemon ^I	Ginger ^I
Clove ^I	Frankincense ^I
Fennel ^I	

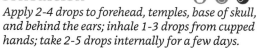

Coma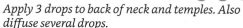

Massage 3-5 drops onto temples and base of skull 3x daily. Also diffuse several drops.

Bergamot ^{AT}	Wild Orange ^{AT}
Lavender ^{AT}	Siberian Fir ^{AT}
Wintergreen ^{AT}	

Concentration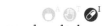

Apply 3 drops to back of neck and temples. Also diffuse several drops.

Frankincense ^{AT}	Vetiver ^{AT}
Peppermint ^{AT}	Rosemary ^{AT}
InTune® ^{AT}	*Protocol on pg. 195*

Concussion

Apply 2-4 drops to forehead, temples, base of skull, and behind the ears; inhale 1-3 drops from cupped hands; take 2-5 drops internally for a few days.

Frankincense ^{ATI}	Copaiba ^{ATI}
Bergamot ^{ATI}	Rosemary ^{ATI}
Cypress ^{ATI}	

Confusion

Apply 3 drops to back of neck and temples. Also diffuse several drops.

Lavender ^{AT}	Bergamot ^{AT}
Peppermint ^{AT}	Lemon ^{AT}
Rosemary ^{AT}	

Congenital Heart Disease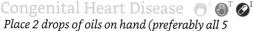

Place 2 drops of oils on hand (preferably all 5 listed) in a capsule and take internally 3x daily. Rub 2-4 drops over chest.

Frankincense ^{TI}	Cinnamon ^{TI}
Ginger ^{TI}	Tea Tree ^{TI}
Clary Sage ^{TI}	

Congestion

Apply 1-3 drops to back of neck, under nose, on bridge of nose, or chest; inhale 1-3 drops from cupped hands as needed. Also gargle a drop.

Breathe ^{ATI}	Cardamom ^{ATI}
Lemon ^{ATI}	Lime ^{ATI}
Rosemary ^{ATI}	

Conjunctivitis (Pink Eye)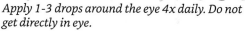

Apply 1-3 drops around the eye 4x daily. Do not get directly in eye.

Tea Tree ^T	Litsea ^T
Myrrh ^T	Lavender ^T
Eucalyptus ^T	

Connective Tissue Injury

Combine 5 drops to carrier oil and apply liberally to affected area as often as desired.

Wintergreen ^T	Helichrysum ^T
Ylang Ylang ^T	Blue Tansy ^T
Deep Blue® ^T	

Constipation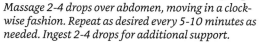

Massage 2-4 drops over abdomen, moving in a clockwise fashion. Repeat as desired every 5-10 minutes as needed. Ingest 2-4 drops for additional support.

DigestZen® ^{TI}	Cilantro ^{TI}
Ginger ^{TI}	Fennel ^{TI}
Celery Seed ^{TI}	*Protocol on pg. 191*

Control Issues

Apply a few drops as often as needed to back of the neck, temples and ears (not inside ears).

Vetiver ^{AT}	Cedarwood ^{AT}
Siberian Fir ^{AT}	Oregano ^{AT}
Lavender ^{AT}	*Protocol on pg. 225*

 Aromatic   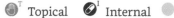 Topical   Internal   N/A

Convulsions

Apply 2-4 drops to bottoms of feet, spine, and back of neck as needed. Also diffuse several drops.

Frankincense ᴬᵀ	Sandalwood ᴬᵀ
Wintergreen ᴬᵀ	Rosemary ᴬᵀ
Vetiver ᴬᵀ	

Cough

Apply 1-3 drops to chest, back of neck, under nose, or on bridge of nose, as needed; inhale from cupped hands; gargle a drop.

Breathe ᴬᵀ	Lemon ᴬᵀᴵ
Rosemary ᴬᵀᴵ	Cardamom ᴬᵀᴵ
Peppermint ᴬᵀᴵ	*Protocol on pg. 192*

Cramps

Massage 2-4 drops into affected areas as needed. Use with carrier oil to improve efficacy.

Deep Blue® ᵀ	ClaryCalm® ᵀ
AromaTouch® ᵀ	Peppermint ᵀ
Arborvitae ᵀ	

Croup

Dilute with carrier oil and apply 1-3 drops to baby's chest and back as needed. Diffuse several drops.

Breathe ᴬᵀ	Sandalwood ᴬᵀ
Roman Chamomile ᴬᵀ	Wild Orange ᴬᵀ
Lemon ᴬᵀ	

Cushing's Syndrome

Apply 3-5 drops 3x daily over the lower back and back of neck.

Clary Sage ᵀ	Juniper Berry ᵀ
Fennel ᵀ	Helichrysum ᵀ
Frankincense ᵀ	

Corns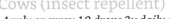

Apply 3-5 drops to affected area 3x daily for a few days, then use pumice stone to remove.

Rosemary ᵀ	Roman Chamomile ᵀ
Tea Tree ᵀ	Oregano ᵀ
Peppermint ᵀ	

Cows (insect repellent)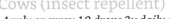

Apply or spray 10 drops 3x daily as needed for insect repellent.

TerraShield® ᵀ	Eucalyptus ᵀ
Citronella ᵀ	Cedarwood ᵀ
Lemon Eucalyptus ᵀ	

Cramps (Menstrual)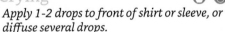

Massage 2-4 drops into abdomen, lower back, and shoulders; apply to a warm compress over uterus area.

ClaryCalm® ᵀ	Peppermint ᵀ
Clary Sage ᵀ	AromaTouch® ᵀ
Frankincense ᵀ	*Protocol on pg. 199*

Crying

Apply 1-2 drops to front of shirt or sleeve, or diffuse several drops.

Lavender ᴬᵀ	Roman Chamomile ᴬᵀ
Wild Orange ᴬᵀ	Peace ᴬᵀ
Calmer ᴬᵀ	

Cuts

Dilute 1-2 drops with a carrier oil and apply to affected area a couple times daily.

Tea Tree ᵀ	Myrrh ᵀ
Lavender ᵀ	Cedarwood ᵀ
Helichrysum ᵀ	

Cortisol (Heightened)

Apply 1-3 drops to back of neck, under nose, on bridge of nose, or chest as needed; ingest 2-4 drops; inhale from cupped hands.

Lavender ᴬᵀᴵ	Marjoram ᴬᵀᴵ
Basil ᴬᵀᴵ	Neroli ᴬᵀ
Bergamot ᴬᵀᴵ	*Protocol on pg. 206*

Cradle Cap

Add 3-5 drops to 30 drops of carrier oil and apply 2x daily.

Tea Tree ᵀ	Lemongrass ᵀ
Lavender ᵀ	Helichrysum ᵀ
Frankincense ᵀ	

Crohn's Disease

Apply 2-5 drops with carrier oil over abdomen as often as needed.

Peppermint ᵀ	Fennel ᵀ
Basil ᵀ	Cardamom ᵀ
Ginger ᵀ	*Protocol on pg. 192*

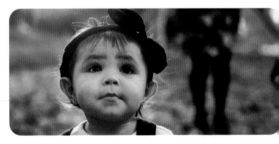

Cutting/Self-Harm

Gargle a few drops. Apply 2-4 drops as often as needed to back of the neck, temples and ears (not inside ears.)

Lavender ᴬᵀ	Bergamot ᴬᵀ
Vetiver ᴬᵀ	Console ᴬᵀ
YlangYlang ᴬᵀ	*Protocol on pg. 239*

 Aromatic   Topical   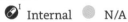 Internal   N/A

Cyst (Ganglion)

Massage 3-5 drops into affected area 3x daily.

Frankincense [T]	Lemongrass [T]
Oregano [T]	Cypress [T]
Thyme [T]	*Protocol on pg. 192*

Cysts

Apply 2-4 drops to affected area 3x daily or as needed.

Oregano [T]	Tangerine [T]
Frankincense [T]	DDR Prime® [T]
Thyme [T]	

Cystic Fibrosis

Apply 1-3 drops to chest and under nose; inhale from cupped hands as needed.

Frankincense [A T]	Eucalyptus [A T]
Breathe [A T]	Tea Tree [A T]
Arborvitae [A T]	

D

Cystitis/Infection

Add 3-5 drops of each to an empty capsule and take after food 3x daily; rub a few drops diluted over affected area.

Clove [T I]	Eucalyptus [T]
Tea Tree [T I]	Cinnamon [T I]
Oregano [T I]	

Dandruf

Dilute 2-6 drops in carrier oil and massage into scalp. Rinse after 60 minutes.

Tea Tree [T]	Myrrh [T]
Cedarwood [T]	Petitgrain [T]
Rosemary [T]	

Dehydrated Skin

Apply 2-4 drops with carrier oil to affected area as needed. Use with lotion for improved efficacy.

Cedarwood [T]	Sandalwood [T]
Beautiful [T]	Immortelle [T]
Myrrh [T]	

Dehydration

Apply 2-4 drops to bottom of feet, spine and back of neck.

Ylang Ylang [T]	Sandalwood [T]
Neroli [T]	Lavender [T]
Roman Chamomile [T]	

Dementia

Apply 2-4 drops to forehead, temples, base of skull; take 2-4 drops internally 3x daily; inhale from cupped hands.

Frankincense [A T I]	Rosemary [A T I]
DDR Prime® [A T I]	Peppermint [A T I]
Rose [A T]	*Protocol on pg. 186*

Deodorant

Add 10 drops with carrier oil to roller bottle or apply a dab with carrier oil to underarms.

Tea Tree [T]	Lemongrass [T]
Arborvitae [T]	Rosemary [T]
Lavender [T]	*Protocol on pg. 192*

Depression

Apply 2-4 drops to forehead and temples; place a drop of Frankincense on thumb and press to roof of mouth; inhale from cupped hands as needed.

Elevation [A T]	Melissa [A T I]
Frankincense [A T I]	Lifelong Vitality Pack® [I]
Cheer [A T]	*Protocol on pg. 193*

Detoxification

Apply 3-5 drops to bottoms of feet and inside of wrists; ingest 2-4 drops a few times daily; supplement regularly for improved cleansing.

Zendocrine® [T I]	Grapefruit [T I]
Cilantro [T I]	Celery Seed [T I]
Lemon [T I]	

Diabetes

Apply a couple drops over pancreas and bottoms of feet daily; take a few drops internally 2-3x daily.

On Guard [T I]	Coriander [T I]
Slim & Sassy® [T I]	Ginger [T I]
Cinnamon [T I]	*Protocol on pg. 193*

Diabetes (Gestational)

Apply a couple drops over pancreas and bottoms of feet daily; take a few drops internally.

On Guard [T I]	Coriander [T I]
Slim & Sassy® [T I]	Ginger [T I]
Cinnamon [T I]	

Diaper Rash

Dilute 1-3 drops with carrier oil and apply to affected area several times daily until rash disappears.

Lavender [T]	Coriander [T]
Roman Chamomile [T]	Cedarwood [T]
Ylang Ylang [T]	

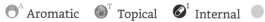 Aromatic   Topical   Internal   N/A

Diarrhea ᴬ ᵀ ᴵ

Ingest 2-4 drops; massage 1-3 drops into abdomen clockwise hourly as needed.

DigestZen® ᵀ ᴵ	Lavender ᵀ ᴵ
Lemon ᵀ ᴵ	Spearmint ᵀ ᴵ
Ginger ᵀ ᴵ	

Digestion Issues ᴬ ᵀ ᴵ

Ingest 2-4 drops; massage 1-3 drops into abdomen clockwise hourly as needed.

Coriander ᵀ ᴵ	Lavender ᵀ ᴵ
Fennel ᵀ ᴵ	Cinnamon ᵀ ᴵ
Ginger ᵀ ᴵ	*Protocol on pg. 194*

Disinfectant ᴬ ᵀ ᴵ

Add 20 drops to glass spray bottle; fill remainder with water.

Tea Tree ᵀ	Lime ᵀ
On Guard ᵀ	Cilantro ᵀ
Purify ᵀ	

Diuretic ᴬ ᵀ ᴵ

Add 3-5 drops with carrier oil and apply over the lower back.

Juniper Berry ᵀ	Cedarwood ᵀ
Cypress ᵀ	Arborvitae ᵀ
Rosemary ᵀ	

Diverticulitis ᴬ ᵀ ᴵ

Ingest 2-4 drops twice daily for ongoing support; massage 1-3 drops into abdomen clockwise as needed.

DigestZen® ᵀ ᴵ	DDR Prime® ᵀ ᴵ
Cypress ᵀ	TerraZyme® ᴵ
Lemon ᵀ ᴵ	

Dizziness ᴬ ᵀ ᴵ

Apply 1-3 drops to back of neck, under nose, or on temples; inhale from cupped hands; ingest 2-4 drops of Zendocrine® as needed.

Balance ᴬ ᵀ	Cedarwood ᴬ ᵀ
Zendocrine® ᴬ ᵀ ᴵ	Arborvitae ᴬ ᵀ
Cypress ᴬ ᵀ	

Dogs: Anxiety ᴬ ᵀ ᴵ

Apply 1-2 drops diluted (25-75% pending weight) to pads of paws or outside of ears 2x daily as needed.

Rose ᴬ ᵀ	Lavender ᴬ ᵀ
Jasmine ᴬ ᵀ	Adaptiv™ ᴬ ᵀ
Copaiba ᴬ ᵀ	

Dogs: Arthritis ᴬ ᵀ ᴵ

Apply 1-2 drops diluted (25-75% pending weight) to affected areas 2x daily as needed.

Turmeric ᵀ	Deep Blue® ᵀ
Frankincense ᵀ	Helichrysum ᵀ
AromaTouch® ᵀ	

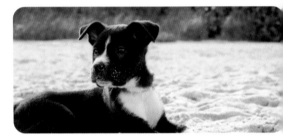

Dogs: Bone Injury ᴬ ᵀ ᴵ

Apply 1-2 drops diluted (25-75% pending weight) to affected areas 2x daily as needed.

Ginger ᵀ	Cypress ᵀ
Helichrysum ᵀ	Wintergreen ᵀ
Frankincense ᵀ	

Dogs: Dermatitis ᴬ ᵀ ᴵ

Apply 1-2 drops diluted (25-75% pending weight) to affected areas 2x daily as needed.

Rose ᵀ	Helichrysum ᵀ
HD Clear® ᵀ	Frankincense ᵀ
Geranium ᵀ	

Dogs: Ear Infection ᴬ ᵀ ᴵ

Apply 1-2 drops diluted (25-75% pending weight) to outside of ears 2x daily as needed.

Rose ᵀ	Helichrysum ᵀ
Purify ᵀ	Frankincense ᵀ
Basil ᵀ	

Dogs: Earache ᴬ ᵀ ᴵ

Apply 1-2 drops diluted (25-75% pending weight) to outside of ears 2x daily as needed.

Copaiba ᵀ	Rosemary ᵀ
Lavender ᵀ	Wintergreen ᵀ
Spearmint ᵀ	

Dogs: Fleas ᴬ ᵀ ᴵ

Add 2-4 drops to dog shampoo and wash 2x daily as needed.

Eucalyptus ᵀ	Lemongrass ᵀ
Lemon Eucalyptus ᵀ	Cedarwood ᵀ
Citronella ᵀ	

Dogs: Heart Issues ᴬ ᵀ ᴵ

Apply 1-2 drops diluted (25-75% pending weight) over chest 2x daily as needed.

Marjoram ᵀ	Wild Orange ᵀ
Helichrysum ᵀ	Roman Chamomile ᵀ
Cypress ᵀ	

ᴬ Aromatic ᵀ Topical 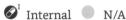ᴵ Internal N/A

Dogs: Sleep

Apply 1-2 drops diluted (25-75% pending weight) to pads of paws or outside of ears 2x daily as needed.

Copaiba ᴬᵀ	Cedarwood ᴬᵀ
Serenity ᴬᵀ	Vetiver ᴬᵀ
Calmer ᴬᵀ	

Dogs: Stroke

Apply 1-2 drops diluted (25-75% pending weight) to pads of paws and back of neck 2x daily as needed.

Cedarwood ᴬᵀ	Rosemary ᴬᵀ
Lavender ᴬᵀ	Roman Chamomile ᴬᵀ
Frankincense ᴬᵀ	

Dry Eyes

Dab a drop diluted with a carrier oil around eyes (do not put directly in eyes). Also apply 2 drops to eye reflex points on bottoms of feet.

Lavender ᵀ	Rosemary ᵀ
Lemon ᵀ	Marjoram ᵀ
Rose ᵀ	

Dry Mouth

Place 1-2 drops on tongue 2x daily.

Peppermint ᴵ	Lemon ᴵ
Lime ᴵ	Ginger ᴵ
Siberian Fir ᴵ	

Dry Skin

Add 3-5 drops to carrier oil and apply to affected area 2-4x daily.

Cedarwood ᵀ	Lavender ᵀ
Frankincense ᵀ	Roman Chamomile ᵀ
Geranium ᵀ	

Dysentery

Massage 1-3 drops into abdomen; ingest 2-4 drops as needed.

Helichrysum ᵀᴵ	Lavender ᵀᴵ
DigestZen® ᵀᴵ	Tea Tree ᵀᴵ
Frankincense ᵀᴵ	

Dysphagia

Apply 1-3 drops to neck or gargle a few drops in water as needed.

Copaiba ᵀᴵ	Peppermint ᵀᴵ
Marjoram ᵀᴵ	Frankincense ᵀᴵ
Lemon ᵀᴵ	

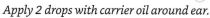

E. Coli

Ingest 1-3 drops every 2-3 hours for systemic and/or internal infections.

Thyme ᵀᴵ	Tea Tree ᵀᴵ
Oregano ᵀᴵ	Arborvitae ᵀ
On Guard ᵀᴵ	

Ear Infection

Apply 1-3 drops around the opening of the ear or apply to a cotton ball and place over ear opening overnight. Do NOT use essential oils in ear. Ingest 2-4 drops as needed.

Tea Tree ᵀᴵ	Helichrysum ᵀᴵ
Lavender ᵀᴵ	Ginger ᵀᴵ
Basil ᵀᴵ	*Protocol on pg. 194*

Ear Mites

Apply 2 drops with carrier oil around ear.

Lemon ᵀ	Sandalwood ᵀ
Lavender ᵀ	Cinnamon ᵀ
Tea Tree ᵀ	

Earache

Apply 1-3 drops around the opening of the ear or apply to a cotton ball and place over ear opening overnight. Do NOT use essential oils in ear.

Helichrysum ᵀ	Tea Tree ᵀ
Basil ᵀ	Frankincense ᵀ
Lavender ᵀ	*Protocol on pg. 194*

Eating Disorder

Apply 3-5 drops as needed to abdomen and inside of legs from knees to ankles.

Bergamot ᴬᵀ	Ginger ᴬᵀ
Lemon ᴬᵀ	Coriander ᴬᵀ
Cinnamon ᴬᵀ	

Ebola Virus

Apply 3-5 drops to back of neck and spine 3x daily; take 3-5 drops in a capsule 2-3x daily as needed.

Oregano ᵀᴵ	Tea Tree ᵀᴵ
Clove ᵀᴵ	Arborvitae ᵀ
Frankincense ᵀᴵ	

Eczema

Apply 2-4 drops to affected area as needed. For improved efficacy, dilute with carrier oil.

HD Clear® ᵀ	Immortelle ᵀ
Helichrysum ᵀ	Magnolia ᵀ
Cedarwood ᵀ	

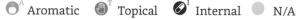 ᴬ Aromatic ᵀ Topical ᴵ Internal N/A

Edema

Massage 2-4 drops into affected area and on bottoms of feet; ingest a couple times daily or as needed.

Lemon ᵀ ᴵ	Slim & Sassy® ᵀ ᴵ
Eucalyptus ᵀ	Grapefruit ᵀ ᴵ
Peppermint ᵀ ᴵ	

Endurance

Massage 2-4 drops on lower back over adrenals, or inhale from cupped hands. Ingest 2-4 drops as needed.

Basil ᴬ ᵀ ᴵ	Geranium ᴬ ᵀ ᴵ
Juniper Berry ᴬ ᵀ ᴵ	Ylang Ylang ᴬ ᵀ ᴵ
Rosemary ᴬ ᵀ ᴵ	*Protocol on pg. 216*

Epstein-Barr Virus

Apply 3-5 drops 3x daily to outside of legs, spine and back of neck. Also take in a capsule 2x daily.

Bergamot ᵀ ᴵ	Marjoram ᵀ ᴵ
Ylang Ylang ᵀ ᴵ	Rosemary ᵀ ᴵ
Lavender ᵀ ᴵ	

Exhaustion

Inhale 1-3 drops from cupped hands; apply a couple drops to feet and back; ingest 2-4 drops Ylang Ylang or Tangerine as needed.

Ylang Ylang ᴬ ᵀ ᴵ	Motivate ᴬ ᵀ
Tangerine ᴬ ᵀ ᴵ	Peppermint ᴬ ᵀ ᴵ
Cheer ᴬ ᵀ	*Protocol on pg. 195*

Emphysema

Apply 1-3 drops to back of neck, under nose, chest, or on bridge of nose as needed; ingest 3-5 drops; inhale from cupped hands.

Breathe ᴬ ᵀ	Eucalyptus ᴬ ᵀ
Frankincense ᴬ ᵀ ᴵ	Lavender ᴬ ᵀ ᴵ
Rose ᴬ ᵀ	

Energy (low)

Apply 2-4 drops to bottoms of feet, under nose, or chest as needed; inhale from cupped hands as needed; use a drop under the tongue.

Wild Orange ᴬ ᵀ ᴵ	Mito2Max® ᴵ
Peppermint ᴬ ᵀ ᴵ	Lifelong Vitality Pack® ᴵ
Spearmint ᴬ ᵀ ᴵ	*Protocol on pg. 195*

Erectile Dysfunction

Apply 2-4 drops to temples, wrists, and back of neck as needed; inhale from cupped hands; add a drop to personal lubricant.

Cypress ᴬ ᵀ	Passion ᴬ ᵀ
AromaTouch® ᴬ ᵀ	DDR Prime® ᴬ ᵀ
Ylang Ylang ᴬ ᵀ	

Eye Support

Apply 2-4 drops diluted around eyes (do not get directly in eyes), lower back, and eye reflex points.

Clary Sage ᵀ	Cypress ᵀ
Frankincense ᵀ	Vetiver ᵀ
Helichrysum ᵀ	

Fainting

Inhale 1-3 drops from cupped hands as needed; apply a drop onto ears and under nose; diffuse several drops.

Peppermint ᴬ ᵀ	Neroli ᴬ ᵀ
Frankincense ᴬ ᵀ	Breathe ᴬ ᵀ
Wild Orange ᴬ ᵀ	

Endometriosis

Apply 3-5 drops to lower abdomen 3x daily.

Clary Sage ᵀ	Ylang Ylang ᵀ
Eucalyptus ᵀ	Patchouli ᵀ
Frankincense ᵀ	*Protocol on pg. 194*

Epilepsy

Apply 1-3 drops to back of neck, under nose, or on temples; inhale from cupped hands; ingest 2-4 drops of Frankincense or DDR Prime® 3-5x daily.

Frankincense ᴬ ᵀ ᴵ	DDR Prime® ᴬ ᵀ ᴵ
Spikenard ᴬ ᵀ	Lifelong Vitality Pack® ᴵ
Copaiba ᴬ ᵀ ᴵ	

Estrogen Imbalance

Apply 2-4 drops to feet, abdomen, and lower back; inhale from cupped hands; take 2-4 drops of Clary Sage in a capsule 2x daily.

Clary Sage ᴬ ᵀ ᴵ	Whisper ᴬ ᵀ
Lavender ᴬ ᵀ ᴵ	Phytoestrogen Complex ᴵ
Basil ᴬ ᵀ ᴵ	

Eyes (Swollen)

Apply 1-3 drops diluted around eyes (do not get directly in eyes.)

Geranium ᵀ	Eucalyptus ᵀ
Frankincense ᵀ	Juniper Berry ᵀ
Rose ᵀ	

Fear

Inhale from cupped hands; apply a couple drops to feet and back.

Black Pepper ᴬ ᵀ	Frankincense ᴬ ᵀ
Juniper Berry ᴬ ᵀ	Motivate ᴬ ᵀ
Balance ᴬ ᵀ	

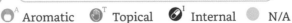 **Aromatic** **Topical** **Internal** N/A

Fever

Apply 2-4 drops to back of neck, under nose, on bridge of nose, or chest; ingest 2-4 drops Oregano every 2-4 hours until symptoms subside.

Peppermint ^{ATI}	Lavender ^{ATI}
Oregano ^{ATI}	Frankincense ^{ATI}
Roman Chamomile ^{ATI}	

Fibrocystic Breasts

Massage 1-3 drops into breasts as needed; ingest 3-5 drops 3x daily.

Frankincense ^{TI}	Rose ^T
Clary Sage ^{TI}	DDR Prime® ^{TI}
Sandalwood ^{TI}	

Fibroids (Uterine)

Apply 2-4 drops to abdomen 3x daily; ingest 3-5 drops.

Sandalwood ^{TI}	DDR Prime® ^{TI}
Thyme ^{TI}	Helichrysum ^{TI}
Frankincense ^{ATI}	

Fibromyalgia

Apply 2-4 drops to affected area; ingest 2-4 drops 3x daily; use full protocol for most profound results.

DDR Prime® ^{ATI}	Frankincense ^{ATI}
Deep Blue® ^{AT}	Turmeric ^{ATI}
Copaiba ^{ATI}	*Protocol on pg. 195*

Flu (Influenza)

Apply 2-4 drops to chest, bottoms of feet, and back over lungs; ingest 2-4 drops every 2-3 hours as desired for antiviral and immune-boosting support.

Breathe ^{AT}	Lemon Eucalyptus ^{AT}
On Guard ^{ATI}	Black Pepper ^{ATI}
Oregano ^{ATI}	*Protocol on pg. 195*

Focus

Apply 1-3 drops to forehead, temples, back of neck, and behind the ears; inhale from cupped hands; diffuse several drops.

Peppermint ^{AT}	Frankincense ^{AT}
InTune® ^{AT}	Green Mandarin ^{AT}
Rosemary ^{AT}	*Protocol on pg. 195*

Food Poisoning

Apply 1-3 drops to stomach and rub clockwise; ingest 2-4 drops every 2-4 hours as needed

Oregano ^{TI}	On Guard ^{TI}
DigestZen® ^{TI}	GX Assist® ^I
Pink Pepper ^{TI}	

Fragile Hair

Apply 3-5 drops to a carrier oil and apply to hair at bedtime or 30 minutes before showering.

Lavender ^T	Cedarwood ^T
Peppermint ^T	Lemongrass ^T
Rosemary ^T	

Frozen Shoulder

Apply 2-4 drops to affected area. Massage with carrier oil for improved efficacy.

Deep Blue® ^T	Siberian Fir ^T
AromaTouch® ^T	Lemongrass ^T
Cypress ^T	

Fungal Skin

Apply 1-3 drops to affected area several times daily.

Tea Tree ^T	Arborvitae ^T
HD Clear® ^T	Cedarwood ^T
Oregano ^T	

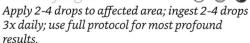

G

Gallbladder Issues

Massage 2-4 drops over gallbladder several times daily; ingest 2-4 drops as needed.

Juniper Berry ^{TI}	Helichrysum ^{TI}
Zendocrine® ^{TI}	Tangerine ^{TI}
Tea Tree ^{TI}	

Gallbladder Stones

Apply 2-4 drops over gallbladder several times daily; ingest 2-4 drops as needed.

Lemon ^{TI}	Bergamot ^{TI}
Cilantro ^{TI}	Zendocrine® ^{TI}
Rosemary ^{TI}	

Gangrene

Combine 3-5 drops with a carrier oil and apply to affected area hourly.

Lavender ^T	Copaiba ^T
Tea Tree ^T	Arborvitae ^T
Frankincense ^T	

Gas (Flatulence)

Massage 1-3 drops into stomach area; ingest 1-3 drops as needed.

DigestZen® ^{TI}	Ginger ^{TI}
Fennel ^{TI}	Celery Seed ^{TI}
Peppermint ^{TI}	*Protocol on pg. 194*

  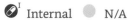

^A Aromatic   ^T Topical   ^I Internal   N/A

Gastritis

Massage 1-3 drops into stomach area; ingest 2-4 drops diluted in carrier oil inside a veggie cap as needed.

Lavender [T I]	Lemon [T I]
Peppermint [T I]	Coriander [T I]
Roman Chamomile [T I]	*Protocol on pg. 194*

Gastroesophageal Reflux Disease

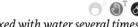

Apply 3 -5 drops to upper chest and back before meals.

Lavender [T]	Ginger [T]
Lemon [T]	Fennel [T]
Peppermint [T]	

Genital Warts

Dilute heavily with a carrier oil and apply 1-3 drops to affected area 3x daily.

Oregano [T]	Tea Tree [T]
Frankincense [A T]	Lemon [T]
Melissa [T]	

Giardia

Massage 1-3 drops clockwise onto stomach and chest area; ingest 1-3 drops as needed.

DigestZen® [T I]	Spearmint [T I]
Oregano [T I]	Tea Tree [T I]
Rosemary [T I]	

Gingivitis

Gargle 1-3 drops mixed with water several times daily; ingest 1-3 drops as needed

On Guard [I]	Tea Tree [I]
Myrrh [I]	Arborvitae [I]
Clove [I]	

Glaucoma

Dab a drop diluted around eye (do not get directly in eyes); combine 2-5 drops into a capsule and take 3x daily.

Rosemary [T I]	Lemon [T I]
Clary Sage [T I]	Eucalyptus [I]
Cypress [T]	

Gluten Sensitivity

Ingest 1-3 drops as needed. Ingest TerraZyme® 20-30 minutes before eating, or immediately after or during consumption. Rub 2-4 drops over stomach.

TerraZyme® [I]	Zendocrine® [T I]
DigestZen® [T I]	TriEase® Softgels [I]
Lemon [T I]	

Gout

Ingest 2-4 drops twice a day; massage 1-3 drops gently into affected joints as needed.

Lemongrass [T I]	Spearmint [T I]
Deep Blue® [T]	Lavender [T I]
Black Spruce [T]	*Protocol on pg. 196*

Grave's Disease

Apply 1-3 drops to front of neck. Dilute with carrier oil for easier application. Ingest 1-3 drops a few times daily or as needed.

Frankincense [T I]	Zendocrine® [T I]
Myrrh [T I]	Lifelong Vitality Pack® [I]
DDR Prime® [T I]	*Protocol on pg. 207*

Greasy/Oily Hair

Apply 3-5 drops to a carrier oil and apply to hair at bedtime or 30 minutes before showering.

Basil [T]	Eucalyptus [T]
Roman Chamomile [T]	Lemongrass [T]
Cedarwood [T]	

Growing Pains

Massage 2-4 drops into affected areas as needed.

Deep Blue® [T]	Wintergreen [T]
Marjoram [T]	Spikenard [T]
Lemongrass [T]	

Gum Disease

Apply 1-3 drops to gums; gargle a few drops in water as needed.

On Guard [I]	Tea Tree [I]
Myrrh [I]	Lavender [I]
Clove [I]	

Gums (Bleeding)

Apply 1-3 drops to gums; gargle a few drops in water as needed.

Helichrysum [I]	Tea Tree [I]
Myrrh [I]	Clove [I]
Geranium [I]	

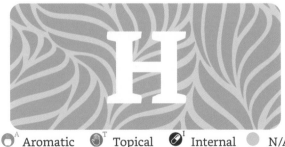

H. Pylori

Massage 2-4 drops into stomach area; ingest 1-3 drops as needed.

Fennel [T I]	Ginger [T I]
Peppermint [T I]	Tangerine [T I]
DigestZen® [T I]	

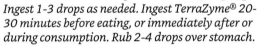

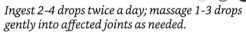

A-Z Ref.

38

Legend: ⬤[A] Aromatic   ⬤[T] Topical   ⬤[I] Internal   ⬤ N/A

Hair Loss

Dilute 5 drops in 20 drops of carrier oil. Massage into scalp every night or 30 minutes before showering.

Rosemary [T]	Spikenard [T]
Peppermint [T]	Lifelong Vitality Pack® [I]
Geranium [T]	

Halitosis

Gargle a few drops mixed with water several times daily or as needed; ingest 1-3 drops Cilantro twice daily.

On Guard [I]	Zendocrine® [I]
Cilantro [I]	Spearmint [I]
Peppermint [I]	

Hand, Foot, & Mouth

Apply 1-3 drops to affected areas (dilute for increased effectiveness); ingest as needed.

On Guard [T I]	Copaiba [T I]
Rose [T]	Melissa [T I]
DDR Prime® [T I]	

Hands Tingling

Apply 3-5 drops to the affected area, lower back, and spine.

Peppermint [T]	Frankincense [T]
Eucalyptus [T]	Lavender [T]
Rosemary [T]	

Hangover

Add 4-6 drops to warm bath; massage into back of neck and over liver; ingest 2-4 drops as needed.

DigestZen® [A T I]	Zendocrine® [A T I]
PastTense® [A T]	Lemon [A T I]
Grapefruit [A T I]	

Hashimoto's

Apply 1-3 drops to front of neck. Dilute with carrier oil for easier application. Ingest 1-3 drops a few times daily or as needed.

Clove [T I]	Peppermint [T I]
Lemongrass [T I]	Rosemary [T I]
Myrrh [T I]	*Protocol on pg. 207*

Hay Fever

Apply 1-3 drops to bridge of nose and over sinuses or chest as needed; use a drop of Lavender under the tongue; inhale from cupped hands; diffuse several drops.

Breathe [A T]	Purify [A T]
Lavender [A T I]	TriEase® Softgels [I]
Peppermint [A T I]	*Protocol on pg. 186*

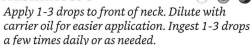

Head Lice

Dilute 1-3 drops and apply to entire scalp, shampoo, and rinse 30 minutes later. Repeat daily for several days.

Tea Tree [T]	Rosemary [T]
Arborvitae [T]	Eucalyptus [T]
TerraShield® [T]	

Headache (Sinus)

Massage 2-4 drops into forehead, temples, and back of neck; inhale from cupped hands.

PastTense® [A T]	Frankincense [A T]
Breathe [A T]	Rosemary [A T]
Peppermint [A T]	*Protocol on pg. 205*

Headache (Tension)

Massage 1-3 drops into forehead, temples, and back of neck; inhale from cupped hands.

PastTense® [A T]	Lavender [A T]
Peppermint [A T]	AromaTouch® [A T]
Frankincense [A T]	*Protocol on pg. 196*

Hearing Issues

Apply 1-3 drops to temples and around the opening of the ear; apply to a cotton ball and place over ear opening overnight. Do not apply into ear.

Helichrysum [T]	Rose [T]
Basil [T]	Tea Tree [T]
Frankincense [T]	

Heart Disease

Apply 2-4 drops over chest; ingest 3-5 drops as a daily supplement.

Geranium [T I]	DDR Prime® [T I]
Helichrysum [T I]	Lifelong Vitality Pack® [I]
Marjoram [T I]	

Heartburn

Massage 1-3 drops into abdomen; ingest 1-3 drops as needed.

DigestZen® [T I]	Ginger [T I]
Peppermint [T I]	Fennel [T I]
Slim & Sassy® [T I]	*Protocol on pg. 196*

Heat Exhaustion

Apply 1-3 drops to forehead, back of neck, inside of wrists, and bottom of feet; add Lemon or Peppermint to mineral water and sip slowly.

Peppermint ᴬᵀᴵ	Siberian Fir ᴬᵀᴵ
Lemon ᴬᵀᴵ	Lavender ᴬᵀᴵ
PastTense® ᴬᵀ	

Heatstroke

Apply 1-3 drops to forehead, temples, back of neck, and chest; ingest 1-3 drops as needed.

Peppermint ᴬᵀᴵ	Spearmint ᴬᵀᴵ
Frankincense ᴬᵀᴵ	Copaiba ᴬᵀᴵ
PastTense® ᴬᵀ	

Heavy Metal Detox

Ingest 2-4 drops 2x daily; massage 2-4 drops into bottoms of feet.

Cilantro ᵀᴵ	Zendocrine® ᴵ
Frankincense ᵀᴵ	Lemon ᵀᴵ
DDR Prime® ᵀᴵ	

Hematoma

Apply 1-3 drops to affected areas 2-3x daily or as needed; take 3-5 drops in a capsule 2x daily.

Cypress ᵀ	Marjoram ᵀᴵ
AromaTouch® ᵀ	Lemon ᵀᴵ
Geranium ᵀᴵ	

Hemorrhoids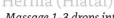

Dilute 2-4 drops with carrier oil and apply directly to affected areas daily or as needed.

Geranium ᵀ	Siberian Fir ᵀ
Cypress ᵀ	Myrrh ᵀ
Rose ᵀ	*Protocol on pg. 196*

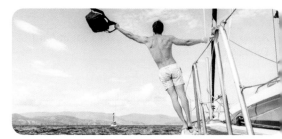

Hepatitis

Ingest 1-3 drops; use several drops topically with a warm compress over the liver area.

Copaiba ᵀᴵ	Helichrysum ᵀᴵ
Myrrh ᵀᴵ	Lavender ᵀᴵ
Zendocrine® ᵀᴵ	*Protocol on pg. 197*

Hernia (Hiatal)

Massage 1-3 drops into affected area as needed; Take 2-3 TerraZyme® as needed.

Helichrysum ᵀ	DigestZen® ᵀ
Frankincense ᵀ	TerraZyme® ᴵ
Arborvitae ᵀ	

Herniated Disc

Massage 2-4 drops into affected area as often as needed (at least 3x daily.)

Deep Blue® ᵀ	Copaiba ᵀ
AromaTouch® ᵀ	Wintergreen ᵀ
Lemongrass ᵀ	*Protocol on pg. 197*

Herpes Simplex

Ingest 1-3 drops; use topically with a warm compress over the kidney area; apply on the right and left side of throat daily.

Tea Tree ᵀᴵ	Oregano ᵀᴵ
Melissa ᵀᴵ	Rose ᵀ
On Guard ᵀᴵ	*Protocol on pg. 197*

Hiccups

Inhale 1-3 drops from cupped hands; massage into chest and stomach area as needed.

Arborvitae ᴬᵀ	DigestZen® ᴬᵀ
Lemon ᴬᵀ	Neroli ᴬᵀ
Copaiba ᴬᵀ	

HIV

Apply 1-3 drops to bottoms of feet; ingest 3-5 drops 3x daily; inhale from cupped hands for emotional support.

Melissa ᴬᵀᴵ	DDR Prime® ᴬᵀᴵ
Oregano ᴬᵀᴵ	Thyme ᴬᵀᴵ
Helichrysum ᴬᵀᴵ	*Protocol on pg. 185*

Hives

Apply 1-3 drops diluted to affected area; ingest 2-4 drops twice daily as needed.

Tea Tree ᵀᴵ	Tulsi ᵀ
Frankincense ᵀᴵ	Magnolia ᵀ
Lavender ᵀᴵ	

Hoarse Voice

Gargle 1-3 drops in water as needed; apply diluted to outside of throat.

Lemon ᵀᴵ	On Guard ᵀᴵ
Myrrh ᵀᴵ	Arborvitae ᵀ
Lavender ᵀᴵ	

Hormone Balance (Female)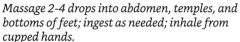

Massage 2-4 drops into abdomen, temples, and bottoms of feet; ingest as needed; inhale from cupped hands.

ClaryCalm® ᴬᵀ	Frankincense ᴬᵀᴵ
Clary Sage ᴬᵀᴵ	Sandalwood ᴬᵀᴵ
Ylang Ylang ᴬᵀᴵ	

 Aromatic   Topical Internal N/A

Hormone Balance (Male)

Combine 2-5 drops and apply to bottom of feet and inside of legs; take a few drops in a capsule daily.

Fennel ᴬ ᵀ ᴵ	Clary Sage ᴬ ᵀ ᴵ
Geranium ᴬ ᵀ ᴵ	Sandalwood ᴬ ᵀ ᴵ
Frankincense ᴬ ᵀ ᴵ	

Horse: Anxiety/Nervousness

Apply 3-5 drops of these oils to remedy physical conditions (digestive, hormones, pain) that would cause horse anxiety.

Copaiba ᴬ ᵀ	Peppermint ᴬ ᵀ
Fennel ᴬ ᵀ	Whisper ᴬ ᵀ
Slim & Sassy® ᴬ ᵀ	

Horse: Hoof Rot

Mix 3-5 drops with hot water and soak hoof for several minutes.

Oregano ᵀ	Helichrysum ᵀ
Cinnamon ᵀ	Thyme ᵀ
Clove ᵀ	

Horse: Infection

Apply 3-5 drops to the affected area 5x daily. Dilute for sensitive skin.

On Guard ᵀ	Rosemary ᵀ
Tea Tree ᵀ	Thyme ᵀ
Lavender ᵀ	

Horse: Leg Fracture

Apply 3-5 drops to the affected area 5x daily. Dilute for sensitive skin.

Ginger ᵀ	Cypress ᵀ
Helichrysum ᵀ	Wintergreen ᵀ
Frankincense ᵀ	

Horse: Muscle Tissue

Massage 3-5 drops to the affected area 3x daily. Dilute for sensitive skin.

Marjoram ᵀ	Helichrysum ᵀ
Copaiba ᵀ	Lemongrass ᵀ
AromaTouch® ᵀ	

Horse: Wounds

Allow horse to smell the oil. Apply 3-5 drops to the affected area 2-3x daily. Dilute for sensitive skin.

Helichrysum ᴬ ᵀ	Roman Chamomile ᴬ ᵀ
Stronger ᴬ ᵀ	Myrrh ᴬ ᵀ
Clove ᴬ ᵀ	

Hot Flashes

Massage 2-4 drops into chest, neck, and face as needed; ingest 2-5 drops Clary Sage and Ylang Ylang 2x daily.;

ClaryCalm® ᴬ ᵀ	Ylang Ylang ᴬ ᵀ ᴵ
Peppermint ᴬ ᵀ ᴵ	Whisper ᴬ ᵀ
Clary Sage ᴬ ᵀ ᴵ	*Protocol on pg. 199*

Hyperactivity

Apply 1-3 drops on back of neck and bottoms of feet; inhale from cupped hands; diffuse several drops.

InTune® ᴬ ᵀ	Adaptiv™ ᴬ ᵀ
Balance ᴬ ᵀ	Lavender ᴬ ᵀ
Vetiver ᴬ ᵀ	

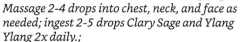

Hypersomnia

Apply 2-4 drops to chest area, bottoms of feet, or inside of wrists; inhale 1-3 drops from cupped hands; supplement regularly for long-term benefits.

Melissa ᴬ ᵀ ᴵ	Mito2Max® ᴵ
Lemon ᴬ ᵀ ᴵ	Lifelong Vitality Pack® ᴵ
Basil ᴬ ᵀ ᴵ	

Hypertension

Apply 1-2 drops behind ears; inhale from cupped hands; use a drop under the tongue; diffuse several drops.

Adaptiv™ ᴬ ᵀ	Rose ᴬ ᵀ
Balance ᴬ ᵀ	Lemon ᴬ ᵀ ᴵ
Yarrow|Pom ᴬ ᵀ ᴵ	

Hyperthyroid

Apply 1-3 drops diluted to front of neck. Ingest 3-5 drops a few times daily or as needed.

Myrrh ᵀ ᴵ	Zendocrine® ᵀ ᴵ
Frankincense ᵀ ᴵ	Lifelong Vitality Pack® ᴵ
DDR Prime® ᵀ ᴵ	*Protocol on pg. 207*

Hypoglycemia

Apply 1-3 drops to chest, bottoms of feet, and inside of wrists; ingest 2-4 drops a few times daily or as needed.

Slim & Sassy® ᵀ ᴵ	Zendocrine® ᵀ ᴵ
Cinnamon ᵀ ᴵ	DDR Prime® ᵀ ᴵ
Coriander ᵀ ᴵ	

Hypothyroid

Apply 1-3 drops to front of neck. Dilute with carrier oil for easier application. Ingest 3-5 drops a few times daily or as needed.

Peppermint ᵀ ᴵ	Myrrh ᵀ ᴵ
Lemongrass ᵀ ᴵ	Lifelong Vitality Pack® ᴵ
Clove ᵀ ᴵ	*Protocol on pg. 207*

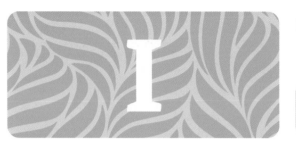

Hysteria

Apply 3-5 drops of each with carrier oil to back of neck, temples and spine; inhale a few drops from cupped hands; diffuse several drops.

Vetiver ᴬᵀ	Sandalwood ᴬᵀ
Lavender ᴬᵀ	Cypress ᴬᵀ
Console ᴬᵀ	

Impetigo

Combine 2 drops of each with carrier oil and apply to affected area 5x daily.

Lavender ᵀ	Helichrysum ᵀ
Tea Tree ᵀ	Sandalwood ᵀ
Myrrh ᵀ	

Indigestion

Massage 1-3 drops into stomach area clockwise as needed; drink 1-3 drops with water or in a capsule.

DigestZen® ᵀ ᴵ	Cardamom ᵀ ᴵ
Ginger ᵀ ᴵ	DigestTab® ᴵ
Lemon ᵀ ᴵ	*Protocol on pg. 184*

Infertility

Apply 2-4 drops to abdomen, wrists, and lower back daily; ingest 2-4 drops 2x daily.

Clary Sage ᵀ ᴵ	Fennel ᵀ ᴵ
DDR Prime® ᵀ ᴵ	Lifelong Vitality Pack® ᴵ
Ylang Ylang ᵀ ᴵ	*Protocol on pg. 198*

Ingrown Toenail

Apply 1-3 drops to affected toenail 3x daily. Soak toenail in warm water for 15 minutes and gently work out over time.

Tea Tree ᵀ	Lavender ᵀ
On Guard ᵀ	Oregano ᵀ
Zendocrine® ᵀ	

Impotence

Rub 3-5 drops on lower back and outside of legs; add 1-2 drops to personal lubricant; diffuse several drops.

Ylang Ylang ᴬᵀ	Lavender ᴬᵀ
Passion ᴬᵀ	Cinnamon ᴬᵀ
Rosemary ᴬᵀ	*Protocol on pg. 198*

Infant Reflux

Apply 1-2 drops diluted to stomach area and chest as needed.

Tamer ᵀ	DigestZen® ᵀ
Lavender ᵀ	Ginger ᵀ
Fennel ᵀ	

Inflammation

Apply 2-4 drops to affected areas as needed. For systemic inflammation, ingest 2-4 drops 2x daily.

Deep Blue® ᴬᵀ	Turmeric ᴬᵀ ᴵ
Frankincense ᴬᵀ ᴵ	Wintergreen ᴬᵀ
Copaiba ᴬᵀ ᴵ	

Injury (Muscle, Bone)

Apply 3-5 drops liberally to affected area as often as desired. Dilute for sensitive tissues.

Wintergreen ᵀ	Helichrysum ᵀ
Ylang Ylang ᵀ	Blue Tansy ᵀ
Deep Blue® ᵀ	

Immune Boost

Apply 2-4 drops to bottoms of feet; ingest 3-5 drops 2x daily; inhale from cupped hands as needed.

On Guard ᴬᵀ ᴵ	Black Pepper ᴬᵀ ᴵ
Tea Tree ᴬᵀ ᴵ	Black Spruce ᴬᵀ
Oregano ᴬᵀ ᴵ	

Incontinence

Massage 2-4 drops over bladder and kidneys before bedtime as needed.

Cypress ᵀ	Lemongrass ᵀ
Black Pepper ᵀ	Roman Chamomile ᵀ
Ylang Ylang ᵀ	

Infected Wounds

Apply 1-3 drops to affected areas 2-3x daily as needed; dilute for sensitive skin

Tea Tree ᵀ	Lavender ᵀ
Helichrysum ᵀ	On Guard ᵀ
Tulsi ᵀ	

Inflammatory Bowel Disease

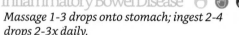

Massage 1-3 drops onto stomach; ingest 2-4 drops 2-3x daily.

DigestZen® ᵀ ᴵ	TerraZyme® ᴵ
Frankincense ᵀ ᴵ	Deep Blue® Complex ᴵ
Lavender ᵀ ᴵ	*Protocol on pg. 198*

Insect Bites

Apply 1-2 drops to insect bite hourly or as needed.

Lavender ᵀ	Roman Chamomile ᵀ
Tea Tree ᵀ	Frankincense ᵀ
Purify ᵀ	

 A Aromatic **T** Topical **I** Internal **N/A**

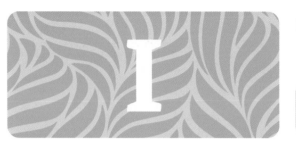

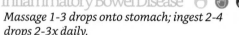

Insect Repellent

Apply liberally over exposed skin areas; combine with carrier oil to spread easily.

TerraShield®ᵀ	Forgiveᵀ
Arborvitaeᵀ	Citronellaᵀ
Peppermintᵀ	

Insomnia

Apply 1-3 drops to forehead, temples, base of skull, and behind the ear; diffuse several drops.

Serenity ᴬᵀ	Cedarwood ᴬᵀ
Vetiver ᴬᵀ	Petitgrain ᴬᵀ
Lavender ᴬᵀ	*Protocol on pg. 205*

Insulin Imbalance

Apply 2-4 drops to bottoms of feet; take 3-5 drops internally 2x daily.

Cinnamon ᵀ ᴵ	Clove ᵀ ᴵ
On Guard ᵀ ᴵ	Slim & Sassy® ᵀ ᴵ
Lavender ᵀ ᴵ	*Protocol on pg. 193*

Irritable Bowel Syndrome

Apply 1-3 drops to bottoms of feet or over stomach; take 2-4 drops internally as needed.

DigestZen® ᵀ ᴵ	Frankincense ᵀ ᴵ
Ginger ᵀ ᴵ	Peppermint ᵀ ᴵ
Turmeric ᵀ ᴵ	*Protocol on pg. 198*

Itchy Skin

Apply 1-3 drops to affected areas as needed. Use with carrier oil or lotion for improved efficacy.

Tea Tree ᵀ	Cedarwood ᵀ
Lavender ᵀ	Frankincense ᵀ
HD Clear® ᵀ	

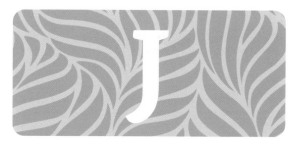

Jaundice

Massage 1-3 drops diluted over the liver; diffuse several drops nearby.

Lavender ᴬᵀ	Rose ᴬᵀ
Myrrh ᴬᵀ	Grapefruit ᴬᵀ
Neroli ᴬᵀ	

Jet Lag

Apply 1-3 drops to forehead, temples, back of neck, and chest; inhale from cupped hands as needed.

Peppermint ᴬᵀ	On Guard ᴬᵀ
Tangerine ᴬᵀ	DDR Prime® ᴬᵀ
Lemon ᴬᵀ	

Jock Itch

Apply 1-3 drops to affected areas as needed with carrier oil; ingest 3-4 drops 3x daily.

Tea Tree ᵀ ᴵ	Purify ᵀ
HD Clear® ᵀ	Thyme ᵀ ᴵ
Lavender ᵀ ᴵ	

Joint Pain

Massage 1-3 drops into affected areas as needed; use carrier oil for improved efficacy.

Deep Blue® ᵀ	Copaiba ᵀ
Lemongrass ᵀ	Frankincense ᵀ
Wintergreen ᵀ	

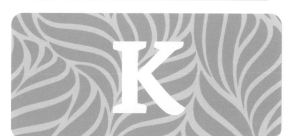

Kidney Infection

Apply 2-4 drops diluted over kidneys 3-5x daily; ingest 1-3 drops 3-5x daily.

Juniper Berry ᵀ ᴵ	On Guard ᵀ ᴵ
Lemongrass ᵀ ᴵ	Clove ᵀ ᴵ
Oregano ᵀ ᴵ	

Kidney Stones

Massage 2-4 drops over kidneys 3-5x daily; ingest 1-3 drops 3-5x daily.

Lemon ᵀ ᴵ	Wintergreen ᵀ
Juniper Berry ᵀ ᴵ	Wild Orange ᵀ ᴵ
Helichrysum ᵀ ᴵ	

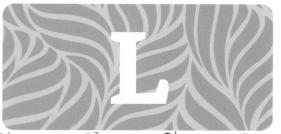

Lactose Intolerance

Ingest 2-4 drops or massage over stomach as needed.

DigestZen® ᵀ ᴵ	TerraZyme® ᴵ
Coriander ᵀ ᴵ	Deep Blue® Complex ᴵ
Lemongrass ᵀ ᴵ	

ᴬ Aromatic ● ᵀ Topical ● ᴵ Internal ● N/A

Laryngitis

Diffuse several drops throughout the day; ingest 3-5 drops 3x daily; massage 1-3 drops onto outside of throat.

On Guard ᴬᵀᴵ	Lemon ᴬᵀᴵ
Tea Tree ᴬᵀᴵ	Rosemary ᴬᵀᴵ
Pink Pepper ᴬᵀᴵ	

Leg Cramps

Massage several drops into legs as needed; use carrier oil for improved efficacy

Deep Blue® ᵀ	Marjoram ᵀ
Cypress ᵀ	Black Pepper ᵀ
AromaTouch® ᵀ	

Lice

Apply 3-5 drops with carrier oil to scalp 4x daily.

Tea Tree ᵀ	Lemon Eucalyptus ᵀ
Lavender ᵀ	Eucalyptus ᵀ
Purify ᵀ	

Lockjaw (Tetanus)

Massage 2-3 drops into jaw joint as needed.

Lavender ᵀ	Copaiba ᵀ
Cypress ᵀ	AromaTouch® ᵀ
Frankincense ᵀ	

Lupus

Ingest 2-4 drops 3-5x daily during flare ups; massage 2-4 drops into inflamed areas; diffuse several drops for emotional support.

Frankincense ᴬᵀᴵ	Copaiba ᴬᵀᴵ
DDR Prime® ᴬᵀᴵ	Turmeric ᴬᵀᴵ
Deep Blue® ᴬᵀ	*Protocol on pg. 198*

Leukemia

Ingest 2-4 drops 3x daily; massage 2-4 drops into bottoms of feet and spine 3-5x daily.

DDR Prime® ᵀᴵ	Sandalwood ᵀᴵ
Frankincense ᵀᴵ	Myrrh ᵀᴵ
Lemongrass ᵀᴵ	*Protocol on pg. 190*

Lipoma

Massage 3-5 drops to affected area 3x daily.

Grapefruit ᵀ	Frankincense ᵀ
Ginger ᵀ	Tea Tree ᵀ
Patchouli ᵀ	

Lou Gehrig's Disease

Apply 3-5 drops to spine and back of legs 3x daily.

Frankincense ᵀ	Geranium ᵀ
Myrrh ᵀ	Tea Tree ᵀ
Lavender ᵀ	

Lyme Disease

Massage 2-4 drops into lower back 3x daily; take 3-5 drops in a capsule 3x daily.

Melissa ᵀᴵ	Geranium ᵀᴵ
Thyme ᵀᴵ	Lifelong Vitality Pack® ᴵ
Oregano ᵀᴵ	*Protocol on pg. 199*

Leaky Gut Syndrome

Combine 3-5 drops in a capsule and take 3x daily after food.

Fennel ᴵ	Ginger ᴵ
Coriander ᴵ	Tea Tree ᴵ
Helichrysum ᴵ	*Protocol on pg. 227*

Libido (Low)

Apply 1-3 drops to abdomen, bottoms of feet, and wrists as needed; inhale from cupped hands; diffuse several drops.

Passion ᴬᵀ	ClaryCalm® ᴬᵀ
Ylang Ylang ᴬᵀ	Rose ᴬᵀ
Jasmine ᴬᵀ	*Protocol on pg. 198*

Liver Disease

Apply 3-5 drops over the liver 3x daily.

Clove ᵀ	Rosemary ᵀ
Grapefruit ᵀ	Frankincense ᵀ
Geranium ᵀ	

Lumbago

Apply 3-5 drops liberally to affected area as often as needed; use carrier oil for improved efficacy.

Deep Blue® ᵀ	Helichrysum ᵀ
Wintergreen ᵀ	Blue Tansy ᵀ
Ylang Ylang ᵀ	*Protocol on pg. 188*

Lymphatic Support

Apply 3-5 drops to sides of neck and sides of rib cage 2x daily.

Grapefruit ᵀ	Basil ᵀ
Lemon ᵀ	Frankincense ᵀ
Juniper Berry ᵀ	

 Aromatic Topical Internal N/A

Lymphoma (Non-Hodgkin's)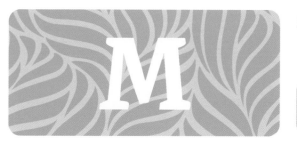

Ingest 3-5 drops 2-4x daily; rub 2-4 drops to sides of throat; supplement for added support.

DDR Prime® ᵀ ᴵ	Arborvitae ᵀ
Frankincense ᴬ ᵀ ᴵ	Lifelong Vitality Pack® ᴵ
Sandalwood ᴬ ᵀ ᴵ	

Malaria

Take 3-5 drops in a capsule 4x daily; rub 2-4 drops onto spine and bottoms of feet.

Ginger ᵀ ᴵ	Basil ᵀ ᴵ
Grapefruit ᵀ ᴵ	Thyme ᵀ ᴵ
Cinnamon ᵀ ᴵ	

Memory Loss

Massage 2-4 drops into forehead, temples, back of neck, and chest as needed; inhale from cupped hands.

Rosemary ᴬ ᵀ	Black Spruce ᴬ ᵀ
Peppermint ᴬ ᵀ	Frankincense ᴬ ᵀ
Bergamot ᴬ ᵀ	*Protocol on pg. 199*

Menstrual Bleeding

Massage 2-4 drops into abdomen and lower back; apply to a warm compress over uterus area; ingest 2-4 drops as needed.

Helichrysum ᵀ ᴵ	ClaryCalm® ᵀ
Geranium ᵀ ᴵ	Lavender ᵀ ᴵ
Clary Sage ᵀ ᴵ	*Protocol on pg. 199*

Mental Fatigue

Massage 1-3 drops into forehead, temples, back of neck, and bottoms of feet; inhale from cupped hands as needed.

Peppermint ᴬ ᵀ	Frankincense ᴬ ᵀ
Basil ᴬ ᵀ	Mito2Max® ᴵ
Green Mandarin ᴬ ᵀ	*Protocol on pg. 222*

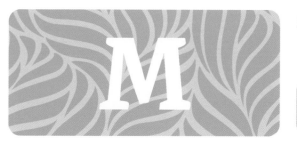

Measles

Dab a few drops onto spots several times daily; add several drops to bath and soak for at least 30 minutes as needed.

Lavender ᵀ	Eucalyptus ᵀ
Roman Chamomile ᵀ	On Guard ᵀ
Oregano ᵀ	

Meningitis

Ingest 2-4 drops 2x daily; massage 2-4 drops into back of neck with carrier oil daily.

On Guard ᵀ ᴵ	Melissa ᵀ ᴵ
Lavender ᵀ ᴵ	DDR Prime® ᵀ ᴵ
Oregano ᵀ ᴵ	

Menstrual Cycle (irregular)

Massage 2-4 drops into abdomen and lower back; ingest 2-4 drops 2x daily.

Clary Sage ᵀ ᴵ	Rose ᵀ
ClaryCalm® ᵀ	Lavender ᵀ ᴵ
Ylang Ylang ᵀ ᴵ	*Protocol on pg. 199*

Metabolism (low)

Apply 1-3 drops to front of neck. Dilute with carrier oil for easier application. Ingest 2-4 drops 3x daily.

Slim & Sassy® ᵀ ᴵ	Basil ᵀ ᴵ
Clove ᵀ ᴵ	Frankincense ᵀ ᴵ
Lemongrass ᵀ ᴵ	*Protocol on pg. 209*

Macular Degeneration

Apply 2-4 drops to lower back and temples.

Sandalwood ᵀ	Lavender ᵀ
Juniper Berry ᵀ	Frankincense ᵀ
Rose ᵀ	

Melanoma

Apply 2-4 drops to affected areas 3-5x daily; ingest 2-4 drops 3x daily.

Frankincense ᵀ ᴵ	Rose ᵀ
DDR Prime® ᵀ ᴵ	Clove ᵀ ᴵ
Sandalwood ᵀ ᴵ	

Menopause

Apply 2-4 drops topically to abdomen, bottoms of feet, and back of neck daily; ingest 2-4 drops Clary Sage and Siberian Fir as needed.

Clary Sage ᵀ ᴵ	Geranium ᵀ ᴵ
ClaryCalm® ᵀ	Rose ᵀ
Siberian Fir ᵀ ᴵ	*Protocol on pg. 199*

Menstrual Pain

Massage 1-3 drops into abdomen, lower back, and shoulders; apply to a warm compress over uterus area; ingest 2-4 drops as needed.

ClaryCalm® ᵀ	Clary Sage ᴬ ᵀ ᴵ
Frankincense ᴬ ᵀ ᴵ	Marjoram ᴬ ᵀ ᴵ
Peppermint ᴬ ᵀ ᴵ	*Protocol on pg. 199*

Migraine

Apply 1-3 drops to forehead, temples, base of skull, back of neck, and bottoms of feet; inhale from cupped hands as needed.

PastTense® ᴬ ᵀ	Deep Blue® ᴬ ᵀ
Peppermint ᴬ ᵀ	Copaiba ᴬ ᵀ
Frankincense ᴬ ᵀ	*Protocol on pg. 200*

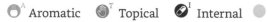

○ᴬ Aromatic   ●ᵀ Topical   ●ᴵ Internal   ● N/A

Milk Supply (Low)

Massage 3-5 drops into breast as often as needed.

Basil [T]	Fennel [T]
Clary Sage [T]	Frankincense [T]
Geranium [T]	

Miscarriage

Apply 3-5 drops to lower abdomen and lower back as often as needed.

Clary Sage [T]	Myrrh [T]
Geranium [T]	Bergamot [T]
Frankincense [T]	

Mold/Mildew

Diffuse several drops where mold is present throughout the day until no longer needed. Mix 20 drops with 4 oz water and apply to area of concern.

Tea Tree [AT]	Oregano [AT]
Purify [AT]	Lemon [AT]
On Guard [AT]	

Moles

Use a toothpick to apply a dab to mole 2-3x daily (avoid surrounding skin with hot oils like Oregano).

Oregano [T]	HD Clear® [T]
Frankincense [T]	Purify [T]
DDR Prime® [ATI]	

Mononucleosis

Ingest 3-5 drops 3x daily; apply 2-4 drops to bottoms of feet; diffuse several drops.

Thyme [ATI]	Oregano [ATI]
Melissa [ATI]	On Guard [ATI]
Bergamot [ATI]	*Protocol on pg. 200*

Mood Swings

Inhale 1-3 drops from cupped hands; apply a few drops to forehead, temples, back of neck, and bottoms of feet; diffuse several drops.

Balance [AT]	Tulsi [AT]
Cheer [AT]	Wild Orange [AT]
Frankincense [AT]	*Protocol on pg. 200*

Motion Sickness

Apply 1-3 drops behind the ears and over navel; inhale from cupped hands; use a drop under the tongue.

DigestZen® [ATI]	Balance [AT]
Peppermint [ATI]	Basil [ATI]
Ginger [ATI]	

Mouth Ulcers

Gargle 1-3 drops mixed with water several times daily; apply a dab to affected area 2-3x daily.

On Guard [TI]	Tulsi [T]
Clove [TI]	Tea Tree [TI]
Myrrh [TI]	*Protocol on pg. 190*

MRSA

Apply 3-5 drops with carrier oil 3-5x daily to affected areas.

On Guard [T]	Geranium [T]
Zendocrine® [T]	Grapefruit [T]
Patchouli [T]	

Mucus

Apply 3-5 drops over the nose and sinuses (avoid the eyes).

Arborvitae [T]	Tea Tree [T]
Eucalyptus [T]	Lime [T]
Peppermint [T]	

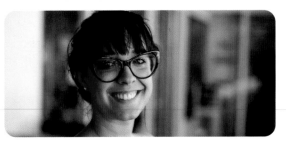

Multiple Sclerosis

Apply 3-5 drops to the bottoms of feet and spine 3x daily.

Frankincense [T]	Neroli [T]
Lavender [T]	Black Pepper [T]
Rose [T]	*Protocol on pg. 200*

Muscle Cramps

Massage 3-5 drops with carrier oil into affected area as often as desired.

Deep Blue® [T]	Helichrysum [T]
Wintergreen [T]	Blue Tansy [T]
Ylang Ylang [T]	*Protocol on pg. 201*

Muscle Injury

Massage 2-4 drops into affected muscles 3x daily or as needed.

Deep Blue® [T]	AromaTouch® [T]
Marjoram [T]	Yarrow|Pom [T]
Helichrysum [T]	

Muscle Pain

Massage 2-4 drops into affected muscles 3x daily or as needed; use a drop under the tongue for pain relief.

Deep Blue® [T]	AromaTouch® [T]
Marjoram [T]	Copaiba [TI]
Helichrysum [T]	*Protocol on pg. 201*

Muscle Spasms

Massage 2-4 drops into affected muscles as needed; use a drop under the tongue.

Black Pepper ᵀ ᴵ   Blue Tansy ᵀ
Deep Blue® ᵀ ᴵ   Yarrow|Pom ᵀ ᴵ
Copaiba ᵀ ᴵ

Muscle Stiffness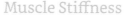

Massage 2-4 drops into affected muscles 2-3x daily.

AromaTouch® ᵀ   Lemongrass ᵀ
Deep Blue® ᵀ   Marjoram ᵀ
Cypress ᵀ

Muscular Dystrophy

Apply 3-5 drops with carrier oil to spine and back of neck 3x daily.

Frankincense ᵀ   Neroli ᵀ
Lavender ᵀ   Helichrysum ᵀ
Rose ᵀ

N

Nails/Nail Beds

Apply 1 drop to nails of concern.

Tea Tree ᵀ   Eucalyptus ᵀ
Frankincense ᵀ   Lavender ᵀ
Myrrh ᵀ

Nasal Congestion

Apply 1-3 drops over bridge of nose, under nose, and rub over sinuses; diffuse several drops.

Breathe ᴬ ᵀ   Eucalyptus ᴬ ᵀ
Siberian Fir ᴬ ᵀ   Peppermint ᴬ ᵀ
Lime ᴬ ᵀ

Nasal Polyps

Apply 1-3 drops over bridge of nose and under nose.

Frankincense ᵀ   Breathe ᵀ
Tea Tree ᵀ   Oregano ᵀ
Melissa ᵀ

Nausea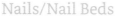

Apply 1-3 drops behind ears and over navel hourly; use a drop under the tongue; inhale from cupped hands.

DigestZen® ᴬ ᵀ ᴵ   Cardamom ᴬ ᵀ ᴵ
Ginger ᴬ ᵀ ᴵ   Balance ᴬ ᵀ
Peppermint ᴬ ᵀ ᴵ

Neck Pain

Massage 2-4 drops onto neck several times daily; use carrier oil to improve efficacy; use a drop of Copaiba under the tongue for pain.

Deep Blue® ᵀ   Wintergreen ᴬ ᵀ
Lemongrass ᵀ   Douglas Fir ᴬ ᵀ
Copaiba ᵀ ᴵ   *Protocol on pg. 201*

Nervous Fatigue

Inhale from cupped hands; apply 1-3 drops to temples, behind ears, and on back of neck as needed; diffuse several drops.

Balance ᴬ ᵀ   Vetiver ᴬ ᵀ
Lemon ᴬ ᵀ   Tangerine ᴬ ᵀ
Cedarwood ᴬ ᵀ

Nervousness

Apply 1-3 drops over the forehead, back of neck and top of head as needed; diffuse several drops

Peace ᴬ ᵀ   Balance ᴬ ᵀ
Rose ᴬ ᵀ   Jasmine ᴬ ᵀ
Lavender ᴬ ᵀ   *Protocol on pg. 186*

Neuromuscular Disorder

Apply 3-5 drops with carrier oil to spine and back of neck 3x daily.

Frankincense ᵀ   Neroli ᵀ
DDR Prime® ᵀ   Helichrysum ᵀ
Rose ᵀ   *Protocol on pg. 201*

Neuropathy

Apply 2-4 drops to affected areas several times daily; ingest 1-3 drops as needed.

Deep Blue® ᵀ   Roman Chamomile ᵀ ᴵ
Frankincense ᵀ ᴵ   Peppermint ᵀ ᴵ
AromaTouch® ᵀ   *Protocol on pg. 201*

Night Sweats

Apply 2-4 drops to abdomen and back of neck before sleeping.

Zendocrine® ᵀ   Lavender ᵀ
DDR Prime® ᵀ   Lime ᵀ
Peppermint ᵀ

Nightmares

Apply 2-4 drops to abdomen and back of neck before sleeping; diffuse several drops.

Juniper Berry ᴬ ᵀ   Lavender ᴬ ᵀ
Serenity ᴬ ᵀ   Peace ᴬ ᵀ
Calmer ᴬ ᵀ

 Aromatic   Topical   Internal   N/A

Nosebleeds

Apply 1-3 drops to the bridge and sides of nose and back of neck as needed.

Helichrysum [T]	Lavender [T]
Geranium [T]	Cypress [T]
Frankincense [T]	

Obsessive Compulsive Disorder

Massage 2-4 drops with carrier oil into spine and neck; inhale from cupped hands; diffuse several drops.

Frankincense [A T]	Ylang Ylang [A T]
Lavender [A T]	Clary Sage [A T]
Roman Chamomile [A T]	*Protocol on pg. 201*

Olfactory Loss

Apply 1-2 drops over nose (avoid eyes) and back of neck 3x daily.

Rose [A T]	Vetiver [A T]
Eucalyptus [A T]	Bergamot [A T]
Lemon [A T]	

Ovarian Cysts

Blend 1-3 drops with carrier oil and soak tampon to insert overnight; apply 3-5 drops with warm compress over abdomen; take 3-5 drops internally.

Frankincense [T I]	Oregano [T I]
Clary Sage [T I]	Sandalwood [T I]
DDR Prime® [T I]	

Overeacting

Apply 1-3 drops to stomach; take 2-4 drops internally; inhale from cupped hands as needed.

Slim & Sassy® [A T I]	Forgive [A T]
Peppermint [A T I]	Cinnamon [A T I]
Grapefruit [A T I]	

O

Odors

Diffuse several drops; apply 2-3 drops with a carrier oil to surface odors; ingest 3-5 drops twice daily for body odors.

Purify [A T]	Lemon Eucalyptus [A T]
Tea Tree [A T I]	Abōde™ [A T]
Cilantro [A T I]	

Osteoarthritis

Massage 2-4 drops into affected areas daily; use carrier oil for improved efficacy.

Deep Blue® [T]	Copaiba [T]
Frankincense [T]	DDR Prime® [T]
Lemongrass [T]	*Protocol on pg. 187*

Overactive Bladder

Take 2-4 drops internally or apply over abdomen as needed.

Peppermint [T I]	Lavender [T I]
DigestZen® [T I]	Lemon [T I]
Ginger [T I]	

Overwhelm

Apply 2-4 drops to back of neck and temples; inhale from cupped hands; diffuse several drops.

Cedarwood [A T]	Lavender [A T]
Spearmint [A T]	Lemongrass [A T]
Frankincense [A T]	*Protocol on pg. 224*

Obesity

Add 2-5 drops to water to manage cravings and encourage metabolism. Inhale from cupped hands to satisfy cravings.

Slim & Sassy® [A T I]	Green Mandarin [A T I]
Grapefruit [A T I]	Lemon [A T I]
Peppermint [A T I]	*Protocol on pg. 209*

Oily Skin

Apply 3-5 drops to affected areas at bedtime.

Basil [T]	Eucalyptus [T]
Roman Chamomile [T]	Lemongrass [T]
Cedarwood [T]	

Osteoporosis

Massage 2-4 drops onto spine and affected areas daily; take 2-4 drops DDR Prime® internally 2x daily.

Wintergreen [T]	DDR Prime® [T I]
Birch [T]	Bone Nutrient Complex [I]
Frankincense [T I]	

Oxytocin Production

Inhale 1-3 drops from cupped hands 3x daily.

Clary Sage [A T]	
Thyme [A T]	
Sandalwood [A T]	

 Aromatic   Topical   Internal   N/A

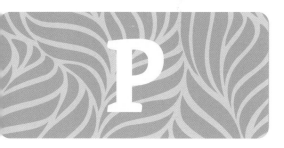

P

Pain

Combine 3-5 drops with carrier oil and apply liberally to affected area as often as desired; use a drop under the tongue.

Deep Blue® ᴬ ᵀ	Copaiba ᴬ ᵀ ᴵ
Frankincense ᴬ ᵀ ᴵ	Turmeric ᴬ ᵀ ᴵ
Helichrysum ᴬ ᵀ ᴵ	*Protocol on pg. 201*

Palpitations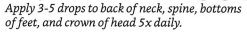

Apply 1-3 drops over heart 3x daily; inhale from cupped hands.

Marjoram ᴬ ᵀ	Ylang Ylang ᴬ ᵀ
Lavender ᴬ ᵀ	Wild Orange ᴬ ᵀ
Geranium ᴬ ᵀ	

Pancreatitis

Ingest 1-3 drops 3x daily; massage 1-3 drops over abdomen as needed.

Zendocrine® ᵀ ᴵ	Coriander ᵀ ᴵ
Marjoram ᵀ ᴵ	Rosemary ᵀ ᴵ
Lemon ᵀ ᴵ	

Panic Attacks

Inhale 1-3 drops from cupped hands; apply to back and front of neck; diffuse several drops.

Cedarwood ᴬ ᵀ	Lavender ᴬ ᵀ
Spearmint ᴬ ᵀ	Lemongrass ᴬ ᵀ
Frankincense ᴬ ᵀ	*Protocol on pg. 186*

Paralysis

Apply 3-5 drops to back of neck, spine, bottoms of feet, and crown of head 5x daily.

Frankincense ᴬ ᵀ	DDR Prime® ᴬ ᵀ
Cypress ᴬ ᵀ	Lemongrass ᴬ ᵀ
Vetiver ᴬ ᵀ	

Parasites

Ingest 3-5 drops 3x daily; apply in a warm compress over intestinal area 2-3x daily.

Zendocrine® ᵀ ᴵ	Clove ᵀ ᴵ
Oregano ᵀ ᴵ	Thyme ᵀ ᴵ
Geranium ᵀ ᴵ	

Parathyroid Disorder

Apply 1-3 drops to front of neck; dilute with carrier oil for easier application; ingest 1-3 drops a few times daily or as needed.

Frankincense ᵀ ᴵ	Zendocrine® ᵀ ᴵ
Myrrh ᵀ ᴵ	Lifelong Vitality Pack® ᴵ
DDR Prime® ᵀ ᴵ	

Parkinson's Disease

Apply 3-5 drops to spine and back of neck 3x daily; inhale from cupped hands; diffuse several drops throughout the day.

Frankincense ᴬ ᵀ	Neroli ᴬ ᵀ
Lavender ᴬ ᵀ	Pink Pepper ᴬ ᵀ
Rose ᴬ ᵀ	

Pelvic Pain Syndrome

Apply 3-5 drops to lower abdomen 3x daily.

Clary Sage ᵀ	Ylang Ylang ᵀ
Eucalyptus ᵀ	Patchouli ᵀ
Frankincense ᵀ	

Perforated Ear Drum

Apply 1-2 drops behind ear 2-3x daily.

Helichrysum ᵀ	Rosemary ᵀ
Basil ᵀ	Cypress ᵀ
Balance ᵀ	

Perimenopause

Massage 2-4 drops into abdomen, lower back, and shoulders.

ClaryCalm® ᴬ ᵀ	Peppermint ᴬ ᵀ
Frankincense ᴬ ᵀ	Marjoram ᴬ ᵀ
Clary Sage ᴬ ᵀ	

Pernicious Anemia

Take 2-4 drops internally 3x daily; apply to stomach area as needed.

Lemon ᵀ ᴵ	Cinnamon ᵀ ᴵ
Lime ᵀ ᴵ	DDR Prime® ᵀ ᴵ
Helichrysum ᵀ ᴵ	

Pests

Apply 3-5 drops with carrier oil to skin; add oils to a 20 oz glass spray bottle and spray pest-ridden areas as needed.

Peppermint ᵀ	Basil ᵀ
Eucalyptus ᵀ	Tea Tree ᵀ
Clove ᵀ	

Phantom Pains

Combine 3-5 drops with carrier oil and apply liberally to affected area as often as desired; inhale from cupped hands.

Wintergreen ᴬ ᵀ	Helichrysum ᴬ ᵀ
Ylang Ylang ᴬ ᵀ	BlueTansy ᴬ ᵀ
Deep Blue® ᴬ ᵀ	

 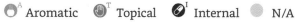

Pineal Gland

Inhale 1-3 drops for 30 seconds from cupped hands 3x daily; apply to pineal gland reflexology point.

Bergamot ᴬ ᵀ	Lemon ᴬ ᵀ
Clary Sage ᴬ ᵀ	Ginger ᴬ ᵀ
Lavender ᴬ ᵀ	

Pink Eye/ Conjunctivitis

Apply 1-2 drops around (but not in) eyes 3x daily; dilute for sensitive skin.

Tea Tree ᵀ	Clary Sage ᵀ
Rosemary ᵀ	Purify ᵀ
Arborvitae ᵀ	

Pituitary Gland

Apply 1-3 drops to front of neck; dilute with carrier oil for easier application; ingest 1-3 drops a few times daily or as needed.

Clove ᴬ ᵀ ᴵ	Lemongrass ᴬ ᵀ ᴵ
Frankincense ᴬ ᵀ ᴵ	Basil ᴬ ᵀ ᴵ
Sandalwood ᴬ ᵀ ᴵ	

Plantar Fasciitis

Combine 3-5 drops with carrier oil and apply liberally to affected area 3x daily or as desired.

Deep Blue® ᵀ	Helichrysum ᵀ
Wintergreen ᵀ	Blue Tansy ᵀ
Ylang Ylang ᵀ	

Plantar Warts

Apply 1-3 drops to wart several times daily (avoid surrounding skin with hot oils like Oregano.)

Oregano ᵀ	Melissa ᵀ
Frankincense ᵀ	Rose ᵀ
DDR Prime® ᵀ	

Pleurisy

Apply 3-5 drops over chest 3x daily; diffuse several drops.

Breathe ᴬ ᵀ	Blue Tansy ᴬ ᵀ
Eucalyptus ᴬ ᵀ	Clove ᴬ ᵀ
Roman Chamomile ᴬ ᵀ	

Pneumonia

Apply 2-4 drops to chest, neck, and bottoms of feet 3-5x daily; gargle a drop hourly; inhale from cupped hands as needed; diffuse several drops.

Breathe ᴬ ᵀ	Bergamot ᴬ ᵀ ᴵ
On Guard ᴬ ᵀ ᴵ	Roman Chamomile ᴬ ᵀ ᴵ
Arborvitae ᴬ ᵀ	*Protocol on pg. 202*

Poison Ivy/Oak

Apply 1-3 drops to affected area with carrier oil a couple times daily or as needed.

Lavender ᵀ	Patchouli ᵀ
Frankincense ᵀ	Petitgrain ᵀ
Geranium ᵀ	

Polio

Apply 3-5 drops to spine, back of neck, and bottoms of feet; inhale from cupped hands often.

Frankincense ᴬ ᵀ ᴵ	Neroli ᴬ ᵀ
Lavender ᴬ ᵀ ᴵ	Black Pepper ᴬ ᵀ ᴵ
Rose ᴬ ᵀ	

Polycystic Ovary Syndrome

Apply 3 -5 drops to lower abdomen 3 x daily.

Clary Sage ᵀ	Ylang Ylang ᵀ
Eucalyptus ᵀ	Patchouli ᵀ
Frankincense ᵀ	

Polyps

Add 4-6 drops to capsule and take after eating 3x daily.

Frankincense ᵀ	Oregano ᵀ
Patchouli ᵀ	Peppermint ᵀ
Myrrh ᵀ	

Post-Traumatic Stress Disorder

Apply 2-4 drops to forehead, temples, back of neck, chest, and bottoms of feet; inhale from cupped hands as needed.

Peace ᴬ ᵀ	Console ᴬ ᵀ
Sandalwood ᴬ ᵀ	Forgive ᴬ ᵀ
Frankincense ᴬ ᵀ	

Pre-Workout

Massage 2-4 drops with carrier oil into appropriate muscles and joints; apply a drop over the chest; inhale from cupped hands.

Deep Blue® ᴬ ᵀ	Lime ᴬ ᵀ
Bergamot ᴬ ᵀ	Rosemary ᴬ ᵀ
Lemon ᴬ ᵀ	*Protocol on pg. 216*

Preeclampsia

Apply 3-5 drops to lower back and neck.

Lavender ᵀ	Clary Sage ᵀ
Ylang Ylang ᵀ	Cedarwood ᵀ
Roman Chamomile ᵀ	

 Aromatic Topical Internal N/A

Pregnancy: Delivery

Apply 1-3 drops to hips, lower back, and back of neck; inhale from cupped hands; diffuse several drops.

Balance ^{AT}	Basil ^{AT}
Lavender ^{AT}	Frankincense ^{AT}
Jasmine ^{AT}	

Pregnancy: Labor (During)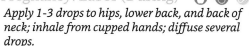

Apply 1-3 drops to hips, lower back, and back of neck; inhale from cupped hands; diffuse several drops.

Lemon ^{AT}	Rosemary ^{AT}
Bergamot ^{AT}	Jasmine ^{AT}
Lavender ^{AT}	

Pregnancy: Lactation

Massage 1-3 drops with carrier oil over breasts and apply to bottoms of feet; ingest 1-3 drops.

Fennel ^{TI}	Lifelong Vitality Pack® ^I
Clary Sage ^{TI}	Bone Nutrient ^I
Basil ^{TI}	

Pregnancy: Mastitis

Apply 3-5 drops to affected area 3x daily.

Lavender ^T	Arborvitae ^T
Frankincense ^T	Helichrysum ^T
Tea Tree ^T	

Pregnancy: Sore Nipples

Apply 1-2 drops diluted to affected area 3x daily; wipe nipples clean before nursing; monitor baby's response.

Lavender ^T	Helichrysum ^T
Tea Tree ^T	
Sandalwood ^T	

Pregnancy: Hemorrhaging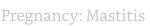

Apply 1-3 drops to spine and lower abdomen.

Clary Sage ^T	Peppermint ^T
Helichrysum ^T	Ginger ^T
Wintergreen ^T	

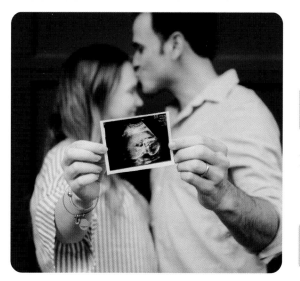

Pregnancy: Morning Sickness

Apply 1-3 drops behind ears and over navel hourly; inhale from cupped hands; ingest 1-3 drops as needed.

DigestZen® ^{ATI}	Clary Calm® ^{AT}
Peppermint ^{ATI}	Ylang Ylang ^{ATI}
Ginger ^{ATI}	*Protocol on pg. 203*

Pregnancy: Tender Breasts

Combine 3-5 drops with carrier oil and massage into affected area as often as needed.

Lavender ^T	Peppermint ^T
Frankincense ^T	Yarrow|Pom ^T
Geranium ^T	

Pregnancy: High Blood Pressure

Apply 2-4 drops to bottoms of feet and behind ears 2x daily; inhale from cupped hands; take 2-3 drops in a capsule.

Marjoram ^{ATI}	Manuka ^{ATI}
Lemon ^{ATI}	Rose ^{AT}
Lavender ^{ATI}	

Pregnancy: Labor (post)

Apply 3-5 drops to lower back 3x daily to stimulate regeneration.

Jasmine ^T	Sandalwood ^T
ClaryCalm® ^T	Yarrow|Pom ^T
Balance ^T	*Protocol on pg. 203*

Pregnancy: Low Libido

Apply 3-5 drops to inside of thighs and calves 2x daily; diffuse several drops.

Rose ^{AT}	Clary Sage ^{AT}
Jasmine ^{AT}	Fennel ^{AT}
Ylang Ylang ^{AT}	

Pregnancy: Postpartum Depression

Apply 1-3 drops to forehead and temples; use a drop of Frankincense under the tongue; inhale from cupped hands.

Adaptiv™ ^{AT}	Frankincense ^{AT}
Elevation ^{AT}	Console ^{AT}
Citrus Bliss® ^{AT}	*Protocol on pg. 203*

Pregnancy: Uterine Health

Apply 3-5 drops to lower abdomen 3x daily.

Clary Sage ^T	Ylang Ylang ^T
Eucalyptus ^T	Patchouli ^T
Frankincense ^T	

 ^A Aromatic   ^T Topical   ^I Internal   N/A

Premenstrual Syndrome (PMS)

Add 3-6 drops to warm bath; apply to abdomen; inhale from cupped hands; ingest 1-3 drops as needed.

ClaryCalm® ᴬ ᵀ	Frankincense ᴬ ᵀ ᴵ
Clary Sage ᴬ ᵀ ᴵ	Madagascar Vanilla ᴬ ᵀ ᴵ
Geranium ᴬ ᵀ ᴵ	*Protocol on pg. 199*

Prolapsed Mitral Valve

Apply 3-5 drops to inside of arms and chest 3x daily.

Lemon ᵀ	Marjoram ᵀ
Lavender ᵀ	Yarrow|Pom ᵀ
Ylang Ylang ᵀ	

Prostatitis

Apply 3-5 drops to lower abdomen and lower back 3x daily or as needed.

Rosemary ᵀ	Frankincense ᵀ
Marjoram ᵀ	Myrrh ᵀ
Thyme ᵀ	

Psoriasis

Apply 1-3 drops to affected area a couple times daily with carrier oil; ingest 2-4 drops 2x daily.

Tea Tree ᴬ ᵀ ᴵ	Roman Chamomile ᴬ ᵀ ᴵ
Zendocrine® ᴬ ᵀ ᴵ	Deep Blue® Complex ᴵ
Thyme ᴬ ᵀ ᴵ	*Protocol on pg. 203*

R

Radiation

Ingest 2-4 drops 2x daily; apply 1-3 drops to bottoms of feet with carrier oil as desired.

Sandalwood ᵀ ᴵ	Peppermint ᵀ ᴵ
DDR Prime® ᵀ ᴵ	Patchouli ᵀ ᴵ
Cilantro ᵀ ᴵ	

Rashes

Dilute 1-3 drops with a carrier oil and apply to affected area as needed.

Tea Tree ᵀ	Cedarwood ᵀ
Roman Chamomile ᵀ	Magnolia ᵀ
Lavender ᵀ	*Protocol on pg. 203*

Raynaud's Disease

Apply 3-5 drops to lower back and abdomen and apply a hot compress daily.

Clove ᵀ	Lavender ᵀ
Black Pepper ᵀ	Fennel ᵀ
Geranium ᵀ	

Reaction Attachment Disorder

Apply 3-5 drops to top of head, forehead and back of neck 3x daily.

Hope ᴬ ᵀ	Bergamot ᴬ ᵀ
ClaryCalm® ᴬ ᵀ	Lavender ᴬ ᵀ
Rose ᴬ ᵀ	*Protocol on pg. 219*

Reiter's Arthritis

Massage 1-3 drops into affected areas 3x daily; use a carrier oil for improved efficacy.

Deep Blue® ᵀ	Copaiba ᵀ
Frankincense ᵀ	Turmeric ᵀ
DDR Prime® ᵀ	*Protocol on pg. 187*

Relapse

Apply 2-4 drops as often as needed to back of the neck, temples and ears (not inside ears.)

Hope ᴬ ᵀ	Rosemary ᴬ ᵀ
Motivate ᴬ ᵀ	Cedarwood ᴬ ᵀ
Cinnamon ᴬ ᵀ	*Protocol on pg. 214*

Relaxation

Apply 3-5 drops over the forehead, back of neck and top of head as needed; use 3-6 drops in a hot bath; diffuse several drops.

Peace ᴬ ᵀ	Balance ᴬ ᵀ
Madacascar Vanilla ᴬ ᵀ	Blue Tansy ᴬ ᵀ
Lavender ᴬ ᵀ	*Protocol on pg. 232*

Renal Artery Stenosis

Rub 2-4 drops to bottoms of feet and inner thighs 2x daily; use a carrier oil for improved efficacy.

Cypress ᵀ	Lavender ᵀ
Peppermint ᵀ	Douglas Fir ᵀ
Balance ᵀ	

Respiratory Issues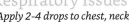

Apply 2-4 drops to chest, neck, under nose, and on bridge of nose; inhale from cupped hands as needed; diffuse several drops.

Breathe ᴬ ᵀ	Cardamom ᴬ ᵀ
Eucalyptus ᴬ ᵀ	Rosemary ᴬ ᵀ
Douglas Fir ᴬ ᵀ	

Respiratory Virus

Apply 3-5 drops 3x daily to chest, outside of arms and nose; diffuse several drops; take 2-4 drops in a capsule 3x daily.

Breathe ᴬ ᵀ	Lime ᴬ ᵀ ᴵ
On Guard ᴬ ᵀ ᴵ	Arborvitae ᴬ ᵀ
Eucalyptus ᴬ ᵀ	

  Aromatic Topical Internal N/A

Restless Leg Syndrome

Massage 2-4 drops onto legs and bottoms of feet; diffuse several drops; use 2 drops Yarrow|Pom under the tongue.

Deep Blue® ᴬ ᵀ	Petitgrain ᴬ ᵀ
Ylang Ylang ᴬ ᵀ	Yarrow|Pom ᴬ ᵀ ᴵ
Cypress ᴬ ᵀ	

Restlessness

Inhale 1-3 drops from cupped hands; apply 2-4 drops to bottoms of feet and back of neck as needed.

Balance ᴬ ᵀ	Vetiver ᴬ ᵀ
Lavender ᴬ ᵀ	Spikenard ᴬ ᵀ
Serenity ᴬ ᵀ	*Protocol on pg. 232*

Rheumatic Fever

Apply 1-3 drops to bottoms of feet; ingest 1-3 drops twice daily; gargle a few drops mixed with water as needed.

Oregano ᵀ ᴵ	Wintergreen ᵀ
Peppermint ᵀ ᴵ	Arborvitae ᵀ
Melissa ᵀ ᴵ	

Rheumatoid Arthritis

Apply 1-3 drops to affected areas daily; dilute for sensitive skin and for easier application.

Deep Blue® ᵀ	Lemongrass ᵀ
Frankincense ᵀ	Copaiba ᵀ
Oregano ᵀ	*Protocol on pg. 204*

Rhinitis

Inhale 1-3 drops from cupped hands several times daily; apply a couple drops to forehead and bridge of nose; ingest 2-4 drops 3x daily; diffuse several drops.

Breathe ᴬ ᵀ	Siberian Fir ᴬ ᵀ ᴵ
Tea Tree ᴬ ᵀ ᴵ	Oregano ᴬ ᵀ ᴵ
Pink Pepper ᴬ ᵀ ᴵ	

Ringworm

Apply 1-3 drops to affected area 3-4x daily; use with carrier oil for improved efficacy; take 2-4 drops in a capsule 3x daily.

Tea Tree ᵀ ᴵ	Petitgrain ᵀ ᴵ
Purify ᵀ	Zendocrine® ᵀ ᴵ
HD Clear® ᵀ	

Rosacea

Combine 2-3 drops with carrier oil and apply to face at bedtime.

Jasmine ᵀ	Patchouli ᵀ
Geranium ᵀ	Roman Chamomile ᵀ
Lavender ᵀ	

Rotator Cuff Issues

Massage 3-5 drops with carrier oil into affected area as often as desired.

Deep Blue® ᵀ	Helichrysum ᵀ
Wintergreen ᵀ	Blue Tansy ᵀ
Ylang Ylang ᵀ	

Runner's Knee

Massage 3-5 drops with carrier oil into affected area as often as desired.

Deep Blue® ᵀ	Helichrysum ᵀ
Lemongrass ᵀ	Blue Tansy ᵀ
Ylang Ylang ᵀ	

S

Scabies

Apply 2 drops 2x daily as needed; add 20 drops to glass water bottle and spray furniture as needed.

Peppermint ᵀ	Purify ᵀ
Tea Tree ᵀ	Roman Chamomile ᵀ
Cedarwood ᵀ	

Scarring

Massage 2-4 drops into scarred area 2x daily.

Immortelle ᵀ	Sandalwood ᵀ
Frankincense ᵀ	Neroli ᵀ
Helichrysum ᵀ	

Schizophrenia

Apply 3-5 drops to back of neck and spine 3x daily; diffuse several drops throughout the day.

Frankincense ᴬ ᵀ	Lavender ᴬ ᵀ
Melissa ᴬ ᵀ	Balance ᴬ ᵀ
Tea Tree ᴬ ᵀ	

Schmidt's Syndrome

Apply 3-5 drops to back of neck, bottoms of feet, and spine 3x daily; ingest 3-5 drops 2x daily; diffuse several drops throughout the day.

Clove ᴬ ᵀ ᴵ	Basil ᴬ ᵀ ᴵ
DDR Prime® ᴬ ᵀ ᴵ	Clary Sage ᴬ ᵀ ᴵ
Rosemary ᴬ ᵀ ᴵ	

Sciatica

Massage 1-3 drops into affected area a couple times daily.

Deep Blue® ᵀ	Copaiba ᵀ
Frankincense ᵀ	Helichrysum ᵀ
Vetiver ᵀ	*Protocol on pg. 204*

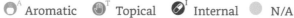 Aromatic   Topical   Internal   N/A

Scleroderma

Apply 1-3 drops to affected areas as needed; use with carrier oil for improved efficacy.

Tea Tree [T]	Zendocrine® [T]
HD Clear® [T]	Frankincense [T]
Cedarwood [T]	

Scurvy

Take 3-5 drops in a capsule 3x daily after eating; apply 2-3 drops to bottoms of feet.

Lime [T I]	Jasmine [T I]
Wild Orange [T I]	Lemongrass [T I]
Bergamot [T I]	

Seizures

Apply 1-3 drops to back of neck and bottoms of feet; inhale from cupped hands as needed; ingest 2-4 drops 2x daily.

Frankincense [A T I]	Yarrow|Pom [A T I]
Balance [A T]	Roman Chamomile [A T I]
Spikenard [A T]	*Protocol on pg. 204*

Shin Splints

Massage 3-5 drops with carrier oil into affected area as often as desired.

Deep Blue® [T]	Helichrysum [T]
Ylang Ylang [T]	Blue Tansy [T]
Wintergreen [T]	

Shock

Apply 1-3 drops on temples, under nose, and on back of neck as needed; inhale from cupped hands; diffuse several drops.

Balance [A T]	Cheer [A T]
Frankincense [A T]	Forgive [A T]
Helichrysum [A T]	*Protocol on pg. 237*

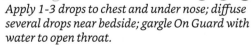

Shingles

Apply 2-4 drops to affected areas, on back of neck, and along the spine 3x daily; take 2-4 drops 3x daily.

Tea Tree [T I]	Yarrow|Pom [T I]
Melissa [T I]	Geranium [T I]
Black Pepper [T I]	*Protocol on pg. 205*

Sickle Cell Anemia

Combine 3-5 drops of oils on hand (preferably all 5 listed) a capsule and take 3x daily after meals.

Lemon [I]	Rosemary [I]
Rose [I]	Geranium [I]
Siberian Fir [I]	

Sinus Infection

Apply 1-3 drops over bridge of nose and sinuses (avoid eyes) 3x daily; diffuse several drops; take 3-5 drops in a capsule 3x daily.

Tea Tree [A T I]	Breathe [A T]
Melissa [A T I]	Rosemary [A T I]
Oregano [A T I]	*Protocol on pg. 205*

Skin Tags

Apply a drop to affected areas 3x daily (dilute hot oils like Oregano and avoid surrounding skin).

Frankincense [T]	Rosemary [T]
Oregano [T]	Basil [T]
Tea Tree [T]	

Skin Ulcers

Apply 1-3 drops diluted into affected area 2-3x daily.

Lavender [T]	Sandalwood [T]
Myrrh [T]	Yarrow|Pom [T]
HD Clear® [T]	

Sleep Issues

Apply 3-5 drops over the forehead, back of neck, and top of head 30 minutes before sleep; diffuse several drops; use a drop under the tongue.

Serenity [A T]	Rose [A T]
Lavender [A T I]	Vetiver [A T I]
Peace [A T]	*Protocol on pg. 205*

Snoring

Apply 1-3 drops to chest and under nose; diffuse several drops near bedside; gargle On Guard with water to open throat.

Breathe [A T]	Eucalyptus [A T]
On Guard [A T I]	Douglas Fir [A T]
Petitgrain [A T]	*Protocol on pg. 206*

Sore Throat

Gargle 1-3 drops with water, then swallow; apply to throat and neck, diluting with carrier oil as needed.

On Guard [T I]	Arborvitae [T]
Oregano [T I]	Melissa [T I]
Lemon [T I]	*Protocol on pg. 206*

 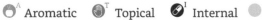 Aromatic Topical Internal N/A

Spasms

Apply 3-5 drops to affected area and bottoms of feet as needed; use a drop under the tongue.

Frankincense ^{TI}	Ylang Ylang ^{TI}
Black Pepper ^{TI}	Lavender ^{TI}
Copaiba ^{TI}	

Spina Bifida

Apply 3-5 drops to spine and back of neck 3x daily; inhale from cupped hands.

Peppermint ^{AT}	Clove ^{AT}
Roman Chamomile ^{AT}	Frankincense ^{AT}
Vetiver ^{AT}	

Sprains

Gently apply 2-4 drops to affected area as needed.

Deep Blue® ^{T}	Spikenard ^{T}
Helichrysum ^{T}	AromaTouch® ^{T}
Lemongrass ^{T}	

Staph Infection

Apply 2-4 drops to the affected 3-5x daily; dilute if necessary.

Zendocrine® ^{T}	Geranium ^{T}
Patchouli ^{T}	Grapefruit ^{T}
Tea Tree ^{T}	

Stenosis (Vessel Narrowing)

Take 1-2 drops of each oil on hand (preferably all 5 listed) in a capsule 3x daily; apply 2-4 drops to bottoms of feet 3x daily.

Frankincense ^{TI}	Cinnamon ^{TI}
Ginger ^{TI}	Tea Tree ^{TI}
Clary Sage ^{TI}	

Stings

Apply 1-2 drops topically to sting or bite several times daily until symptoms cease.

Lavender ^{T}	Roman Chamomile ^{T}
Tea Tree ^{T}	Basil ^{T}
Purify ^{T}	

Stomach Ache

Rub 2-4 drops over stomach as needed; ingest 1-3 drops as needed.

DigestZen® ^{TI}	Roman Chamomile ^{TI}
Ginger ^{TI}	Wild Orange ^{TI}
Peppermint ^{TI}	*Protocol on pg. 194*

Strep Throat

Apply 1-3 drops with a carrier oil to outside of throat 5x daily; ingest 2-5 drops in a capsule 3x daily; gargle a drop with water.

Arborvitae ^{T}	On Guard ^{TI}
Oregano ^{TI}	Tea Tree ^{TI}
Thyme ^{TI}	

Stress

Apply 3-5 drops over the forehead, back of neck, and top of head as needed; inhale from cupped hands; diffuse several drops.

Adaptiv™ ^{AT}	Frankincense ^{AT}
Balance ^{AT}	Peace ^{AT}
Lavender ^{AT}	*Protocol on pg. 206*

Stretch Marks

Massage 1-3 drops to affected areas 2x daily; use a carrier oil for improved efficacy.

Frankincense ^{T}	Neroli ^{T}
Helichrysum ^{T}	Yarrow|Pom ^{T}
Immortelle ^{T}	

Stroke

Apply 2-4 drops to temples, forehead, behind ears, and back of neck 3-5x daily; ingest 2-4 drops 3x daily; diffuse several drops.

Cypress ^{AT}	Fennel ^{ATI}
Frankincense ^{ATI}	Helichrysum ^{ATI}
Basil ^{ATI}	

Sunburn

Apply 1-3 drops to affected area hourly or as needed. Blend 2-3 oils, 2-3 drops each with carrier oil for improved results.

Lavender ^{T}	Frankincense ^{T}
Helichrysum ^{T}	Cedarwood ^{T}
Peppermint ^{T}	*Protocol on pg. 207*

Swimmer's Ear

Apply 2 drops behind ear 2x daily.

Copaiba ^{T}	Rosemary ^{T}
Lavender ^{T}	Wintergreen ^{T}
Spearmint ^{T}	

 ^{A} Aromatic ^{T} Topical ^{I} Internal   N/A

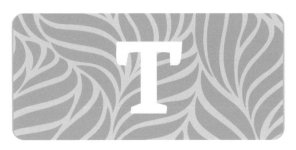

T

A-Z Ref.

Tachycardia ^A ^T ^I

Apply 3 -5 drops to inside of arms and chest 3x daily.

Ylang Ylang ^T	Vetiver ^T
Lavender ^T	Geranium ^T
Neroli ^T	

Taste (loss of) ^A ^T ^I

Apply 1-2 drops directly to tongue 2x daily.

Tangerine ^I	Geranium ^I
Lemon ^I	Lime ^I
Clove ^I	

Teeth Grinding ^A ^T ^I

Massage 2-4 drops into jaw joints, back of neck, and top of head as needed.

Peace ^{A T}	Rose ^{A T}
Lavender ^{A T}	Balance ^{A T}
Frankincense ^{A T}	

Teething Pain ^A ^T ^I

Dilute with carrier oil and gently massage a drop along baby's jawline, reapplying as needed.

Lavender ^T	Frankincense ^T
Clove ^T	Calmer ^T
Magnolia ^T	

Tendinitis ^A ^T ^I

Massage 2-4 drops into affected areas 4-5x daily, or as needed.

Lemongrass ^T	Cardamom ^T
Deep Blue® ^T	Siberian Fir ^T
Marjoram ^T	

Tennis Elbow ^A ^T ^I

Massage 2-4 drops into affected area as needed.

Lemongrass ^T	Blue Tansy ^T
Deep Blue® ^T	Frankincense ^T
Siberian Fir ^T	

Tension ^A ^T ^I

Apply 3-5 drops over the forehead, back of neck and top of head as needed; inhale from cupped hands; diffuse several drops.

PastTense® ^{A T}	Deep Blue® ^{A T}
Lavender ^{A T}	Rose ^{A T}
Frankincense ^{A T}	*Protocol on pg. 206*

Testosterone (low) ^A ^T ^I

Apply 2-4 drops to bottoms of feet and inside of thighs 2x daily; inhale from cupped hands as needed.

Patchouli ^T	InTune® ^T
Sandalwood ^T	Rose ^T
Passion ^T	

Thrombosis, Deep Vein ^A ^T ^I

Place 1-2 drops of oils on hand (preferably all 5 listed) in a capsule and take 3x daily

Frankincense ^I	Cinnamon ^I
Ginger ^I	Tea Tree ^I
Clary Sage ^I	

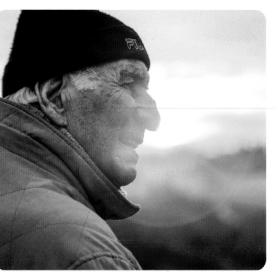

Thrush ^A ^T ^I

Gargle 1-3 drops mixed with water several times daily; apply topically to lower throat and bottoms of feet; ingest 1-3 drops as needed.

Tea Tree ^{T I}	Oregano ^{T I}
Geranium ^{T I}	On Guard ^{T I}
Arborvitae ^T	

Thymus Support ^A ^T ^I

Apply 3-5 drops to throat 2x daily; use carrier oil for improved efficacy.

Frankincense ^T	Basil ^T
Juniper Berry ^T	Tea Tree ^T
Rosemary ^T	

Tick Bites ^A ^T ^I

Apply 1-2 drops to bite frequently for the first hour after carefully removing tick. Dilute Oregano if necessary.

Oregano ^T	Lavender ^T
Tea Tree ^T	TerraShield® ^T
Purify ^T	

^A Aromatic   ^T Topical   ^I Internal   N/A

Tingling

Apply 2-4 drops to affected areas several times daily; ingest 1-3 drops as needed.

Peppermint T I	Deep Blue® T
Roman Chamomile T I	Frankincense T I
AromaTouch® T	

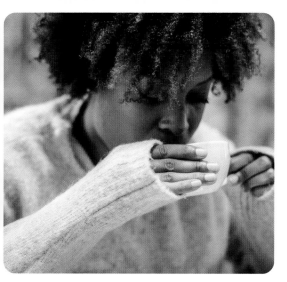

Tinnitus

Apply 1-2 drops behind ear 2-3x daily.

Helichrysum T	Frankincense T
Balance T	Rosemary T
Basil T	*Protocol on pg. 208*

Tonsillitis

Gargle 1-3 drops mixed with water or ingest 3x daily; apply to outside of throat with carrier oil 3x daily.

On Guard T I	Tea Tree T I
Oregano T I	Melissa T I
Arborvitae T	

Tourette's Syndrome

Massage 1-3 drops with carrier oil solution into spine and neck; diffuse several drops.

Frankincense A T	Ylang Ylang A T
Lavender A T	Clary Sage A T
Roman Chamomile A T	*Protocol on pg. 208*

TMJ (Temporomandibular Joint Dysfunction)

Massage 1-3 drops into jaw joint 3x daily.

Deep Blue® T	Eucalyptus T
Wintergreen T	Rosemary T
Sandalwood T	

Toothache

Apply a drop to gums and directly onto tooth; swish 1-3 drops with water.

Clove T I	Copaiba T I
On Guard T I	Wintergreen T
Helichrysum T I	

Toxemia

Gargle a few drops with water several times daily or as needed; take 1-3 drops in a capsule 2x daily; apply 2-4 drops to bottoms of feet 30 minutes before showering.

Cilantro T I	Clove T I
Zendocrine® T I	Thyme T I
Oregano T I	

Trauma (Emotional)

Apply 2-4 drops to forehead, temples, back of neck, and chest; inhale from cupped hands as needed; diffuse several drops.

Console A T	Frankincense A T
Peace A T	Rose A T
Forgive A T	*Protocol on pg. 237*

Tuberculosis (TB)

Apply 1-3 drops to a carrier solution and massage into spine and neck 3x daily.

On Guard T	Frankincense T
Cinnamon T	Arborvitae T
Tea Tree T	

Tumor

Apply 3-5 drops over the affected area 3-5x daily.

Frankincense T	Arborvitae T
DDR Prime® T	Rosemary T
Sandalwood T	

Typhoid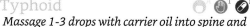

Massage 1-3 drops with carrier oil into spine and neck 2-3x daily; ingest 2-4 drops in a capsule.

On Guard T I	Frankincense T I
Cinnamon T I	Rosemary T I
Tea Tree T I	

U

Ulcers (Stomach)

Ingest 1-3 drops at least once daily; massage gently into abdomen as needed.

Lemongrass T I	Zendocrine® T I
Frankincense T I	Geranium T I
Myrrh T I	

Aromatic   Topical   Internal   N/A

Urinary Support

Massage 1-3 drops over bladder and kidneys before bedtime as needed.

Cypress ^T	Lemongrass ^T
Juniper Berry ^T	Roman Chamomile ^T
Ylang Ylang ^T	

Urinary Tract Infection

Massage 1-3 drops over kidneys and on bottoms of the feet; take 2-4 drops in a capsule 3x daily.

Cypress ^T	Juniper Berry ^{T I}
Basil ^{T I}	Purify ^T
Lemongrass ^{T I}	*Protocol on pg. 208*

Vaginal Infection

Apply 3-5 drops over lower abdomen and to vaginal area 3x daily.

Lavender ^T	Frankincense ^T
Tea Tree ^T	Arborvitae ^T
Rosemary ^T	*Protocol on pg. 209*

Vaginitis

Apply 3-5 drops over lower abdomen and to vaginal area 3x daily.

Bergamot ^T	Lavender ^T
Cedarwood ^T	Myrrh ^T
Tea Tree ^T	*Protocol on pg. 209*

Varicose Veins

Massage 2-4 drops into the affected area several times daily.

Cypress ^T	Zendocrine® ^T
Helichrysum ^T	Celery Seed ^T
Siberian Fir ^T	

Vertigo

Apply 2-4 drops to forehead and back of neck as needed.

Ginger ^{A T}	Basil ^{A T}
Lavender ^{A T}	Rosemary ^{A T}
Clary Sage ^{A T}	

Viruses

Apply 2-4 drops to bottoms of feet, back of neck, and spine 3-5x daily; ingest 2-5 drops 3x daily

On Guard ^{T I}	Black Pepper ^{T I}
Oregano ^{T I}	Lime ^{T I}
Melissa ^{T I}	

Vision Loss

Apply 1-3 drops around eyes (do not get in eyes) and lower back 2x daily.

Clary Sage ^T	DDR Prime® ^T
Helichrysum ^T	Yarrow|Pom ^{A T}
Immortelle ^T	

Vomiting

Apply 1-3 drops over stomach as needed; drink a few drops in water; inhale from cupped hands.

DigestZen® ^{A T I}	Peppermint ^{A T I}
Ginger ^{A T I}	Roman Chamomile ^{A T I}
Bergamot ^{A T I}	

Warts

Apply a dab directly to wart several times daily until the wart disappears. Avoid the surrounding skin with Oregano.

Oregano ^T	HD Clear® ^T
Frankincense ^T	Neroli ^T
Thyme ^T	

Wasp Sting

Apply one drop to sting several times daily or as needed.

Lavender ^T	Purify ^T
Roman Chamomile ^T	Myrrh ^T
Cedarwood ^T	

Water Retention

Massage 2-4 drops over bladder and kidneys before bedtime as needed.

Cypress ^T	Lemongrass ^T
Black Pepper ^T	Roman Chamomile ^T
Ylang Ylang ^T	

Weight Loss

Add 2-4 drops to water to manage cravings and encourage metabolism; inhale from cupped hands to satisfy cravings.

Slim & Sassy® ^{A T I}	Lemon ^{A T I}
Grapefruit ^{A T I}	Mito2Max® ^I
Peppermint ^{A T I}	*Protocol on pg. 209*

 ^A Aromatic   ^T Topical   ^I Internal   ● N/A

Wheezing

Rub 2-4 drops over chest with carrier oil; diffuse several drops.

Eucalyptus ^{A T}	Frankincense ^{A T}
Lavender ^{A T}	Bergamot ^{A T}
Breathe ^{A T}	

Whiplash

Massage 2-4 drops into affected area 2-3x daily; use with carrier oil to improve efficacy.

Deep Blue® ^T	Patchouli ^T
Siberian Fir ^T	Sandalwood ^T
Marjoram ^T	

Whooping Cough

Apply 2-4 drops over chest and on bottoms of feet with carrier oil; diffuse several drops.

Bergamot ^{A T}	Frankincense ^{A T}
Lavender ^{A T}	Eucalyptus ^{A T}
Breathe ^{A T}	

Withdrawal Symptoms

Apply 2-4 drops to wrists, chest, and bottoms of feet as often as needed; diffuse several drops.

Zendocrine® ^{A T}	Juniper Berry ^{A T}
Cilantro ^{A T}	Motivate ^{A T}
Cinnamon ^{A T}	*Protocol on pg. 222*

Worms

Apply 2-4 drops over abdomen, bottoms of feet, and back of neck; add 2-4 drops to water or take in capsule.

Oregano ^{T I}	Basil ^{T I}
Thyme ^{T I}	Clove ^{T I}
Ginger ^{T I}	

Wounds

Apply 2-4 drops to affected area; use a carrier oil if needed.

Helichrysum ^T	Roman Chamomile ^T
Tea Tree ^T	Myrrh ^T
Lavender ^T	

Wrinkles

Apply 1-3 drops to affected areas as needed 2x daily; add a few drops to facial lotion or use with carrier oil for added benefits.

Immortelle ^T	Jasmine ^T
Frankincense ^T	Yarrow|Pom ^T
Myrrh ^T	*Protocol on pg. 209*

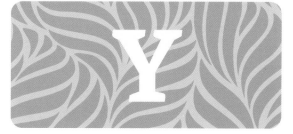

Yeast Infection

Apply 3-5 drops over lower abdomen 3x daily; use with a warm compress; ingest 3-5 drops in a capsule 3x daily.

Tea Tree ^{T I}	Clove ^{T I}
Lemon Eucalyptus ^T	Oregano ^{T I}
Thyme ^{T I}	*Protocol on pg. 209*

 Aromatic   Topical   Internal   ⬤ N/A

A-Z Ref.

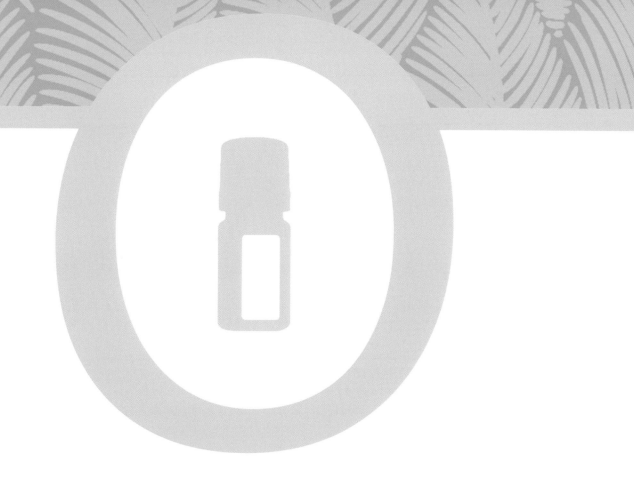

Section 3
Single *Oils*

Arborvitae
Thuja Plicata

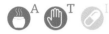 A T I

Scan Here To Experience More

Top *Uses*

Strep Throat
Rub 2 drops over outside of throat, and gargle 2 drops with water.

Bug Repellent
Dilute with several drops of carrier oil, and rub over needed areas.

Skin Cancer
Apply diluted to the affected area often and in small amounts.

Candida
Rub 2 drops over abdomen and bladder several times a day.

Fungal Issues
Apply neat to needed areas.

Furniture Polish
Combine 4 drops with 4 drops lemon oil, and rub in using a clean rag.

Main Properties
Antibacterial, Anticancer Anti-fungal, Astringent, Expectorant

Chemical Constituents
α, β, γ-Thujaplicin, Methyl thujate, Thujic acid

Other Uses
Colds, Cold Sores, Cysts, Fevers, Intestinal Parasites, Meditation, Respiratory Viruses

Emotional Use
Esters in Arborvitae like Methyl thujate make it a restorative oil. Use it to restore spiritual balance and to open receptivity to guidance.

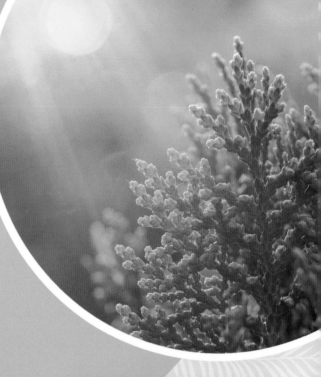

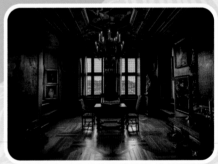

 Wooded Bliss Diffuser Blend

4 drops Frankincense
2 drops Arborvitae
2 drops Cedarwood

Diffuse this special blend to inspire feelings of peace and calm along with a woody, earth scent.

 Decay Away Wood Protector

4 drops Arborvitae
2 drops Lemon

Mix the oils together and use on wood to keep it fresh and preserved for long-time use.

Basil

Ocimum Basilicum

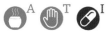

**Scan Here To
Experience More**

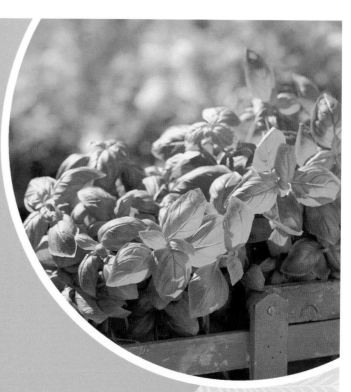

Top Uses

Adrenal Fatigue
Apply 1-2 drops directly to the adrenal areas or to the bottoms of the feet.

Mental Fatigue
Inhale from cupped hands, or diffuse.

Earache
Place a drop on a cotton ball, and rest over the ear for 15 minutes.

Muscle Spasms
Massage into muscles with carrier oil.

Carpal Tunnel
Massage into wrists & joints.

Cramps (abdominal)
Rub a drop clockwise over abdomen.

Cooking
Use a toothpick to add to dishes according to taste.

Main Properties
Antibacterial, Anti-infectious, Antispasmodic, Carminative, Nervine

Chemical Constituents
Linalool, 1,8-Cineole (eucalyptol), Bergamotene, Methyl chavicol

Other Uses
Bee Stings, Bronchitis, Dizziness, Frozen Shoulder, Gout, Greasy Hair, Infertility, Lactation (increase milk supply), Loss of Sense of Smell, Migraines, Nausea, Viral Hepatitis

Emotional Use
Alcohols in Basil like Linalool make it a renewing and calming oil. Use it to feel rejuvenated and renewed in your commitment to a higher life.

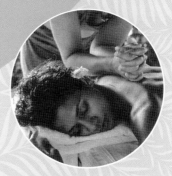

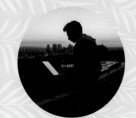

Focus Focused Diffuser Blend

2 drops Basil
2 drops Ginger
2 drops Grapefruit

Combine the essential oils with water and diffuse to boost clear thinking and mental alertness.

Spirit-Relaxing Oil Massage

3 drops Basil
2 drops Geranium
3 drops Wild Orange
1 oz. FCO

Blend oils together and use for an uplifting, aromatic massage.

Bergamot
Citrus Bergamia

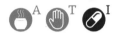 A T I

Scan Here To Experience More

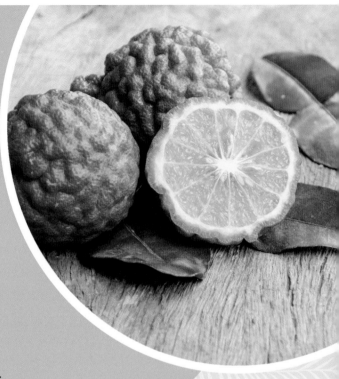

Top *Uses*

Psoriasis
Dilute 1-2 drops heavily with carrier oil, and apply frequently to affected area.

Sadness
Inhale from cupped hands or diffuse.

Appetite Loss
Drink 1-2 drops in 8 oz. water throughout the day, or diffuse.

Addictions
Apply to bottoms of feet, or diffuse.

Acne
Apply small amount to affected areas. Avoid sun for 12 hours after.

Self-Confidence/Self-Worth
Apply over sacral (belly button).

Insomnia
Use 1 drop under tongue or in water

Main Properties
Antidepressant, Carminative, Neuroprotective, Sedative, Stomachic

Chemical Constituents
δ-Limonene, Linalyl acetate, Linalool, Terpinene, β-Pinene

Other Uses
Brain Injury, Colic, Depression, Fungus Issues, Irritability, Low Energy, Muscle Cramps, Oily Skin, Stress

Safety
Avoid sun for 12 hours after topical application.

Emotional Use
Esters like Linalyl acetate in Bergamot make it a powerful calming oil, perfect for reflecting on and connecting to Self.

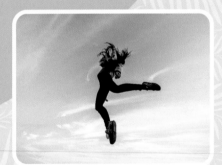

Happy Feet Diffuser Blend

5 drops Bergamot
3 drops Cassia
2 drops Spearmint
2 drops Lime

Diffuse this energizing blend while doing your dance workout!

Oh-So-Soft Body Oil Blend

3 drops Bergamot
2 drops Clary Sage
2 drops Sandalwood
3 tsp. FCO

Combine oils and FCO in a small glass jar. Apply generously to skin after showering for a luxurious, nourishing treatment.

Black Pepper

Piper Nigrum

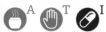 A T I

Scan Here To Experience More

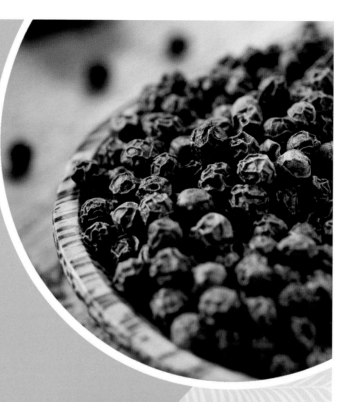

Top Uses

Cold & Flu
Take 2 drops in a capsule, or apply to the bottoms of feet.

Smoking (quitting)
Apply to bottoms of feet (big toes) several times a day to curb cravings.

Circulation
Apply to bottoms of feet.

Sprains
Massage into muscles with carrier oil.

Congestion
Apply diluted over chest and upper back.

Airborne Viruses
Diffuse to cleanse the air.

Cooking
Add a drop to soups, sauces, and other dishes.

Main Properties
Analgesic, Anticatarrhal, Anti-microbial, Antiviral, Immunostimulant

Chemical Constituents
β-caryophyllene, ι-limonene, Sabinene, α-pinene, ß-Pinene, δ-3-carene, Caryophyllene oxide

Other Uses
Antioxidant, Anxiety, Cellular Oxygenation, Diarrhea, Digestion, Gas, Emotional Repression, Inflammation, Laxative

Safety
Dilute for use on sensitive skin.

Emotional Use
Sesquiterpenes like Caryophyllene make Black Pepper a soothing oil that can unmask repressed emotions.

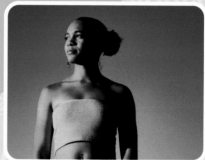

Rest and Ease Bath Soak

1 drop of Black Pepper
1 drop of Melissa
2 drops of Copaiba
2 drops of Frankincense

1 Tbsp FCO
1/2 cup of Epsom salts

Combine together and add to a full tub to enjoy a relaxing and relieving bath soak.

Happy Tummy Massage Oil

3 drops Black Pepper
3 drops Spearmint
3 drops Cardamom
2 ounces FCO
3 drops Green Mandarin

Mix all the oils in a BPA-free squeeze bottle and fill it with FCO. Shake well. Apply a teaspoon over the stomach and massage in a downward motion.

Black Spruce
Picea Mariana

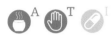

Scan Here To Experience More

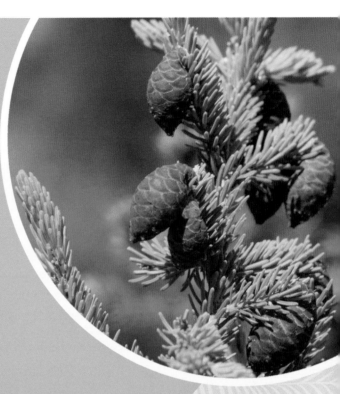

Top Uses

Memory
Apply 1-2 drops over forehead and behind ears; diffuse several drops.

Muscle Tension
Massage 2-4 drops with carrier oil.

Immune Support
Apply 1-3 drops to bottoms of feet; diffuse several drops.

Respiratory Infection
Rub 2-4 drops over chest and upper back; diffuse several drops.

Mental Stress
Apply 1-2 drops to wrists and temples.

Adrenal Fatigue
Massage 1-2 drops with 1-2 drops of Siberian Fir over kidneys.

Immunity During Pregnancy
Apply a drop diluted over lower abdomen.

Main Properties
Analgesic, Anthelmintic, Antifungal, Anti-inflammatory, Expectorant

Chemical Constituents
Bornyl acetate, β-Pinene, α-Pinene, Camphor

Other Uses
Analgesic, Airborne Diseases, Cystitis, Diarrhea, Dry Skin, Emotional Release, Energy, Gingivitis, Leucorrhoea, Mental Stress, Metabolism Regulation, Mucous Colitis, Pharyngitis, Relaxation, Restlessness, Stomatitis

Safety
Use with caution on sensitive skin and during pregnancy.

Emotional Use
Esthers like Bornyl acetate make Black Spruce a restoring oil. Use it to release trauma and to re-attune to universal energy.

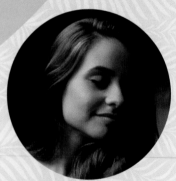

Single Oils

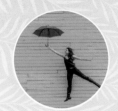

Spirited Roller Perfume
10 drops Black Spruce
10 drops Rose
10 drops Tangerine
FCO

Combine oils in a 10ml roller bottle and top with FCO. Use as needed any time of day for a bright and vibrant mood.

Room Deodorizer Diffuser Blend
8 drops Black Spruce
4 drops Tea Tree
4 drops Lemon

Eliminate unpleasant odor by diffusing this special blend.

Blue Tansy
Tanacetum Annuum

 A T I

Scan Here To Experience More

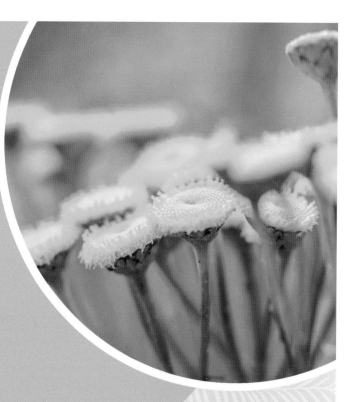

Top Uses

Allergies
Put 1-2 drops under the tongue for 30 seconds, then swish and spit.

Arthritis & Muscle Pain
Add 5-10 drops to a bath, or massage into affected areas with carrier oil.

Anxiety
Apply a drop to pulse points, or diffuse.

Digestive Discomfort
Massage 2 drops clockwise onto stomach.

Dry, Itchy, or Inflamed Skin
Apply heavily diluted to affected skin.

Headaches
Rub a drop into temples and back of skull.

Congestion
Rub 2 drops onto chest and mid-back.

Main Properties
Antihistamine, Anti-parasitic, Anti-rheumatic, Hypotensive, Sedative

Chemical Constituents
Sabinene, Chamazulene, ρ-Cymene, α-Phellandrene, β-Pinene, Camphor

Other Uses
Bacterial Infection, Constipation, Cramping, Eczema, Fungus, Gas, Gout, Indigestion, Insect Repellent, Psoriasis, Rashes, Rheumatism, Sneezing

Safety
Dilute to avoid temporary skin colorizing. Dilute for use on sensitive skin.

Emotional Use
Monoterpenes like Sabinene make Blue Tansy an uplifting oil to conquer procrastination and take inspired action.

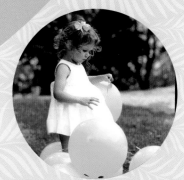

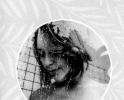

Blue Vanilla Body Scrub

10 drops Blue Tansy
10 drops Madagascar Vanilla
1 cup Raw Sugar
1 cup Argan Oil

Mix everything together in a large bowl and store in a glass jar. Gently massage over skin during a shower or bath at least once weekly.

Insect Shoo! Spray

4 drops Blue Tansy
4 drops Citronella
4 drops Lavender
4 drops Eucalyptus

Use an 8-ounce spray bottle and put all the oils and top with water. Shake well and spray where you want to keep bugs and critters away!

Single Oils

67

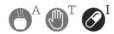

Cardamom
Elettaria Cardamomum

 A T I

Scan Here To Experience More

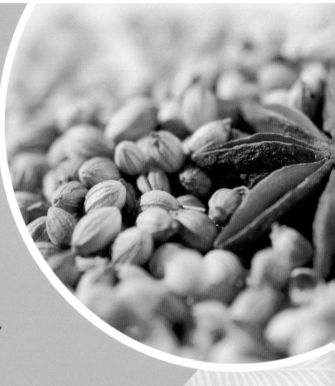

Top *Uses*

Digestive Discomfort
Drink a drop with a glass of water or in a capsule, or rub over stomach.

Congestion
Rub with carrier oil over chest, or diffuse.

Indigestion
Drink a drop with water or in a capsule.

Cough
Rub with carrier oil over chest.

Motion Sickness
Put a drop under the tongue.

Asthma, Shortness of Breath
Apply to bottoms of feet or over chest.

Cooking
Use a toothpick to add to dishes according to taste.

Main Properties
Anti-infectious, Antispasmodic, Aphrodisiac, Decongestant, Expectorant

Chemical Constituents
α-Terpinyl accetate, Linalool, Sabinene, 1,8-Cineole

Other Uses
Colitis, Constipation, Headaches, Inflammation, Menstrual Pain, Muscle Aches, Nausea, Pancreatitis, Respiratory Issues, Sore Throat, Stomach Ulcers

Emotional Use
Ethers like Terpenyl acetate make Cardamom a restoring oil. Use it to replace anger with clear, objective thinking.

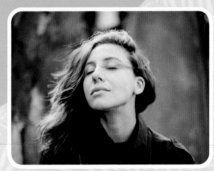

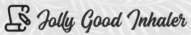 ## *Jolly Good Inhaler*

5 drops Cardamom
5 drops Neroli
5 drops Lemon
Empty EO Inhaler

Add essential oils onto the cotton wick and assemble the inhaler. Deeply inhale the spice and citrus fragrance on the go!

Breathe Eazy Diffuser Blend

3 drops Cardamom
2 drops Eucalyptus
1 drop Lemon
  Eucalyptus

Clear your airways and breathe more easily by diffusing this special blend.

Single Oils

Cassia
Cinnamomum Cassia

   A T I

Scan Here To Experience More

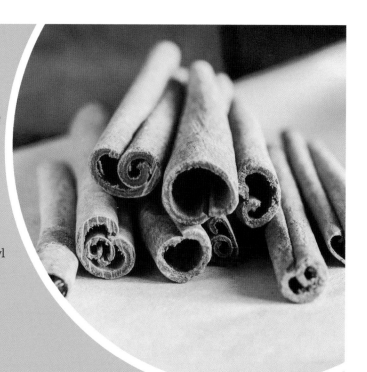

Top Uses

Vomiting
Take 1-2 drops in a capsule to restore proper digestion.

Viruses & Bacteria
Diffuse to cleanse the air, or take 1-2 drops in a capsule to combat internally.

Water Retention
Apply to bottoms of feet, take 1-2 drops in a capsule, or add 2 drops to bath.

Blood Sugar Balance
Take 1-2 drops in a capsule with food.

Sex Drive
Use heavily diluted in massage, or diffuse.

Metabolism Boost
Apply to adrenal reflex points.

Cooking
Use a toothpick to add to dishes.

Main Properties
Antibacterial, Antiviral, Antispasmodic, Cardiotonic, Decongestant

Chemical Constituents
Trans-cinnamaldehyde, Eugenol , Cinnamyl acetate

Other Uses
Antiseptic, Boils, Circulation, Cold Limbs, Upset Stomach, Typhoid

Safety
Dilute heavily for topical use. Avoid during pregnancy.

Emotional Use
Aldehydes like Cinnamaldehyde make Cassia ideal for transforming insecurity and shyness into self-assurance.

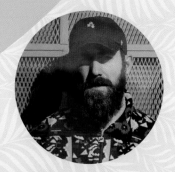

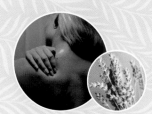

Warm Back Relief

4 drops Cassia
4 drops Lavender
4 drops Turmeric
1 oz. FCO

Combine all the oils together and use it to minimize back pain.

Mighty Man Beard Oil

2 drops Cassia
2 drops Wild Orange
2 drops Tea Tree
1/4 oz. Argan oil
3/4 oz. FCO

Mix all oils in a glass bottle and shake well. Use regularly to maintain a healthy and sweet-smelling beard.

Cedarwood
Juniperus Virginiana

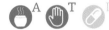

Scan Here To Experience More

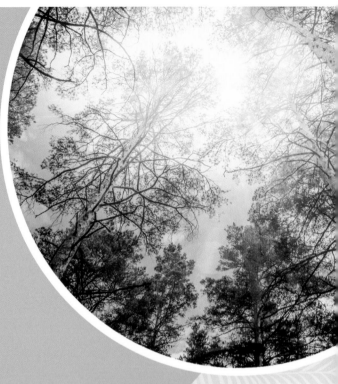

Top Uses

Eczema & Psoriasis
Apply neat and often to affected areas.

ADD/ADHD
Apply to wrists, temples, and back of neck, or diffuse.

Sleep
Rub onto bottoms of feet and back of neck, and diffuse. Blend with Lavender.

Anxiety
Apply to wrists and temples.

Cuts & Scrapes
Apply around wounded area to promote healing.

Urinary & Bladder Infection
Apply over bladder.

Seizures & Stroke
Apply to back of neck and bottoms of feet.

Main Properties
Astringent, Decongestant, Depurative, Diuretic, Sedative

Chemical Constituents
α, β, γ-thujaplicin, α-cedrene, Cedrol, Thujopsene, Methyl thujate, Thujic acid

Other Uses
Blemishes, Cough, Dandruff, Gums, Insect Repellent, Respiratory Function, Sinusitis, Vaginal Infection, Tension

Safety
Cedarwood is very mild, and safe for even the most sensitive skin.

Emotional Use
Alcohols like Cedrol make Cedarwood a Stabilizing oil that takes you from feeling separate to feeling socially connected.

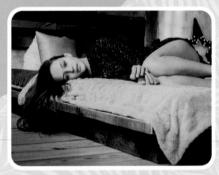

Get the Glow Toner

3 drops Cedarwood
5 drops Ylang Ylang
3 drops Bergamot
1 Tbsp Witch Hazel

Combine all ingredients in an empty glass dropper bottle and use day and night to keep skin healthy and glowing!

Hush Harmony Diffuser Blend

3 drops Cedarwood
2 drops Roman Chamomile
3 drops Clary Sage

Diffuse after a day's work for a relaxing and comforting environment before bedtime.

Celery Seed
Apium Graveolens

 A T I

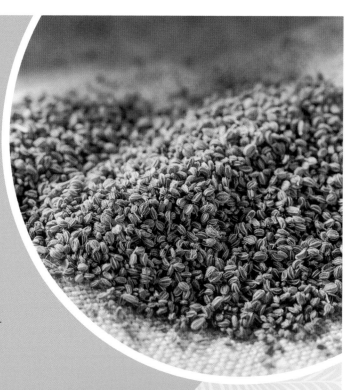

Scan Here To Experience More

Top Uses

Acid Reflux
Add 1-2 drops with 1-2 drops of Lemon or Lime to morning juice or smoothie.

Varicose Veins
Massage 1 drop with 1 drop Cypress diluted into affected areas.

Congestion
Take 2-4 drops in a capsule. Rub with Rosemary or Cardamom over chest.

Hemorrhoids
Apply a dab heavily diluted to affected area 3x daily.

Detox & Urinary Support
Apply 2 drops with 2 drops Cassia over kidneys and the bottoms of feet 30 minutes before showering.

Cooking
Add conservatavely to soups and when preparing poultry.

Main Properties
Antiseptic, Calmative, Circulatory, Depurative, Digestive

Chemical Constituents
Limonene, β, α-Selinene, Butylidene Phthalide, Sedanolide, 3-Butyl Phthalide

Other Uses
Congestion, Depression, Digestive Issues, Gastric Ulcers, Heavy Legs, High Blood Pressure, Hypertension, Inflammation, Insect Repellent, Menstrual Pain

Emotional Use
Monoterpenes like Limonene make Celery Seed an uplifting oil. It increases a sense of spiritual fire and airiness.

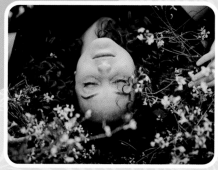

Relaxing Detox Bath

6 drops Celery Seed
4 drops Cedarwood
2 drops Sandalwood
2 drops Rose
1 cup Dead Sea Salt

Completely dissolve the salts in a tub filled with warm, bathing water. Add the oils and mix well. Soak and enjoy a detoxifying and relaxing bath.

Menstrual Relief Blend

3 drops Celery Seed
2 drops Roman Chamomile
2.5ml FCO

Mix together and gently massage onto the lower abdominal area to provide comfort when experiencing period cramps.

Cilantro
Coriandrum Sativum

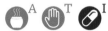 A T I

**Scan Here To
Experience More**

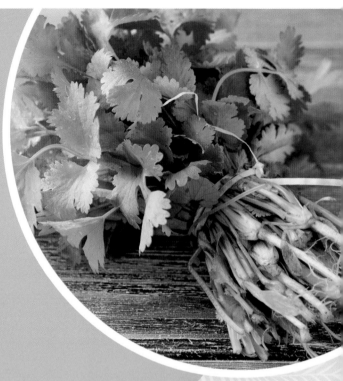

Top *Uses*

Heavy Metal Detox
Apply to the bottoms of feet morning and night.

Halitosis
Take 1-2 drops in a capsule.

Detox
Apply over liver, kidneys, and bottoms of feet.

Fungal Infections
Take 1-2 drops in a capsule for internal issues, or apply topically for external issues.

Body Odor
Use small amounts in food, or take 1-2 drops in a capsule to deodorize internally.

Cooking
Use a toothpick to add to dishes according to taste.

Main Properties
Antibacterial, Anti-fungal, Antimicrobial, Antioxidant, Detoxifier

Chemical Constituents
Linalool, Methyl chavicol, 1, 8-Cineol

Other Uses
Allergies, Antioxidant, Anxiety, Bloating, Gas, Liver Support, Kidney Support

Emotional Use
Alcohols like Linalool make Cilantro a calming oil, perfect for releasing control issues and obsessive compulsive tendencies.

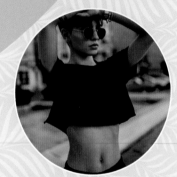

Picnic Vibe Diffuser Blend

3 drops Cilantro
2 drops Black Spruce
2 drops Cedarwood

Diffuse and enjoy a refreshing scent that brings picnic memories!

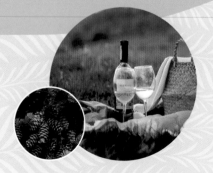

Jolly Belly Rub

5 drops Cilantro
12 drops Spearmint
3 drops Dill
2 drops Helichrysum
FCO

Combine oils in a 10ml roller bottle and top with FCO. Apply over the abdomen and gently massage.

Cinnamon
Cinnamomum Zeylanicum

Scan Here To Experience More

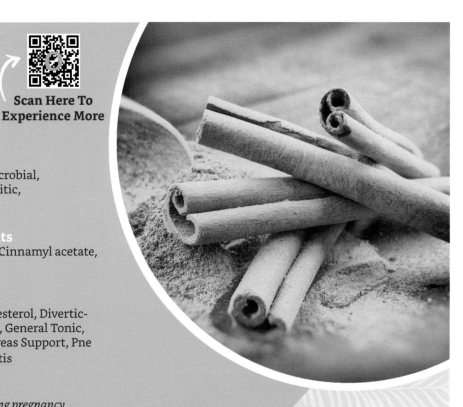

Single Oils

Top Uses

High Blood Sugar
Take 1-2 drops in capsule, or drink with large glass of water.

Bacterial Infection
Apply heavily diluted for external infection, or take 1-2 drops in a capsule for internal infection.

Sex Drive
Use heavily diluted in massage, or diffuse.

Cavities
Swish a drop with water as a mouthwash.

Diabetes
Take 1-2 drops in a capsule daily.

Alkalinity
Drink in water to promote alkalinity.

Cooking
Use a toothpick to achieve desired flavor.

Main Properties
Antidepressant, Antimicrobial, Antioxidant, Anti-parasitic, Immune stimulant

Chemical Constituents
Transcinnamaldehyde, Cinnamyl acetate, Eugenol, Linalool

Other Uses
Airborne Bacteria, Cholesterol, Diverticulitis, Fungal Infections, General Tonic, Immune Support, Pancreas Support, Pnemonia, Typhoid, Vaginitis

Safety
Dilute heavily. Avoid during pregnancy. Repeated use can cause sensitivity.

Emotional Use
Aldehydes like Cinnamaldehyde make Cinnamon a restoring oil. Use it to restore sexual harmony and expression.

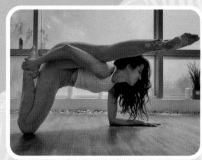

Chase-Away Bug Spray

5 drops Cinnamon
15 drops Citronella
15 drops Eucalyptus
6 oz. Witch Hazel
2 oz. FCO

Combine all ingredients in an 10oz. spray bottle. Shake well before each application.

Bouncing Spirit Roller Blend

4 drops Cinnamon
4 drops Frankincense
2 drops Neroli
FCO

Combine oils in a 10ml roller bottle and fill with FCO. Shake well and use as needed to energize the body and mind!

Citronella
Cymbopogon Nardus

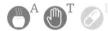

Scan Here To Experience More

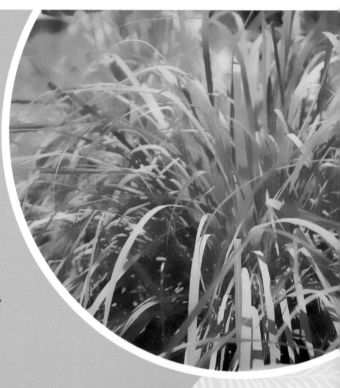

Top *Uses*

Insect Repellent
Rub or spray several drops with carrier oil over exposed skin every hour; diffuse several drops.

Airborne Bacteria
Diffuse 3 drops with 3 drops Rosemary.

Lice
Work 3-5 drops into scalp with shampoo 3x daily.

Toenail Fungus
Apply 1 drop with 1 drop Tea tree to affected areas 2x daily.

Body Odor
Apply 2-4 drops with carrier oil to underarms and bottoms of feet.

Healthy Hair
Massage 2 drops with 2 drops Lavender into hair with conditioner to protect against sun damage and remove tangles.

Main Properties
Antibacterial, Antifungal, Anti-inflammatory, Antiphlogistic, Febrifuge

Chemical Constituents
Citronellal, Geraniol, Limonene, Methyl Isoeugenol, Camphene

Other Uses
Athlete's Foot, Circulation Issues, Colds, Dry Skin, Flu, Fungus, Gas, Immunity Boost, Pain, Parasites, Spasms, Surface Cleaning, Swelling, Weight Loss, Wounds

Safety
May irritate sensitive skin. Topical use recommended during pregnancy.

Emotional Use
Aldehydes like Citronellol make Citronella a restoring oil. It eases fight or flight feelings and relaxes autonomic responses.

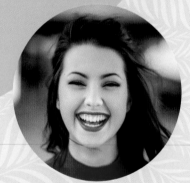

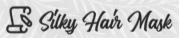 **Silky Hair Mask**

5 drops Citronella
2 Tbsp Argan Oil

Mix the oils in a small dish and apply onto towel-dried hair from the scalp to the tips. Leave on for 15 minutes and rinse well with regular shampoo. Style as usual.

 Fresh and Clean Facial Solution

5 drops Citronella
1 tsp Witch Hazel
1/5 cup distilled water

Using a clean cotton pad, apply the solution to the face to soothe and boost the skin.

Clary Sage
Salvia Sclarea

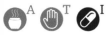

Scan Here To Experience More

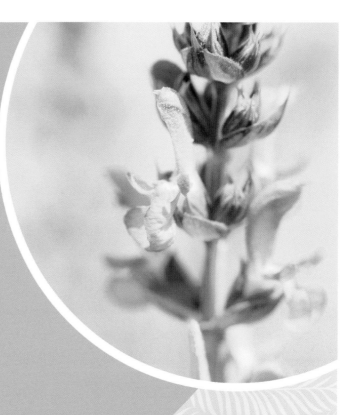

Top *Uses*

Hormone Balance
Apply to wrists and behind ears.

PMS
Apply to bottoms of feet, or take 1-2 drops in capsule.

Postpartum Depression
Diffuse or apply over heart area.

Abdominal Cramps
Massage over abdomen.

Pink Eye
Apply carefully around edge of eye.

Infertility
Apply to abdomen & uterine reflex points, or take 1-2 drops in capsule.

Breast Cancer
Apply diluted to breasts, or take 1-2 drops in capsule to regulate estrogen levels.

Main Properties
Anticonvulsant, Antiseptic, Antispasmodic, Nerve tonic, Tonic

Chemical Constituents
Linalyl acetate, Linalool, Sclareol

Other Uses
Aneurysm, Breast Enlargement, Cholesterol, Convulsions, Endometriosis, Epilepsy, Fragile Hair, Hot Flashes, Impotence, Lactation, Parkinson's, Premenopause, Seizure

Emotional Use
Esters like Linalyl acetate make Clary Sage a calming oil, ideal for calming confusion and bringing about clarified vision.

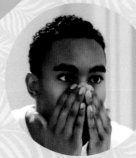

Inner Stillness Diffuser Blend

3 drops Clary Sage
2 drops Wild Orange
2 drops Cinnamon
1 drop Lemon

Diffuse this special blend to release stress and feel inner calmness.

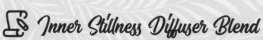

Shine and Shimmer Face Oil

5 drops Clary Sage
2 drops Geranium
1 oz. FCO

Mix together and put in a dark glass bottle. Apply a few drops on a clean face and gently pat.

Clove
Eugenia Caryophyllata

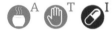

Scan Here To Experience More

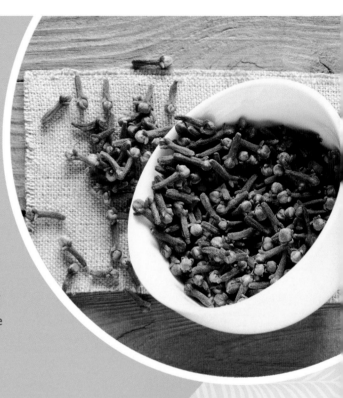

Top Uses

Thyroid (hypo, Hashimoto's)
Apply diluted over thyroid or to thyroid reflex point, or take 1-2 drops in capsule.

Toothache
Apply directly to problematic tooth.

Smoking Addiction
Rub onto bottom of big toe.

Immune Support
Take 1-2 drops in a capsule.

Antioxidant
Take 1-2 drops in a capsule, or use in cooking.

Liver Detox
Rub over liver or on liver reflex point.

Rheumatoid Arthritis
Massage diluted into affected area.

Main Properties
Analgesic, Anti-infectious, Anti-parasitic, Antiviral, Antioxidant

Chemical Constituents
Eugenol, Eugenyl acetate, β-Caryophyllene

Other Uses
Addictions, Blood Clots, Candida, Cataracts, Fever, Herpes Simplex, Hodgkin's Disease, Glaucoma, Gingivitis, Lipoma, Lupus, Lyme Disease, Macular Degeneration, Memory Loss, Parasites, Termites

Safety
Can irritate sensitive skin. Use with caution during pregnancy.

Emotional Use
Phenols like Eugenol make Clove a restoring oil, perfect for defeating victim mentality and holding healthy boundaries.

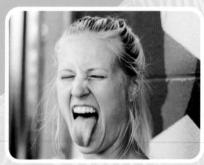

Sweet & Spicy Body Scrub

4 drops Clove
2–4 drops Ginger
4 drops Cinnamon
¾ cup Brown Sugar
½ cup Almond Oil

Combine sugar and Almond Oil in a bowl. Add the essential oils and blend well until you reach the desired texture. Use once a week to exfoliate and soften skin.

Minty Clove Mouthwash

15 drops Clove
5 drops Peppermint
1.5 cup of filtered water

Fill a jar with the filtered water and add the oils. Shake well. Use about 1-2 Tbsps of the mixture twice daily. Swish around your mouth for 30 seconds, spit, and rinse.

Copaiba
Copaifera Officinalis

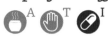

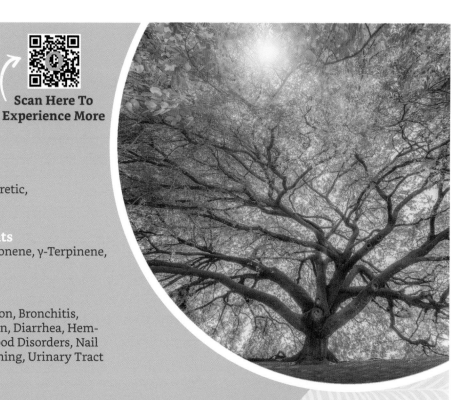

Single Oils

Scan Here To
Experience More

Top *Uses*

Headaches & Migraine
Massage gently onto temples, scalp, and the back of the neck

Pain & Inflammation
Inhale or diffuse, or apply topically to affected areas.

Mood Disorders, Panic Attacks
Massage a drop into the webs of hands and the base of skull.

Wrinkles, Pimples, Blisters
Apply daily with a carrier oil.

High Blood Pressure
Apply to the bottoms of feet twice daily.

Athlete's Foot
Apply several drops to clean, dry feet

Detox
Apply over bladder to stimulate detox through urination.

Main Properties
Analgesic, Anti-fungal, Anti-inflammatory, Diuretic, Expectorant

Chemical Constituents
β-Caryophyllene, δ-Limonene, γ-Terpinene, Linalyl acetate

Other Uses
Anxiety, Bladder Infection, Bronchitis, Congestion, Consitpation, Diarrhea, Hemmorhoids, Infection, Mood Disorders, Nail Fungus, Skin Strengthening, Urinary Tract Infection

Emotional Use
Sesquiterpenes like β-Caryophyllene make Copaiba a soothing oil, powerful for unveiling the falseness in shame and guilt.

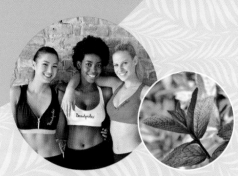

Quiet Mind Diffuser Blend

5 drops Copaiba
3 drops Grapefruit
2 drops Lavender
2 drops Clary Sage

Diffuse before going to sleep to relax the mind and release negative emotions.

After Workout Ointment

10 drops Copaiba
10 drops Peppermint
5 drops Lavender
8 oz. Coconut oil

Melt coconut oil over medium heat. Once melted, remove from heat and mix in the oils. Place inside the fridge to harden. Rub on sore muscles after exercise.

Coriander
Coriandrum Sativum

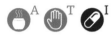 A T I

Scan Here To Experience More

Top Uses

Diabetes (high blood sugar)
Combine with 1 drop Cinnamon & Juniper Berry in capsule daily.

Food Poisoning
Drink 2 drops in water, or take in capsule.

Body Odor
Drink 2 drops in water, or take in a capsule.

Cartilage Injury
Massage into affected area with carrier oil.

Rashes
Apply diluted to affected area

Muscle Aches
Take a drop in a capsule, or massage with carrier oil onto affected muscles.

Cooking
Use a toothpick to add desired flavor.

Main Properties
Anti-rheumatic, Carminative, Regenerative, Sedative, Stomachic

Chemical Constituents
Linalool, α-Pinene, Geranyl

Other Uses
Alzheimer's, Itchy Skin, Joint Pain, Low Energy, Measles, Muscle Tone, Muscle Spasms, Nausea, Neuropathy, Stiffness, Whiplash

Emotional Use
Alcohols like Linalool make Coriander a calming oil. Use it to turn self-betrayal into integrity.

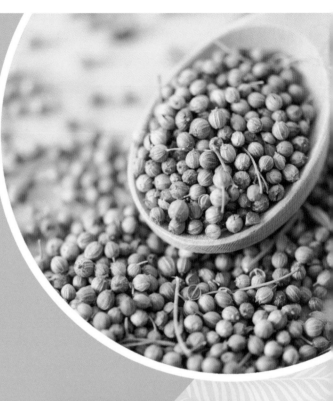

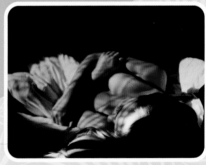

Misty Mind Booster

5 drops Coriander
3 drops Lemon
2 drops Melissa

Add the oils in your personal inhaler and use it whenever you need to concentrate.

Before Bedtime Massage Oil

8 drops Coriander
2 drops Bergamot
2 drops Ylang Ylang
1 oz. Jojoba Oil

Blend all oils in a 2oz. glass bottle. Use to massage neck, shoulders, arms, legs, and feet before going to sleep. This will help soothe and relax tense muscles.

Cypress
Cupressus Sempervirens

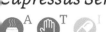

Scan Here To Experience More

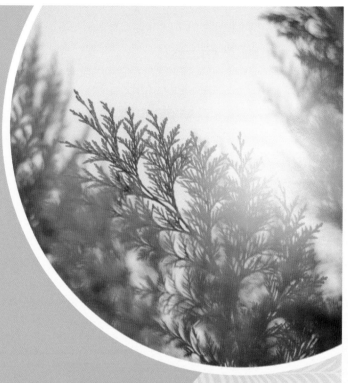

Top Uses

Circulation (poor)
Apply 2 drops to the bottoms of each foot morning and night.

Bladder/Urinary Tract Infection
Massage 2 drops with carrier oil over bladder. Repeat every 2 hours as needed.

Bone Spurs
Apply directly onto affected area

Concussion
Massage 2 drops with carrier oil into back of neck, back of skull, and shoulders.

Restless Leg Syndrome
Massage 2 drops with carrier oil into bottoms of feet, calves, and upper legs.

Bed Wetting
Apply 2 drops neat over bladder before bed.

Main Properties
Antibacterial, Anti-infectious, Diuretic, Lymphatic, Vasodilator

Chemical Constituents
α-Pinene, Cedrol, α-Terpinyl acetate

Other Uses
Aneurysm, Bunions, Edema, Hemorrhoids, Flu, Incontinence, Lou Gehrig's Disease, Ovary Issues, Prostate Issues, Raynaud's Disease, Tuberculosis, Varicose Veins, Whooping Cough

Safety
Can irritate sensitive skin. Use with caution during pregnancy.

Emotional Use
Monoterpenes like α-Pinene make Cypress a restoring oil. It creates motion and flow where energy was once stuck or stagnant.

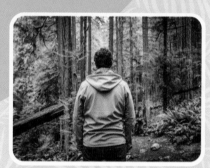

Garden-Fresh Toner

2 drops Cypress
2 drops Helichrysum
1.5 Ounces Witch Hazel
1/4 teaspoon Vitamin E

Fill a 2 ounce bottle with Witch Hazel, then add the oils and shake well. Use to help reduce skin blemishes and improve oily faces.

Earthly Zest Diffuser Blend

6 drops Cypress
2 drops Lemon
2 drops Wild Orange

Invigorate your senses with this woody and zesty blend!

Douglas Fir
Pseudotsuga Menziesil

 A T I

Scan Here To Experience More

Top Uses

Muscle Soreness
Rub 2-4 drops with carrier oil onto sore muscles.

Congestion
Rub 1-2 drops over chest, or diffuse.

Headaches & Migraine
Rub a drop into temples.

Focus & Mental Clarity
Inhale from cupped hands, or diffuse.

Skin Irritations
Apply heavily diluted to irritated skin.

Household Cleansing
Use with Lemon oil for a refreshing household cleaner.

Cough
Apply 1-2 drops to chest or lung reflex points.

Main Properties
Antioxidant, Analgesic, Diuretic, Expectorant, Tonic

Chemical Constituents
β-Pinene, α-Pinene, δ-3-Carene, Sabinene

Other Uses
Arthritis, Constipation, Depression, Emotional Congestion, Energy, Generational Patterns, Weight Gain, Sinus Issues

Emotional Use
Monoterpenes like β-Pinene make Douglas Fir an uplifting oil that lifts you from dysfunctional generational patterns.

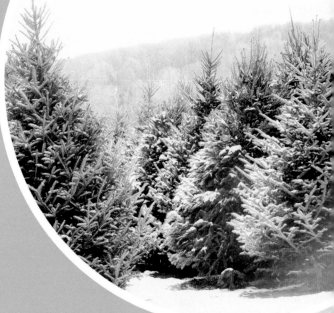

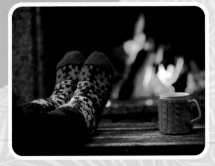

Skin Healing Facial Oil

2 drops Douglas Fir
5 drops Jasmine
5 drops Geranium
5 drops Myrrh
5 drops Copaiba
Rosehip oil

Combine all the oils in a 2ml glass dropper bottle. Fill the rest with rosehip oil. Apply morning and night to a clean dry face, avoiding the eyes.

Festive Home Spray

10 drops Douglas Fir
10 drops Peppermint
10 drops Grapefruit
5 drops Sandalwood
1/4 cup Distilled Water

Add water and oils in an 8 oz. glass spray bottle and shake well. Spray in any part of your home to enjoy a wonderful holiday smell anytime of the year.

Eucalyptus
Eucalyptus Radiata

Scan Here To Experience More

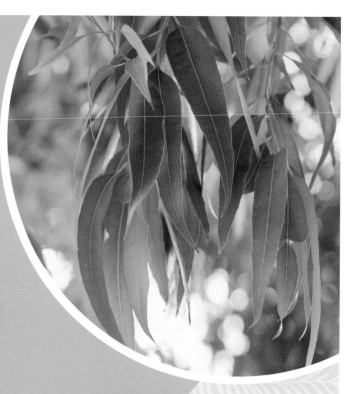

Top *Uses*

Congestion & Cough
Apply 2-4 drops to chest, or diffuse

Bronchitis & Pneumonia
Apply 2-4 drops to chest & mid-back, or diffuse.

Sinusitis
Apply heavily diluted to sinuses, carefully avoiding eyes.

Asthma
Inhale 2 drops from cupped hands, and apply to lung reflex points.

Menstrual Cramps
Rub 1-2 drops with carrier oil over abdomen.

Mental Fatigue
Inhale 1-2 drops from cupped hands, or diffuse.

Main Properties
Antiphlogistic, Antispasmodic, Antiussive, Antiviral, Vermifuge

Chemical Constituents
Eucalyptol , 1,8-Cineole, α & β-Pinene, α-Terpineol

Other Uses
Colds, Fever, Flu, Headache, Earaches, Insect Bites & Stings, Kidney Stones, Muscle Aches, Neuralgia, Rheumatism, Rhinitis

Safety
Not for use topically on newborns.

Emotional Use
Ethers like 1,8-Cineole make Eucalyptus a restoring oil. It's perfect to release attachment to illness, and to shift into a sense of wellness.

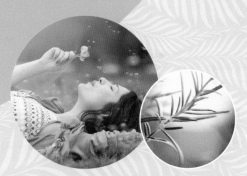

Muscle Soothing Bath Salt

6 drops Eucalyptus
12 drops Lavender
2 cups Epsom salts

Mix all ingredients and store in an airtight container. Put 1/2 cup of the mixture in a warm bath and soak for up to 30 minutes.

Sinus Solace Massage Oil

8 drops Eucalyptus
5 drops Cardamom
5 drops Rosemary
2 oz. FCO

Combine all the oils in an amber glass bottle and shake well. Massage a few drops on temples, chest, and back.

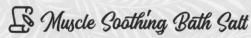

Fennel
Foeniculum Vulgare

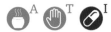 A T I

Scan Here To Experience More

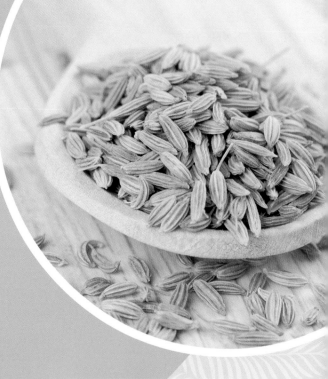

Top Uses

Flatulence
Rub 1-2 drops over outside of stomach, or drink with water.

Milk Supply (low)
Massage 1 drop diluted around nipples 2-3 times daily.

Digestive Disorders
Drink 1-2 drops in water or a capsule.

Nausea
Rub 1-2 drops over stomach, or drink a drop in water.

Menstrual Discomfort
Rub a drop over abdomen.

Parasites
Take 2-4 drops in a capsule.

Colic
Rub a drop diluted over stomach.

Main Properties
Carminative, Depurative, Diuretic, Emmenagogue, Stomachic

Chemical Constituents
Trans-anethole, Trans-ocimene, Fenchone

Other Uses
Blood Sugar Imbalance, Constipation, Digestive Disorders, Edema, Fertility Issues, Fluid Retention, Intestinal Parasites, Menopause, PMS, Spasms, Stroke

Safety
Use with caution if pregnant. Avoid if epileptic.

Emotional Use
Phenylpropenes like Anethole make Fennel an energizer to bring life to sluggish desires and embolden a sense of responsibility.

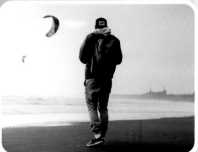

Sweet Calming Body Butter

10 drops Fennel
10 drops Lemon
10 drops Lavender
1/4 cup FCO
1/4 cup Argan oil
1/2 cup Shea Butter

Mix FCO, Argan oil, and shea butter over medium heat until combined. Add oils. Whip hot mixture in mixer until stiff peaks form. Store in an airtight glass container away from heat.

Ache Away Foot Soak

3 drops Fennel
5 drops Petitgrain
4 drops Tea Tree
2 drops Cinnamon
1 drop Ylang Ylang
1 tsp FCO

Fill a shallow wash bin with warm water and mix the oils. Soak your feet for several minutes and rinse with clean water afterwards.

Frankincense
Boswellia Frereana

   A T I

Scan Here To Experience More

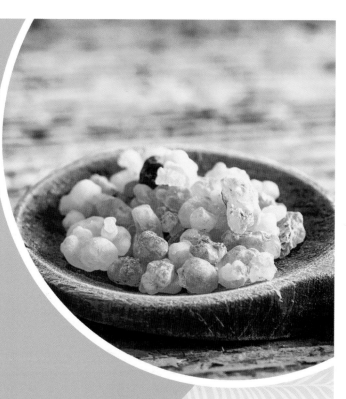

Top Uses

Depression & Anxiety
Use a drop under the tongue, apply to pulse points, or diffuse.

Alzheimer's & Dementia
Apply 2 drops to bottoms of feet and base of skull twice daily.

Cellular Function
Take 1-2 drops in a capsule.

Pain & Inflammation
Use a drop under the tongue, or massage into inflamed areas.

Parkinson's
Apply 1-2 drops to brain reflex points, and diffuse.

Cancer
Take 1-2 drops in a capsule, and apply close to the affected area frequently.

Main Properties
Analgesic, Antidepressant, Antiseptic, Cicatrizing, Cytophylactic

Chemical Constituents
α-Phellandrenes, Geranial, Neral, Geraniol, β-Elemene, Cis-verbenol

Other Uses
ADHD, Aneurysm, Asthma, Balance, Brain Health, Coma, Concussion, Fibroids, Genital Warts, Immune Support, Lou Gehrig's Disease, Memory, Moles, MRSA, Multiple Sclerosis, Scarring, Sciatica, Warts, Wrinkles

Emotional Use
Monoterpenes like α-Pinene make Frankincense a restoring oil, revealing falseness and restoring awareness of the truth.

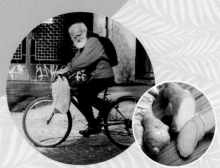

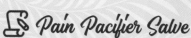

Revitalizing Night Serum

5 drops Frankincense
3 drops Neroli
2 drops Rose
4 tsp Evening Primrose

Mix all ingredients and store in a glass bottle.

Pain Pacifier Salve

25 drops Frankincense
10 drops Ginger
25 drops Myrrh
8 Tbsp Coconut oil (unrefined)

Mix all ingredients into a bowl until well blended. Store in a glass jar with a lid. Massage the salve into aching muscles and joints.

Geranium
Pelargonium Graveolens

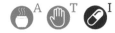

Scan Here To Experience More

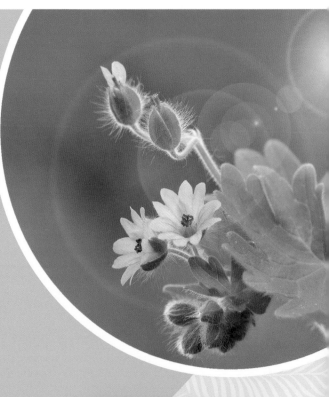

Top Uses

Liver & Kidney Support
Rub a drop directly over liver and kidneys.

Autism
Apply 1-2 drops to bottoms of feet, or diffuse.

Jaundice
Apply 1 drop diluted to bottoms of feet, and diffuse.

PMS & Hormone Balance
Apply a drop to pulse points.

Hemorrhoids
Apply heavily diluted to affected areas.

Reproductive Disorders (female)
Apply 1-2 drops to reproductive reflex points.

Varicose Veins
Massage diluted into affected areas.

Main Properties
Antidepressant, Carminative, Diaphoretic, Vermifuge, Hypertensive

Chemical Constituents
Citronellol, Citronellyl formate, Isomenthone, Geraniol

Other Uses
Bleeding, Circulation, Depression, Diarrhea, Gastric Ulcers, Hernia, Low Libido, Menstrual Cramps, Menopause, Neuralgia, Raynaud's Disease, Spasms, Vertigo

Safety
Possible skin sensitivity.

Emotional Use
Alcohols like Geraniol make Geranium a clarifying oil, reopening the heart to healing, love, and trust.

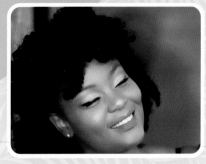

Lovely Skin Clay Mask

3 drops Geranium
2 drops Melissa
1 Tbsp Bentonite Clay
1 tsp Apple Cider Vinegar
1 Tbsp Honey

Mix all the ingredients in a bowl with just enough water to make a paste. Apply on a clean face and let it sit for 20 minutes. Rinse off with warm water.

Luscious Locks Hair Mask

5 drops Geranium
1-2 Eggs (depends on hair length)
2 Tbsp Honey
2 Tbsp Jojoba Oil

Mix all ingredients in a bowl. Apply the mixture to hair from roots to tips. Wrap in a shower cap and leave on for half an hour. Rinse well with shampoo and conditioner.

Ginger
Zingiber Officinale

 A T I

Scan Here To Experience More

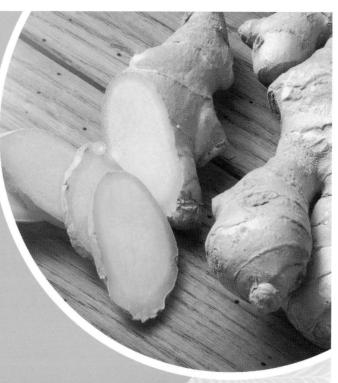

Top Uses

Nausea & Stomach Upset
Drink 1-2 drops in a capsule.

Vomiting
Rub a drop heavily diluted over stomach.

Constipation
Apply 1-2 drops diluted over stomach, or take in a capsule.

Immune Support
Apply 1-2 drops to bottoms of feet, or drink in a capsule.

Congestion & Cough
Diffuse 3-6 drops.

Cold & Flu
Apply 1-2 drops to bottoms of feet, or drink in a capsule.

Cooking
Use toothpick to achieve desired taste.

Main Properties
Antiseptic, Antispasmodic, Antitussive, Expectorant, Stomachic

Chemical Constituents
α-Zingiberene, β-Sesquiphellandrene, Zingiberene, Camphene, Nonanol

Other Uses
Aneurysm, Breast Enlargement, Cholesterol, Convulsions, Endometriosis, Epilepsy, Fragile Hair, Hot Flashes, Impotence, Lactation, Parkinson's, Premenopause, Seizure

Safety
Possible skin sensitivity.

Emotional Use
Sesquiterpenes like Zingiberene make Ginger a calming oil to soothe victim mentality and revitalize a sense of empowerment.

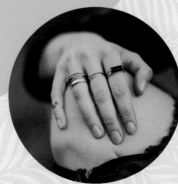

Silky Skin Scrub

10 drops Ginger
5 drops Lemon
½ cup Brown Sugar
½ cup FCO

Blend all ingredients in a bowl then transfer the mixture to an airtight container. Gently massage onto the face. Rinse off with warm water.

Throbbing Joint Blend

12 drops Ginger
10 drops Peppermint
8 drops Eucalyptus
FCO

Mix oils in a 10ml roller bottle and top with FCO. This cool and refreshing blend will help calm and soothe joint pains.

Grapefruit
Citrus X Paradisi

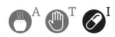

Scan Here To Experience More

Top Uses

Detox
Drink 1-3 drops in water.

Weight Loss
Apply 10 drops diluted with carrier oil over cellulite and fatty areas.

Smoking Addiction
Drink 1-3 drops in water after meals.

Antiviral Support
Apply 1-2 drops to bottoms of feet, or drink in water.

Appetite Suppressant
Diffuse several drops, or drink in water.

Gallbladder Stones
Drink 1-3 drops in water 3 times daily.

Food & Cooking
Use in smoothies, dressings, and sauces.

Main Properties
Anti-infectious, Cholagogue, Depurative, Digestive, Tonic

Chemical Constituents
δ-Limonene, Nonanal, Nootketone

Other Uses
Anorexia, Bulimia, Dry Throat, Edema, Energy, Hangovers, Jet Lag, Lymphatic Congestion, Miscarriage Recovery, Obesity, Overeating

Safety
Avoid sun exposure for 12 hours after topical use.

Emotional Use
Monoterpenes like Limonene make Grapefruit an uplifting oil to lift one out of body shame and into honoring the body.

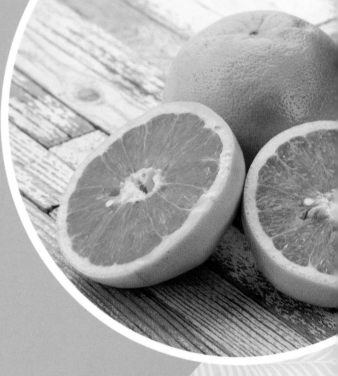

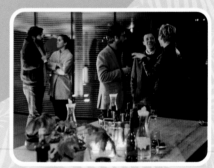

Hydrating Hair Serum

15 drops Grapefruit
5 drops Lavender
4 tsp Argan oil

Combine all oils in a glass bottle and shake well. Apply a few drops on wet hair and massage from roots to tips.

Cheerful Visits Diffuser Blend

5 drops Grapefruit
2 drops Geranium
1 drop Lime

Diffuse for a joyous ambience when you invite guests over!

Lavender
Lavandula Angustifolia

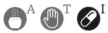 A T I

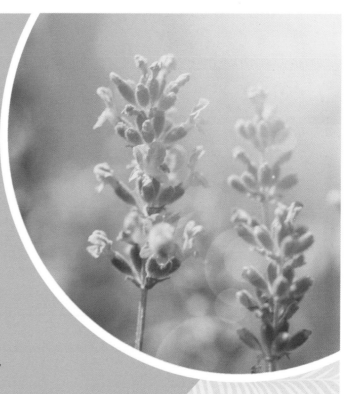

Scan Here To Experience More

Top *Uses*

Stress & Anxiety
Apply 1-2 drops to temples, or diffuse.

Sleep
Apply 2 drops to bottoms of feet and temples, or diffuse near bedside.

Skin Irritations & Burns
Apply 1-2 drops with carrier oil.

Allergies & Hay Fever
Put a drop under tongue for 30 seconds, then swallow with water.

Cuts, Blisters, & Scrapes
Apply diluted to affected areas.

Irritability
Apply 1-2 drops to pulse points.

Headaches & Migraines
Apply 1-2 drops to temples and base of skull.

Main Properties
Antibacterial, Anti-inflammatory, Anti-venomous, Calmative, Cytophylactic

Chemical Constituents
Linalool, Linalyl acetate, β-Ocimene, Ocimene

Other Uses
Allergies, Bee Stings, Bites, Blisters, Chicken Pox, Club Foot, Colic, Convulsions, Crying, Dandruff, Diaper Rash, Gangrene, Giardia, Impetigo, Insomnia, Poison Ivy & Oak, Seizures, Stings, Tachycardia, Teething Pain, Ticks

Emotional Use
Alcohols like Linalool make Lavender a calming oil. Use it to feel certain and collected through challenging communication.

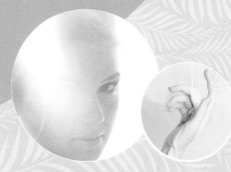

Sleepy Babe Massage Blend

2 drops Lavender
1 drop R. Chamomile
5ml FCO
25ml Argan oil

Put the essential oils in a glass dropper bottle and then fill the rest with the carrier oils. Shake well. Use to massage your baby at night for a peaceful sleep. Spot check before use.

Lavender Face Mask

4 drops Lavender
1 drop Lemon
1 Tbsp Natural Plain Yogurt
2 tsp Honey

Mix all the ingredients in a bowl. Apply on a clean face and leave for at least 20 minutes. Rinse with warm water.

Lemon
Citrus Limon

  A T I

**Scan Here To
Experience More**

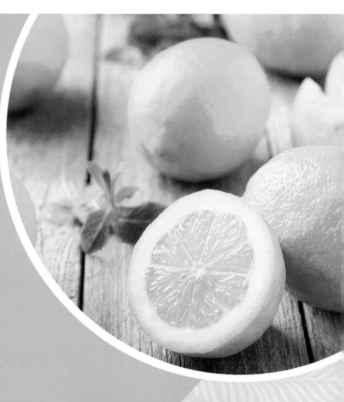

Top Uses

Energy
Inhale 1-2 drops from cupped hands.

Detox
Drink 1-3 drops in water, or apply to bottoms of feet.

Permanent Marker
Rub several drops with clean rag.

Sore Throat
Take 1-2 drops with a spoonful of honey.

Increase Alkalinity
Drink 1-3 drops in water.

Household Cleaner
Use several drops with water in glass spray bottle.

Food & Cooking
Use in smoothies, juices, and sauces.

Main Properties
Antimicrobial, Antiseptic, Antiviral, Astringent Stimulant

Chemical Constituents
δ-Limonene, Citral, β-Pinene, γ-Terpinene

Other Uses
Anxiety, Cold Sores, Colds, Concentration, Constipation, Depression, Disinfectant, Dysentery, Flu, Furniture Polish, Greasy Hair, High Blood Pressure, Kidney Stones, MRSA, Pancreatitis, Parasites, Tonsillitis

Safety
Avoid sun exposure for 12 hours after topical use.

Emotional Use
Monoterpenes like Limonene make Lemon an uplifting oil, making it easier to overcome mental fatigue and focus.

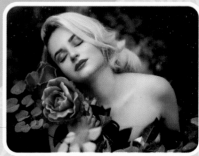

Zesty Energy Bath Blend

1 drop Lemon
3 drops Grapefruit
2 drops Lime
1 Tbsp Jojoba oil

Combine all the oils into warm bath water for a burst of refreshing energy and a feeling of invigoration.

Fairy Glow Skin Serum

8 drops Lemon
4 drops Sandalwood
30ml Rosehip Oil

Combine all the ingredients in a glass serum bottle. Gently shake to blend the oils together. To use, apply a few drops while the skin is still damp and massage gently.

Lemon Eucalyptus
Eucalyptus Citriodora

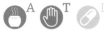

Scan Here To Experience More

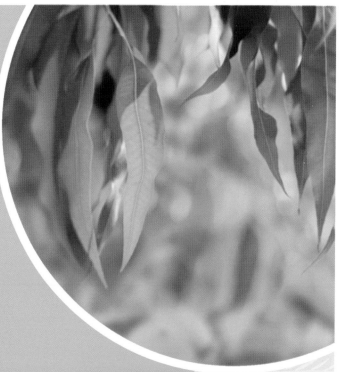

Top Uses

Bathroom Odors
Drop 2 drops into toilet bowl before use.

Mosquito Repellent
Apply 2-4 drops with FCO over exposed skin ever 2 hours for 97% mosquito coverage.

Candida
Apply 1 drop with 1 drop Tea Tree and 1 drop Clove diluted over lower abdomen 6x daily.

Surface Cleaner
Combine 5 drops with 10 drops Lemon in 10oz. glass spray bottle with water.

Air Purifier
Diffuse 2 drops with 2 drops Purify.

Muscle Injury
Massage 1-2 drops diluted into affected areas.

Main Properties
Analgesic, Antibacterial, Antifungal, Antiseptic, Antispasmodic

Chemical Constituents
Citronellal, Citronellol, Isopulegol, β-Caryophyllene

Other Uses
Asthma, Bacterial Skin Infection, Fever, Insect Bites, Respiratory Infection, Skin Fungus, Sores, Wounds

Emotional Use
Aldehydes like Citronellal make Lemon Eucalyptus a restoring oil. It brings about a sense of optimistic concentration.

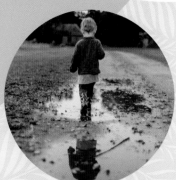

Fresh and Minty Antimicrobial Blend
5 drops Lemon Eucalyptus
5 drops Peppermint
3 drops Lavender

Diffuse as needed to help kill microorganisms or stop their growth.

Bugs Away Garden Spray
10 drops Lemon Eucalyptus
10 drops Citronella
2 oz. Distilled Water
2 oz. of White Vinegar

Mix the ingredients in a glass spray bottle and gently shake. Spray around your house or yard to repel bugs and insects. You can also use indoors.

Lemongrass
Cymbopogon Flexuosus

 A T I

Scan Here To Experience More

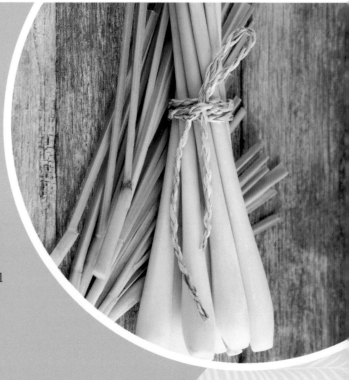

Top *Uses*

Thyroid Support (hypo & hyper)
Apply a drop diluted over thyroid.

High Cholesterol
Take 1-2 drops in a capsule.

Ligament & Tendon Issues
Apply 1-2 drops diluted to painful areas.

Stomach Ulcers
Take 1 drop in a capsule.

Immune Support
Apply 1-2 drops to bottoms of feet.

Lactose Intolerance
Take 1 drop in a capsule.

Cooking
Use toothpick to achieve desired flavor.

Main Properties
Analgesic, Anthelmintic, Antiseptic, Astringent, Tonic

Chemical Constituents
Geranial, Neral, Geraniol, α-Terpineol

Other Uses
Airborne Bacteria, Bladder Infection, Carpal Tunnel, Charley Horses, Connective Tissue Injury, Frozen Shoulder, Lymphatic Drainage, Sprains, Urinary Tract Infection

Safety
Possible skin sensitivity. Use with caution when using internally more than 10 days in a row.

Emotional Use
Aldehydes like Geranial make Lemongrass a restoring oil, ideal for cleansing toxic and negative energy.

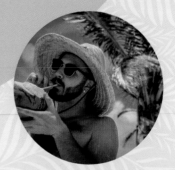

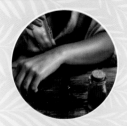

Lovely Lace Body Oil
18 drops Lemongrass
18 drops Jasmine
12 drops Helichrysum
2oz. Jojoba Oil

Mix all ingredients in a glass bottle and gently shake. Apply a few drops onto damp skin after showering to keep it hydrated and silky smooth.

Summer Day Diffuser Blend
4 drops Lemongrass
3 drops Wild Orange
3 drops Spearmint

Diffuse during sunny days to create a refreshing atmosphere and promote positive feelings.

Lime
Citrus Aurantifolia

  A T I

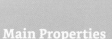 **Scan Here To Experience More**

Top Uses

Chronic Cough
Apply 2-4 drops over chest, mid-back, and lung reflex points.

Colds
Drink 1-3 drops in water, and diffuse.

Sore Throat
Gargle 2 drops with water.

Cold Sores
Apply 1 drop diluted to affected area.

Antioxidant
Drink 1-3 drops in water.

Bacterial Infection
Apply 1-2 drops with carrier oil to affected area.

Mental Clarity
Diffuse 3-6 drops, or inhale from cupped hands.

Main Properties
Anthelmintic, Antimicrobial, Antiviral, Digestive, Restorative

Chemical Constituents
δ-Limonene, 1,8 Cineol, β-Pinene, γ-Terpinene, Geranial

Other Uses
Antiviral Support, Blood Pressure, Cellulite, Depression, Detox, Energy, Exhaustion, Fever, Gallstones, Gum Removal, Herpes, Memory, Water Purification

Safety
Avoid sun exposure for 12 hours after topical use.

Emotional Use
Monoterpenes like Limonene make Lime an uplifting oil that dissipates apathy and restores a zest for life.

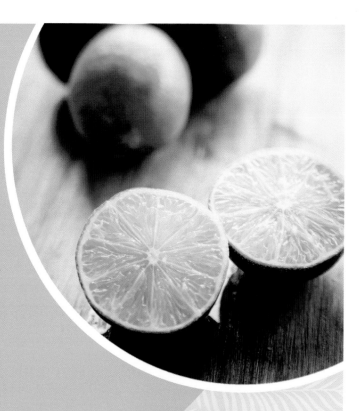

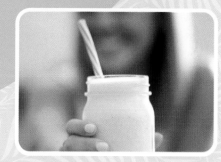

Clean & Clear Clay Mask

2 drops Lime
1 drop Lemon
1 Tbsp Bentonite Clay
1 tsp raw Apple Cider Vinegar

Mix the ingredients and add enough water to make a paste. Apply on your face and let it sit and dry for at least 15 minutes. Remove with warm water.

Yellow Lime Milkshake

2 drops Lime
1 cup Orange juice
3 cups Fresh Mango
3 scoops Vanilla Ice Cream

Blend all ingredients until smooth.

Litsea
Litsea Cubeba

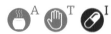

Scan Here To Experience More

Top *Uses*

Emotional Balance
Diffuse several drops, or wear on scarf or sleeve throughout the day.

Mental Rejuvenation
Inhale 1-2 drops from cupped hands.

Postpartum Depression
Diffuse, or apply over heart area.

E. Coli
Apply 1-2 drops diluted to affected areas

Internal Bacterial Infections
Drink 2-4 drops in water or in a capsule.

Aging
Apply 1-2 drops in facial lotion to combat age-promoting free radicals.

Athlete's Foot
Apply 1-2 drops to clean feet.

Main Properties
Antibacterial, Antidepressant, Antiseptic, Antiviral, Hypotensive

Chemical Constituents
Geranial, Neral, Limonene, Methyl heptenone, β-Myrcene

Other Uses
Anxiety, Cold, Cough, Disinfectant, Household Cleaning, Insect Repellent, Odors, Perspiration, Sleep, Stress

Safety
Possible skin sensitivity. Use with caution during pregnancy.

Emotional Use
Alcohols like Geranial make Litsea a clarifying oil. Use it to clear self-doubt and fear of rejection, and to expedite manifestations.

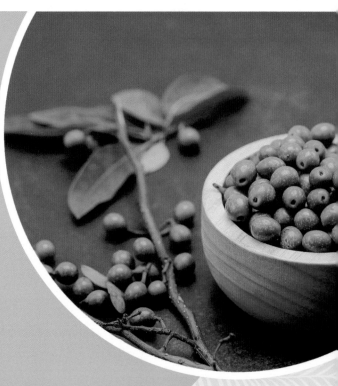

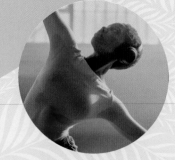

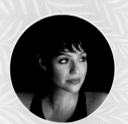

Spice and Nice Diffuser Blend

3 drops Litsea
3 drops Black Pepper
3 drops Bergamot

Diffuse while working out to promote an energizing ambiance.

Sweat Controlling Deodorant

10 drops Litsea
4 Tbsp raw Coconut Oil
4 Tbsp Corn Starch
10 drops Tea Tree
4 Tbsp Baking Soda

Combine all ingredients and mix well. You may add coconut oil to achieve desired consistency. Store in an airtight container and apply to underarms with fingers.

Madagascar Vanilla
Vanilla Planifolia

Scan Here To Experience More

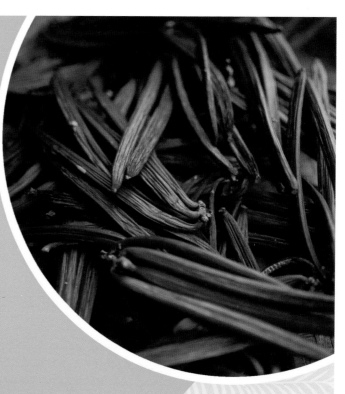

Top *Uses*

Hair Health
Add a drop to regular conditioner.

Sleep Quality
Apply 1-2 drops to bottoms of feet and back of neck 30 minutes before bedtime; diffuse several drops; use a drop under the tongue.

Respiratory Health
Rub 1-3 drops over the chest and upper back; diffuse several drops.

PMS Symptoms
Rub a drop over the abdomen.

Relaxation
Apply a few drops into a warm bath and massage into back of neck.

Low Libido
Rub a drop onto pulse points or diffuse several drops.

Main Properties
Antioxidant, Antidepressant, Anticarcinogenic, Sedative, Aphrodisiac, Antiseptic

Chemical Constituents
Vanillin, 4-Hydroxybenzaldehyde

Other Uses
Blood pressure , Febrifuge, Fine Lines, Infections, Inflammation, Minor burns, Premature Aging, Scrapes, Wrinkles

Emotional Use
The dominant aldehyde Vanillin makes Vanilla a restoring oil, bringing with it an inspiring sense of abundance and prosperity.

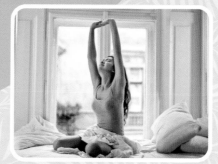

 ## *Vanilla Fantasy Diffuser Blend*

2 drops Madagascar Vanilla
2 drops Geranium
4 drops Jasmine

Diffuse near bedside to enjoy luxurious, dreamy sleep. (Recipe uses diluted Jasmine.)

 ## *Sweet and Sexy Perfume Roll-on*

10 drops Madagascar Vanilla
15 drops Rose
15 drops Jasmine
FCO

Mix essential oils in a 10ml roller bottle and top off with FCO. Shake well to blend the oils together. (Recipe uses diluted Rose & Jasmine.)

Magnolia
Michelia X Alba

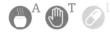

Scan Here To Experience More

Top *Uses*

Stress & Anxiety
Apply to wrists and temples, taking deep breaths.

Menstrual Cramping
Apply over lower abdomen and to wrists.

Sore Muscles
Massage onto affected muscles with carrier oil.

Depression
Apply over heart in the morning and afternoon.

Hives & Rashes
Apply with carrier oil to affected skin.

Cough
Apply over chest and mid-back.

Chronic Pain
Diffuse 3-6 drops or apply to wrists, spine, and bottoms of feet.

Main Properties
Analgesic, Anti-Inflammatory, Calming, Expectorant, Sedative

Chemical Constituents
Linalool, β-Caryophyllene, Selinene, (E)-β-Ocimene

Other Uses
Anger Issues, Bronchitis, Excess Mucus, Heart Health, Motion Sickness, Nervous System Support

Emotional Use
Alcohols like Linalool make Magnolia a calming oil that enhances the heavenly feeling of genuine connection with others.

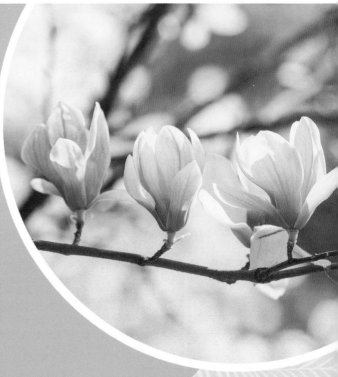

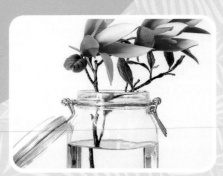

Floral Escape Roller Blend

5 drops Magnolia
4 drops Ylang Ylang
2 drops Sandalwood
3 drops Jasmine
FCO

Combine the oils in a 10ml roller bottle and fill the remainder with FCO. Apply to wrists and pulse points.

Flower Garden Room Freshener

4 drops Magnolia
3 drops Geranium
15ml 70% alcohol
1 drop Rose
Distilled water

Put the oils in a 2 oz. glass spray bottle. Add the alcohol and shake well. Fill the remainder with distilled water and shake again.

Manuka

Leptospermum Scoparium

 A T I

Scan Here To Experience More

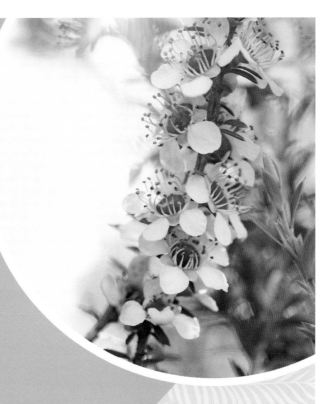

Top Uses

Blemishes & Complexion
Add a couple drops to skincare products, or apply diluted to affected areas.

Hypertension
Apply 1-2 drops to pulse points, or diffuse.

Air Purification
Diffuse 4-8 drops.

Sleep
Graze pillows with a drop of oil, and diffuse near bedside.

Bronchial Infection
Inhale 1-2 drops from cupped hands, or diffuse.

Ringworm & Parasites
Apply 1-2 drops diluted to affected areas.

Main Properties
Cytophylactic, Expectorant, Immunostimulant, Spasmolytic, Vulnerary

Chemical Constituents
Eugenol, Eugenyl acetate, β-Caryophyllene

Other Uses
Athlete's Foot, Bronchitis, Catarrh, Contusions, Cough, Fungal Skin Infections, Head Lice, Influenza, Scabies, Skin Infection, Ulceration

Safety
Possible skin sensitivity. Use with caution when pregnant.

Emotional Use
Phenols like Eugenol make Manuka a restoring oil, providing energetic safety and protection so you never feel abandoned.

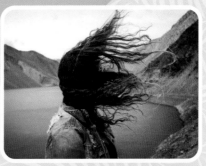

Clear the Cough Roller Blend

3 drops Manuka
3 drops Lemon
2 drops Tea Tree
FCO

Place the essential oils first in a 10ml roller bottle and then top with FCO. Apply to chest and back and bottoms of feet.

Healthy Scalp Treatment

10 drops Manuka
5 drops Tea Tree
5 drops Rosemary
¼ cup FCO

Combine oils together and rub into scalp. Let sit for 15 minutes. Wash well with regular shampoo and conditioner.

Marjoram
Origanum Majorana

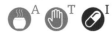

Scan Here To Experience More

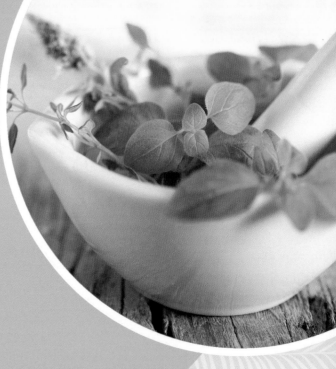

Top Uses

Muscle Injury
Massage 2 drops with carrier oil into injured muscles.

Carpal Tunnel & Arthritis
Apply 1-2 drops neat to affected area.

High Blood Pressure
Apply 2 drops to bottoms of feet, or take in a capsule.

Irritable Bowel Syndrome
Take 1-2 drops in a capsule, or rub over abdomen.

Diverticulitis
Take 1-2 drops in a capsule.

Pancreatitis
Apply 1-2 drops neat over pancreas area.

Chronic Stress
Rub 1-2 drops onto back of neck.

Main Properties
Analgesic, Antibacterial, Antispasmodic, Circulatory, Nervine

Chemical Constituents
α & γ-Terpinene, α-Terpineol, Terpinen-4-ol, Trans-sabinene hydrate

Other Uses
Arterial Vasodilator, Bruises, Colic, Constipation, Croup, Headache, Gastrointestinal Disorders, Insomnia, Menstrual Problems, Parkinson's, Prolapsed Mitral Valve, Ringworm, Sprains, Whiplash

Safety
Use with caution during pregnancy.

Emotional Use
Alcohols like Terpinen-4-ol make Marjoram a clarifying oil, bringing closeness and connection where distrust may have been.

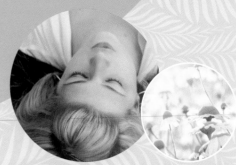

Soak Away Bath Salts

3 drops Marjoram
2 drops Lavender
1 drop Frankincense
1 Tbsp Argan oil
1/4 cup Pink Himalayan Salt

Combine oils together then mix in pink salt. Add into warm bath water and soak to relax after a day's work.

Doze Off Diffuser Blend

3 drops Marjoram
3 drops Lavender
2 drops Roman Chamomile

Add essential oils to diffuser when you need to nap in the afternoon.

Single Oils

Melissa
Melissa Officinalis

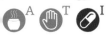 A T I

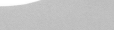

Scan Here To Experience More

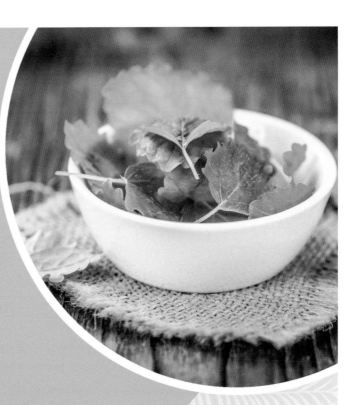

Single Oils

Top *Uses*

Viral Infections
Take 1-2 drops in a capsule.

Cold Sores & Herpes
Apply a drop to affected areas.

Depression
Use thumb to hold a drop to the roof of the mouth.

Bronchitis, Asthma
Apply 1-2 drops diluted over chest

Neurotonic
Apply a drop to the bottoms of feet.

Shock
Apply a drop diluted to back of neck, or diffuse.

Insomnia
Apply a drop to big toe, or use thumb to hold a drop to the roof of mouth.

Main Properties
Antibacterial, Antidepressant, Antiviral, Nervine, Soporific

Chemical Constituents
Geranial, Germacrene-D, Neral

Other Uses
Allergies, Anxiety, Blisters, Colds, Dysentery, Erysipelas, Hypertension, Nervousness, Sleep Disorders, Sterility, Viral Outbreak

Safety
Dilute for sensitive skin.

Emotional Use
Aldehydes like Neral make Melissa a restoring oil. It sparks enthusiasm and shines light where there was despair or darkness.

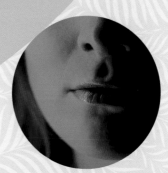

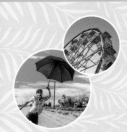

Mood Lifter Roller Blend

2 drops Melissa
1 drop Geranium
1 drop Frankincense
1 drop Lemon
FCO

Combine all oils in a roller bottle and top with FCO. Apply to the back of neck, temples, or wrists to uplift mood.

Healing Lip Balm

15 drops Melissa
2 Tbsps Coconut Oil
3 Tbsps Beeswax
¼ cup Argan Oil

Heat the beeswax and coconut oil until it becomes liquid. Add the other oils and mix well. Pour into a flat metal/glass container. Let it cool to become solid. Use to prevent or help heal cold sores.

Myrrh
Commiphora Myrrha

Scan Here To Experience More

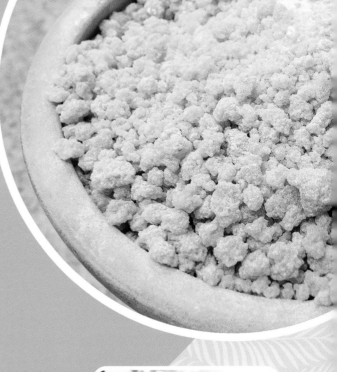

Top Uses

Wrinkles & Fine Lines
Massage into needed areas as desired.

Gum Disease & Issues
Apply 1-2 drops to gums, or swish with water as mouth rinse.

Thyroid Support
Rub 1-2 drops over thyroid.

Anxiety & Depression
Inhale 1-2 drops from cupped hands, or diffuse.

Mucus & Bronchitis
Apply 1-2 drops to chest, or diffuse.

Eczema & Skin Infections
Apply 1-2 drops to affected areas.

Nail Fungus
Apply a drop to affected nails.

Main Properties
Antimicrobial, Antiseptic, Astringent, Cicatrizing, Expectorant

Chemical Constituents
Lindestrene, Methoxyfurogermacrene, Curzenone

Other Uses
Cancer, Chapped Skin, Congestion, Dysentery, Gum Bleeding, Hepatitis, Liver Cirrhosis, Scabies, Stretch Marks

Safety
Use with caution during pregnancy.

Emotional Use
Esters like Curzerene make Myrrh a soothing oil, giving it a maternal nurturing quality. It facilitates trust and safety.

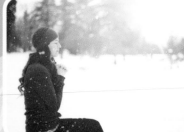

Myrrh-ific Relaxing Massage Oil

7 drops Myrrh
5 drops Lavender
30ml FCO

Add all oils in a glass dropper bottle and gently shake to mix. Use a few drops and massage on neck and shoulders or feet to feel calm and relaxed.

Cold Buster Inhaler

7 drops Myrrh
7 drops Eucalyptus
7 drops Cardamom

Add essential oils onto the cotton wick and assemble the inhaler. Use to relieve colds and promote easy breathing.

Neroli

Citrus Aurantium

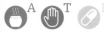 A T I

Scan Here To Experience More

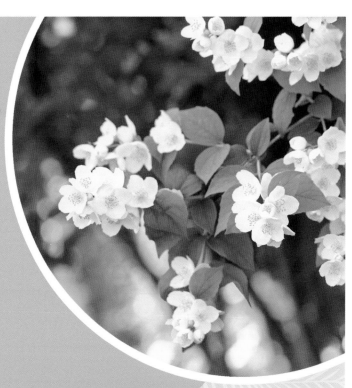

Top Uses

Scar Tissue & Stretch Marks
Massage a few drops with carrier oil into needed areas.

Perfume
Apply 1-2 drops to pulse points.

Cramps & Spasms
Apply neat to affected areas.

Emotional Exhaustion
Inhale from cupped hands, or diffuse.

Nervousness
Apply a drop to pulse points.

Depression
Wear as perfume, inhale from cupped hands, or diffuse.

Skin Regeneration
Apply generously to damaged or worn skin.

Main Properties
Antidepressant, Calmative, Circulatory, Cytophylactic, Regenerative

Chemical Constituents
Linalool, Geraniol, Limonene

Other Uses
Convalescence, Indigestion, Insomnia, Intestinal Cramping, Menopausal Anxiety, Sleep Disorders, Tension

Emotional Use
Alcohols like Linalool make Neroli a calming oil that brings intimacy, trust, and partnership to relationships.

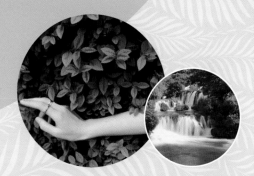

Neroli Facial Oil

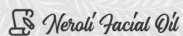

5 drops Neroli
3 drops Frankincense
4 drops Helichrysum
3 Tbsps FCO

Mix the oils into a dark glass dropper bottle and shake well. Use nightly to rejuvenate the skin.

Care-Free Diffuser Blend

4 drops Neroli
3 drops Wild Orange
3 drops Tangerine

Combine and diffuse for a day free of worries and tensions.

Oregano
Origanum Vulgare

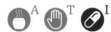

Scan Here To Experience More

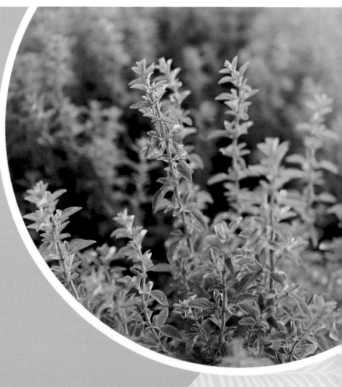

Top Uses

Bacterial & Viral Infection
Take 1-3 drops in a capsule for internal issues.

Warts
Apply directly to wart with toothpick, avoiding surrounding skin.

Candida & Staph Infection
Take 1-3 drops in a capsule.

Pneumonia & Whooping Cough
Diffuse 1-3 drops, sitting nearby the diffuser for several minutes. Also rub onto bottoms of feet.

Rheumatoid Arthritis
Massage 1 drop heavily diluted into affected area. Also take in a capsule.

Strep Throat & Tonsillitis
Gargle a drop in water. Also take 1-3 drops in a capsule.

Main Properties
Antibacterial, Anti-fungal, Antiseptic, Antiviral, Rubefacient

Chemical Constituents
Carvacrol, β-Caryophyllene, Rosmaric acid

Other Uses
Athlete's Foot, Calluses, Canker Sores, Carpal Tunnel, Control Issues, Ebola, Fungal Infections, Intestinal Parasites, MRSA, Nasal Polyps, Plague, Ringworm

Safety
Heavily dilute for topical use. Avoid using internally for more than 10 days in a row.

Emotional Use
Phenols like Carvacrol make Oregano a restoring oil. It brings with it the power of humility and being unattached.

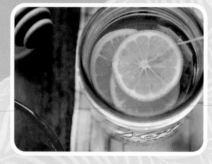

Immunity Booster Shot

2 drops Oregano
1 tsp Raw Honey
Juice of one Fresh Lemon
A piece of Fresh Ginger (1-inch)
2 Tbsp water

Place all ingredients in a blender and process until smooth. Serve in a shot glass and drink in the morning.

Minty Herb Mouthwash

1 drop Oregano
5 drops Peppermint
2 drops Cinnamon
2 cups Spring Water

Combine all ingredients and pour into a clean glass bottle. Shake well to mix. Swish about 10ml or 2 teaspoons for 30 seconds or so and spit. Avoid swallowing. Use daily.

Patchouli
Pogostemon Cablin

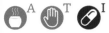

Scan Here To Experience More

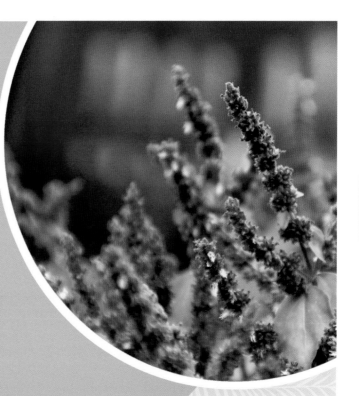

Single Oils

Top Uses

Diuretic
Apply 1-2 drops over lower abdomen.

Wrinkle Prevention
Add a drop to toner or moisturizer.

Shingles
Take 1-2 drops in a capsule, or apply to bottoms of feet.

Dopamine Shortage
Diffuse 2-4 drops, or apply to pulse points.

Dandruff
Massage 1-2 drops into clean, dry scalp after showering.

Weight Loss
Take 1-2 drops with other weight loss essential oils in a capsule.

Main Properties
Antiseptic, Astringent, Cicatrizing, Cytophylactic, Nervine

Chemical Constituents
α-Bulesene, Patchoulol, Pathoulenone

Other Uses
Abscess, Cellulite, Chapped Skin, Depression, Dermatitis, Hemorrhoids, Hives, Irritability, Mastitis, Parasitic Skin Infection, PMS, Weeping Wounds

Emotional Use
Alcohols like Patchoulol make Patchouli a stabilizing oil, which helps with feelings of grounding and body confidence.

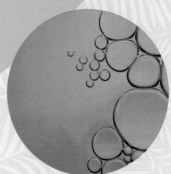

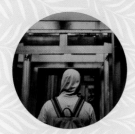

Silent Sanctuary Diffuser Blend

3 drops Patchouli
3 drops Dill
2 drops Cypress

Diffuse this special blend during meditation and feel the grounding and stabilizing effect on your emotions.

Sweet Nourishing Body Oil

8 drops Patchouli
8 drops Wild Orange
8 drops Green Mandarin
2 oz. FCO

Put the oils in a dark glass dropper bottle and roll between palms to blend the body oil together. Use after every bath.

105

Peppermint
Menta Piperita

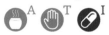 A T I

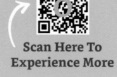

Scan Here To Experience More

Top Uses

Headache & Migraine
Massage 1-2 drops into temples and base of skull, avoiding the eyes.

Digestive Upset
Drink 1-2 drops in water, or massage directly over stomach.

Asthma & Cough
Apply 2 drops with carrier oil over chest and lung reflex points, or diffuse.

Bad Breath
Lick a dab from your finger.

Low Energy & Mental Fog
Drink 1-2 drops in water, or diffuse.

Muscle & Joint Pain
Rub a drop diluted into affected areas.

Fevers
Apply 1-2 drops to back of neck.

Main Properties
Analgesic, Anti-inflammatory, Carminative, Stomachic, Tonic

Chemical Constituents
Menthol, α & β-Pinene, Germacrene-D

Other Uses
Alertness, Allergies, Autism, Burns, Cravings, Gastritis, Hangover, Hot Flashes, Hypothyroidism, Loss of Sense of Smell, Memory, Milk Supply (Decrease), Osteoporosis, Sciatica, Sinusitis, Typhoid

Safety
Possible skin sensitivity.

Emotional Use
Alcohols like Menthol make Peppermint an energizing oil. It brings new life to the heart, and reminds you that life can be happy.

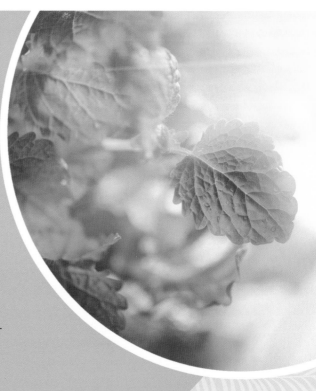

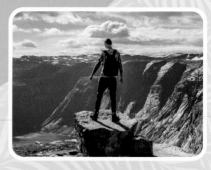

Tension Reliever Blend

10 drops Peppermint
10 drops Eucalyptus
FCO

Place all oils in a roller bottle and shake well to blend. Apply on temples, back of head, neck, and shoulders.

Easy Breathing Ointment

12 drops Peppermint
12 drops Tea tree
12 drops Frankincense
2 Tbsps Shea butter

Melt the shea butter and as soon as it is melted, stir in the oils. Transfer the mixture to a metal or glass container with a lid. Rub on chest for easy and clear breathing.

Petitgrain
Citrus Aurantium

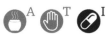 A   T   I

Scan Here To Experience More

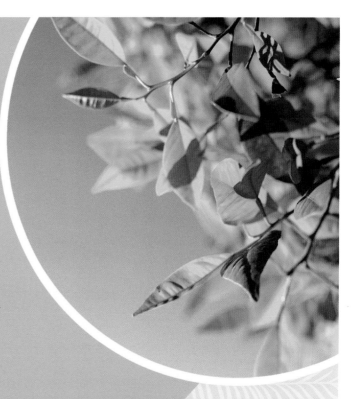

Top Uses

Nervous & Muscular Spasms
Apply 1-2 drops to bottoms of feet, or to area of spasm.

Seizures
Apply 1-2 drops to bottoms of feet and back of neck.

Insomnia
Use a drop under tongue, or on pulse points. Also diffuse.

Irritability & Stress
Apply a drop behind ears, or wear as cologne on pulse points.

Bacterial Infections
Apply topically to affected area, or take 1-3 drops in a capsule.

Spastic Coughing
Apply 1-2 drops with carrier oil over chest and mid-back, or diffuse.

Main Properties
Antidepressant, Antispasmodic, Cicatrizing, Nervine, Relaxant

Chemical Constituents
Linalyl acetate, Linalool, α-Terpineol

Other Uses
Abdominal Cramps/Spasms, Aches, Acne, Convalescence, Depression, Hysteria, Infected Wounds, Nausea, Nervous Asthma, Oily Hair, Shock, Stress-Related Conditions, Tension

Safety
Use with caution during pregnancy.

Emotional Use
Esters like Linalyl acetate make Petitgrain a calming oil, providing a space to form new and healthy traditions.

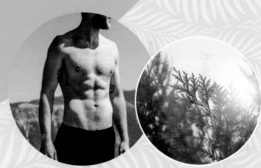

Flawless Skin Toner

2 drops Petitgrain
1 drop Helichrysum
15ml of Micellar Water

Combine and use as a toner to help reduce the appearance of skin imperfections.

Knotty Tummy Massage Oil

2 drops Petitgrain
2 drops Cypress
2 drops Green Mandarin
15ml Grapeseed oil

Blend all oils and place in a dark glass bottle. Use to gently massage into the abdomen when needed.

Pink Pepper
Schinus Molle

 A T 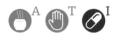 I

↑ Scan Here To Experience More

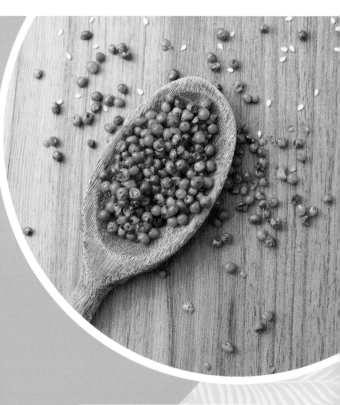

Top Uses

Cancer Prevention
Take 2-4 drops in a veggie capsule or massage with carrier oil 2x daily.

Muscle Spasms
Massage 2-3 drops with carrier oil into affected areas.

Circulatory Disorders
Massage 2 drops with carrier oil into legs.

Pain Relief
Take 2 drops in a capsule as needed.

Convulsions
Use 2-4 drops on the bottoms of feet, or take 5 drops in a capsule.

High Blood Pressure
Apply 3 drops with a carrier oil to chest.

Cough Suppressant
Apply 5 drops with carrier oil to chest and upper back.

Main Properties
Digestive, Circulatory, Anti-tumoral, Antispasmodic, Antimicrobial

Chemical Constituents
β-Myrcene, α-Phellandrene, ρ-Cymene, δ-Cadinene, Limonene, β-Phellandrene

Other Uses
Arthritis, Bee Stings, Cancer, Chest Pain, Colds, Emotional Upset, Flu, Seizures

Emotional Use
Monoterpenes like Myrcene make Pink Pepper an uplifting oil that stimulates capacity to continue giving generously of one's self.

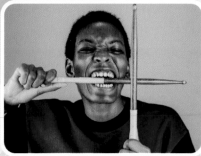

Cramp Relief Roll-On

4 drops Pink Pepper
4 drops Lavender
3 drops Neroli
3 drops Clary Sage
Avocado oil

Blend all oils in a roller bottle and top off with avocado oil. Apply to the abdomen in a circular motion to relieve cramps.

High Spirit Blend

4 drops Pink Pepper
3 drops Eucalyptus
3 drops Spearmint

Combine in a diffuser for an invigorating aroma.

Roman Chamomile

Anthemis Nobilis

 A T I

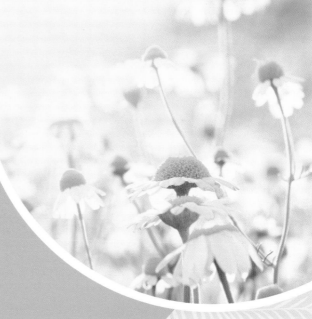

Scan Here To Experience More

Single Oils

Top Uses

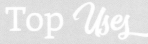

Sleep & Insomnia
Apply 1-2 drops to temples and wrists, or diffuse next to bedside.

Panic Attacks
Carry on person and breathe a drop deeply from cupped hands as needed.

Diaper Rash
Apply 1 drop heavily diluted with carrier oil to baby skin.

Crying
Add a drop to front of shirt or sleeve, or diffuse.

PMS & Cramps
Apply a drop over abdomen.

Parasites & Worms
Apply 1-2 drops over abdomen, and take in a capsule.

Main Properties
Analgesic, Anti-neuralgic, Antispasmodic, Immunostimulant, Sedative

Chemical Constituents
Isobutyl angelate, Butyl angelate, 3-Methyl-pentyl angelate, α & β-Pinene, Pinocarvone

Other Uses
Allergies, Anorexia, Bee/Hornet Stings, Club Foot, Dysentery, Hyperactivity, Menopause, Muscle Spasms, Neuralgia, Rashes, Shock, Sore Nipples

Emotional Use
Esters like Methyl-amylangelate make Roman Chamomile a calming oil that beautifully reminds one of spiritual purpose and the greater good.

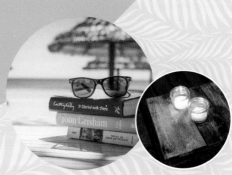

Sleepy Buds Roller Blend

4 drops Roman
 Chamomile
3 drops Ylang Ylang
3 drops Geranium
FCO

Add oils to a 10ml roller bottle and top with FCO. Roll onto chest and shoulders before bedtime.

Sunburn Comforting Oil

3 drops Roman
 Chamomile
1 drop Cedarwood
1 oz. FCO

Mix together and apply it to the affected skin using a cotton ball to reduce swelling and pain.

Rose
Rosa Damascena

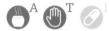

**Scan Here To
Experience More**

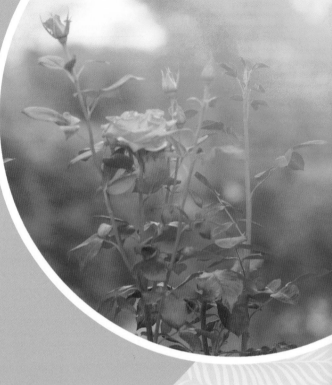

Single Oils

Top *Uses*

Aging Skin
Add a drop to toner or moisturizer, or apply with carrier oil over fine lines, wrinkles, and age spots.

Low Libido & Aphrodisiac
Apply 1-2 drops to pulse points, or to reproductive reflex points.

Scar Tissue
Massage into scar tissue 3 times daily.

Self-Esteem & Depression
Apply 1-2 drops over heart, or diffuse.

MRSA
Apply over affected area 3-5x daily.

Poison Ivy/Oak
Apply 1-2 drops diluted to irritated areas.

Main Properties
Antidepressant, Astringent, Cytophylactic, Hypnotic, Nervine

Chemical Constituents
Citronellol, Stearoptene, Nonadecane

Other Uses
Anxiety, Astringent, Dysmenorrhea, Endometriosis, Grief, Facial Redness, Impotency, Infertility, Irregular Ovulation, Menstrual Cramping, Phobias

Safety
Use with caution during pregnancy.

Emotional Use
Alcohols like Citronellol make Rose a clarifying oil that help connect the mind and soul to divine love and grace.

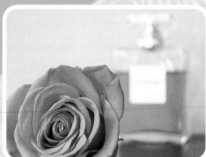

Red Bloom Face Mist

2 drops Rose
10 drops Copaiba
2 Tbsp unscented
   Witch Hazel
Filtered Water

Add the oils first in a glass spray bottle. Add unscented witch hazel, then top with filtered water and gently swirl to blend. Use as a face mist.

Lovely Rose Perfume Blend

3 drops Rose
3 drops Sandalwood
2 drops Tangerine
1 drop Spearmint
Jojoba oil

Combine the oils in a 10ml roller bottle then top with jojoba oil. Apply on wrists and neck as a daily fragrance.

110

Rosemary
Rosmarinus Officinalis

Scan Here To Experience More

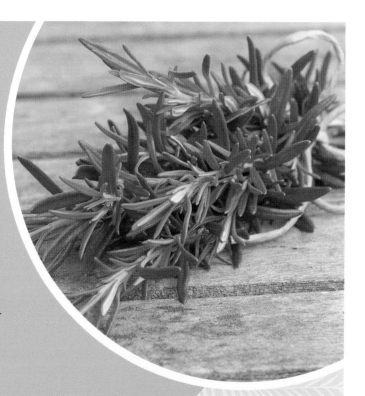

Top Uses

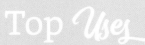

Chronic Cough
Apply 2-4 drops to lung reflex points or diluted over chest, or diffuse.

Mental & Adrenal Fatigue
Inhale 1-2 drops from cupped hands, or take in a capsule.

Focus & Memory Issues
Apply a drop over forehead, or diffuse.

Cold & Flu
Apply 1-2 drops diluted over chest.

Low Blood Pressure
Massage with carrier oil into legs and on bottoms of feet.

Jet Lag
Apply 1-2 drops to temples after flying.

Hair Loss
Work 2 drops into scalp before washing.

Main Properties
Antimicrobial, Decongestant, Depurative, Restorative, Stimulant

Chemical Constituents
1, 8-Cineole, α-Pinene, Camphor

Other Uses
Alcohol Addiction, Adenitis, Arthritis, Bell's Palsy, Cellulite, Club Foot, Constipation, Headaches, Kidney Infection, Lice, Muscular Dystrophy, Osteoarthritis, Schmidt's Syndrome, Sinusitis

Safety
Avoid during pregnancy, if epileptic, or with high blood pressure.

Emotional Use
Ethers like 1,8-Cineole make Rosemary a restoring oil that can fortify knowledge and assist in transitioning to new phases of life.

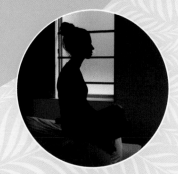

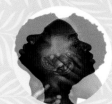

Splitting Head Relief Blend

2 drops Rosemary
2 drops Lavender
1 drop Eucalyptus
1 drop Peppermint

Diffuse when you need to relieve head and neck tension.

Strain and Stress Massage Blend

5 drops Rosemary
2 drops Wintergreen
2 drops Peppermint
2 drops Lavender
FCO

Mix all oils in a 10ml roller bottle then fill up with FCO. Roll on the affected area and massage gently to reduce muscle strain. Apply on temples and the back of your neck for stress.

Sandalwood
Santalum Album

 A T I

 Scan Here To Experience More

Top Uses

Rashes & Skin Conditions
Apply 1-2 drops with carrier oil to affected areas.

Cancer & Tumors
Take 1-2 drops in a capsule, apply diluted to affected area, or diffuse.

Meditation
Apply a drop to temples during meditation.

Low Testosterone
Take 1-2 drops in a capsule, or apply to pulse points and lower abdomen.

Scars
Massage 1-2 drops into scars often.

Alzheimer's Disease
Apply 1-2 drops to base of skull, or take 1-2 drops in a capsule daily.

Main Properties
Antidepressant, Antispasmodic, Calmative, Cicatrizing, Tonic

Chemical Constituents
α & β-Santalols, α & β-Santalenes, Norticycloekasantalic acid, Cis-lanceol

Other Uses
Aphrodisiac, Back Pain, Blemishes, Calming, Cartilage Repair, Coma, Dry Skin/Scalp, Exhaustion, Hiccups, Laryngitis, Lou Gehrig's Disease, Moles, Multiple Sclerosis, UV Radiation, Yoga

Emotional Use
Alcohols like Santalol make Sandalwood a stabilizing oil that grounds one to a higher consciousness and sense of spirituality.

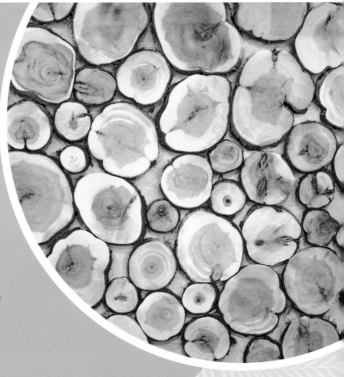

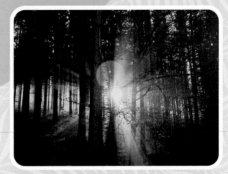

Shiny Tresses Hair Oil

4 drops Sandalwood
1 drop Patchouli
1 Tbsp Sweet Almond Oil

Combine and apply on slightly damp hair. This helps retain moisture and enhance sheen.

Pause and Reflect Diffuser Blend

5 drops Sandalwood
4 drops Lavender
3 drops Lemon
3 drops Geranium

Diffuse when you need to stay in tune with yourself.

Siberian Fir

Abies Sibirica

 A T I

Scan Here To Experience More

Top Uses

Asthma
Apply 1-2 drops with carrier oil over chest or to lung reflex points.

Immune Stimulant
Apply 1-2 drops to bottoms of feet.

Dry Cough, Cold, & Flu
Inhale 1-2 drops from cupped hands, or apply with carrier oil over chest.

Muscle Cramps & Spasms
Massage several drops with carrier oil into affected areas.

Emotional Overwhelm
Inhale 1-2 drops from cupped hands.

Rheumatism
Apply 1-2 drops neat to affected areas.

Mucus
Apply 1-2 drops to throat and chest.

Main Properties
Analgesic, Antiseptic, Antitussive, Expectorant, Tonic

Chemical Constituents
Bornyl acetate, Terpinyl acetate, δ-3-Carene, α-Pinene, Camphene

Other Uses
Anxiety, Bronchitis, Catarrh, Fever, Sinusitis, Sluggish Nerves, Tension, Urinary Infection

Safety
Use with caution during pregnancy. Possible skin sensitivity.

Emotional Use
Esters like Bornyl acetate make Siberian Fir a restoring oil that illuminates the wisdom and purpose of progressing through life.

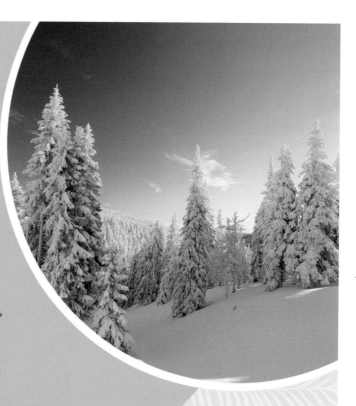

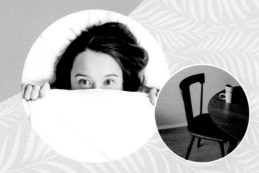

Polished Furniture Spray

6 drops Siberian Fir
1 drop Lemon
1 Tbsp Olive oil
1/2 Tbsp vinegar

Add all ingredients to a 2 oz. spray bottle and shake to combine. Spray on rag then rub onto any wood, metal, or leather surface that needs polishing.

Cold and Flu Supporting Blend

3 drops Siberian Fir
2 drops Cedarwood
2 drops Lemon

Diffuse to help during flu season.

Spearmint
Mentha Spicata

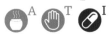 A T I

Scan Here To Experience More

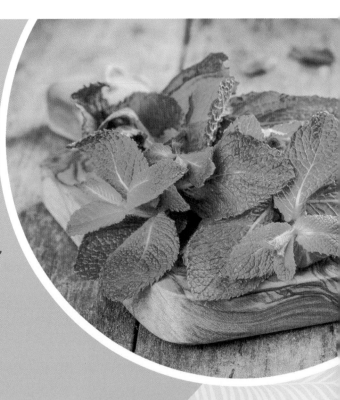

Top Uses

Indigestion
Drink 1-2 drops in water or in a capsule.

Colic
Apply a drop heavily diluted to baby's stomach.

Nausea
Inhale 1-2 drops from cupped hands, or rub over stomach.

Muscle Aches
Massage 1-2 drops diluted over achy muscles.

Bad Breath
Swish 1-2 drops in water as a mouthwash.

Heavy Menstruation
Apply 1-2 drops over back of neck and abdomen, or diffuse.

Main Properties
Antiseptic, Decongestant, Digestive, Nervine, Spasmolytic

Chemical Constituents
ι-Carvone, ι-Limonene, Carveol, 1, 8-Cineole, β-Myrcene

Other Uses
Acne, Bronchitis, Headaches, Focus, Migraines, Nervous Fatigue, Respiratory Infection, Sores, Scars

Emotional Use
Ketones like Carvone make Spearmint an energizing oil. Use it to feel energized when public speaking and voicing opinions.

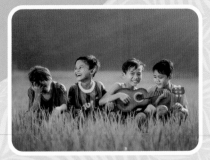

Relaxing Minty Bath Salt

10 drops Spearmint
10 drops Clary Sage
10 drops Lavender
8 oz. Epsom Salt

Combine all ingredients into a sealable glass jar and mix well. Fill your bathtub with warm water and add 2-5 Tbsp of the mixture.

Happy Kids Mist

10 drops Spearmint
10 drops Tangerine
5 drops Geranium

Combine essential oils in a 50ml glass mist bottle and fill with water. Shake and spritz around your children's playroom to brighten their mood.

Single Oils

Spikenard
Nardostachys Jatamansi

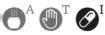 A T I

Scan Here To Experience More

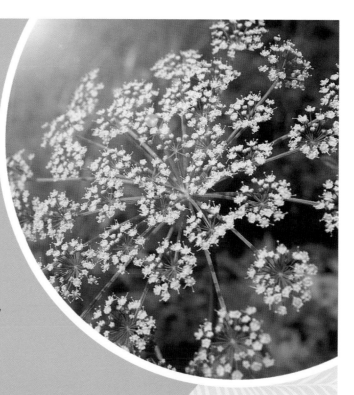

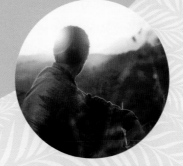

Top Uses

Chronic Fatigue Syndrome
Massage 1-2 drops diluted into adrenals and pulse points.

Insomnia
Apply neat to affected toenail often.

Toenail Fungus
Apply neat to affected toenail often.

Digestive Inflammation
Rub 1-2 drops diluted clockwise over abdomen.

Pancreatitis
Apply 1-2 drops neat over pancreas.

Immune Stimulant
Apply 1-2 drops to bottoms of feet.

Hair Loss
Massage 2 drops into scalp with shampoo daily.

Main Properties
Analgesic, Anti-inflammatory, Nervine, Regenerative, Soporific

Chemical Constituents
Jatamansone, Nardol, α-Selinene

Other Uses
Constipation, Depression, Estrogen Imbalance, Fungal Issues, Mental Fatigue, Pinkeye, PMS Cramping, Progesterone Imbalance, Uterus & Ovaries Detox

Safety
Use with caution during pregnancy.

Emotional Use
Ketones like Jatamansone make Spikenard a stabilizing oil that creates a safe space to indulge in deep, luxurious gratitude.

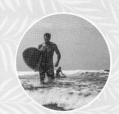

Muscle Spasm Blend

1 drop Spikenard
2 drops of Pink Pepper
2 drops Wintergreen
FCO

Mix the oils together and massage on affected areas.

Spikenard Calming Roll-on

5 drops Spikenard
5 drops Geranium
FCO

Add oils to a 10ml roller bottle and top with FCO. Shake well to combine. Apply to the back of the neck down to the spine and massage downward.

Single Oils

115

Tangerine
Citrus Reticulata

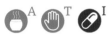 A T I

Scan Here To Experience More

Top *Uses*

Stress-Induced Insomnia
Inhale 1-2 drops during stressful times of the day. Use a drop under the tongue before bedtime.

Cellulite
Massage several drops with carrier oil into cellulite areas.

Nervous Exhaustion
Diffuse 4-8 drops, or wear a drop on pulse points.

Congestion
Rub 2-4 drops over chest and mid-back.

Discouragement
Inhale 1-2 drops from cupped hands. Also add 1-3 drops to water.

Flatulence & Constipation
Rub 1-2 drops clockwise over stomach, or drink with water.

Main Properties
Antiseptic, Cytophylactic, Depurative, Digestive, Tonic

Chemical Constituents
δ-Limonene, β-Carotene, Linalool

Other Uses
Anxious Feelings, Chronic Fatigue, Circulation, Detox, Digestive Problems, Muscle Aches, Muscle Spasms, Parasites, Water Retention

Safety
Avoid sun exposure for 12 hours after topical use.

Emotional Use
Monoterpenes like Limonene make Tangerine an uplifting oil. Use it to bring more cheer and creativity to your day.

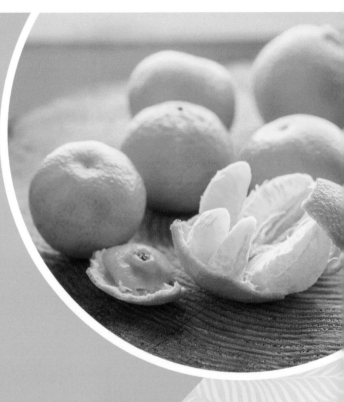

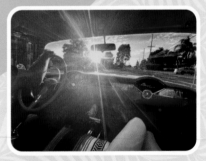

Refreshing Citrus Hand Gel

10 drops Tangerine
8 drops Lemon
2 fl oz. Aloe Vera Gel

Add all ingredients to a glass pump bottle and shake. Cleanse your hands with this mixture.

Tangy Car Diffuser Blend

3 drops Tangerine
3 drops Tea Tree
3 drops Lemon

Drop the oils to a scent pad and place into a diffuser car clip and close lid.

Tea Tree
Melaleuca Alternifolia

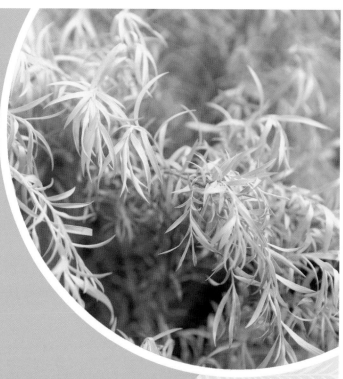

Scan Here To
Experience More

Single Oils

Top Uses

Rashes & Eczema
Apply 1-2 drops diluted to affected areas.

Dandruff
Add 2 drofps to shampoo daily.

Athlete's Foot
Apply 1-2 drops neat to clean feet.

Acne & Blemishes
Apply a dab to affected areas.

Staph Infections
Take 1-2 drops in a capsule*.

Strep Throat & Tonsillitis
Gargle 2 drops with water, and rub 1-2 drops diluted to outside of throat.

Herpes
Apply 1 drop diluted to affected areas

*Truly pure, steam distilled Tea Tree can be used internally

Main Properties
Anthelmintic, Anti-fungal, Antiseptic, Immunostimulant, Vulnerary

Chemical Constituents
α- & γ-Terpinene, Terpinen-4-ol, α- & o-Cadinenes

Other Uses
Aneurysm, Bacterial Infections, Cankers, Candida, Cavities, Cold Sores, Cuts, Dermatitis, Ear Infections, Fungal Infections, Hepatitis, Infected Wounds, MRSA, Nail Fungus, Pink Eye, Rubella, Thrush

Safety
Possible skin sensitivity.

Emotional Use
Alcohols like Terpen4-ol make Tea Tree a clarifying oil, powerful for protecting energetic boundaries.

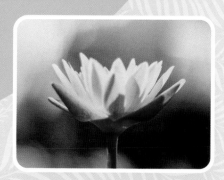

Acne Be Gone Overnight Mask

2 drops Tea Tree
2 Tbsps Aloe Vera Gel
1 tsp FCO

Mix all the ingredients until well blended. Apply a very thin layer to face at bedtime. Rinse with warm water in the morning.

Yoga Mat Cleaning Spray

6 drops Tea Tree
3 drops Frankincense
3 drops Lemongrass
2 tsp Witch Hazel

Combine oils and Witch Hazel in a small spray bottle. Fill the rest with water. Shake before using.

Thyme
Thymus Vulgaris

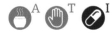

Scan Here To Experience More

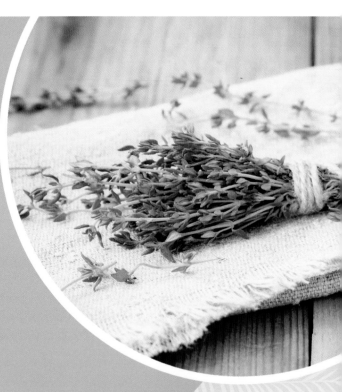

Top Uses

Bacterial Infection
Take 1-2 drops in a capsule, or apply to bottoms of feet.

Mononucleosis
Take 2 drops in a capsule 3 times daily. Also apply to bottoms of feet.

Cough, Cold, & Flu
Diffuse 1-2 drops, and take in a capsule.

Bronchitis
Apply 1-2 drops heavily diluted over chest and lung reflex points.

Skin Infections
Apply a drop heavily diluted to affected area.

Chronic Fatigue
Take 1-2 drops in a capsule, or apply heavily diluted over adrenal glands. Also use one drop in a hot bath.

Main Properties
Anthelmintic, Antimicrobial, Antiputrescent, Immunostimulant, Vermifuge

Chemical Constituents
Thymol, ρ-Cymene, Linalool, Paracymene

Other Uses
Antioxidant, Asthma, Bites/Stings, Blood Clots, Croup, Eczema/Dermatitis, Fragile Hair, Fungal Infections, Greasy Hair, Hair Loss, Laryngitis, Mold, Numbness, Parasites, Prostatitis, Tendinitis, Tuberculosis

Safety
Possible skin sensitivity. Use with caution during pregnancy or with high blood pressure.

Emotional Use
Phenols like Thymol make Thyme a restoring oil that can aid in releasing grudges and injured feelings. Use it to release and forgive.

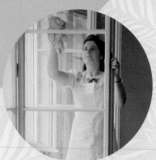

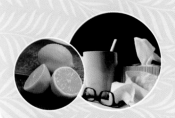

Cold Support Blend

5 drops Thyme
15 drops Lemon
15ml FCO

Combine all the oils in a glass dropper bottle. Apply a small amount to the throat, chest, and back of the neck at least 2-3 times daily.

Thyme Disinfectant Spray

20 drops Thyme
2 cups Hot Water
¼ cup Citric Acid Powder

Combine ingredients into a plastic spray bottle and shake well before use. Spray onto surfaces and wipe with a dry cleaning towel.

Tulsi (Holy Basil)
Ocimum Sanctum

 A T I

Scan Here To Experience More

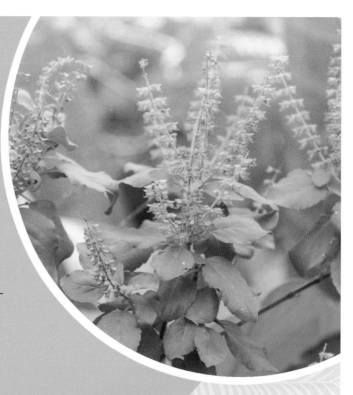

Top Uses

Muscle Spasms
Massage 1-2 drops with FCO into affected areas 2x daily.

Intestinal Spasms
Rub 1-2 drops with FCO in a clockwise fashion over stomach.

Earache/Ear Infection
Place 1-2 drops on a cotton ball and rest over ear for 20 minutes 2-3x daily until symptoms subside.

Mental Fatigue
Rub 1-2 drops into temples and back of neck and shoulders. Diffuse several drops.

Headache & Migraine
Rub 1-2 drops into temples and base of skull.

Constricted Breathing
Rub 1-2 drops with FCO over chest and upper back. Diffuse several drops.

Main Properties
Antibacterial, Antiviral, Anti-fungal, Anti-inflammatory, Analgesic

Chemical Constituents
Eugenol, 1,8-Cineole, Estragole, β-Bisabolene, α-Bisabolene, β-Ocimene

Other Uses
Acne, Anxiety, Arthritis, Bad Breath, Depression, Earache, Environmental Stress (loud volume-induced), Exhaustion, High Cholesterol, Fibromyalgia, Forgetfulness, Insulin Resistance, Joint Pain, Menstrual Cramps, Metabolism Boost, Mouth Ulcers, Peptic Ulcers, Scars, Sexual Problems, Sleep Issues, Stress

Emotional Use
Phenols like Eugenol make Tulsi a restoring essential oil. It's known in Chinese medicine as the herb for nourishing the spirit, drawing the user closer to awareness of his infinite nature.

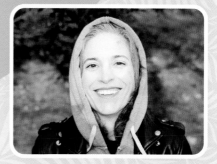

Sunrise Paradise Diffuser Blend

2 drops Tulsi (Holy Basil)
2 drops Clary Sage
2 drops Lemon

Diffuse in the morning for a warm, uplifting mood.

Youthful Glow Facial Oil

5 drops Tulsi (Holy Basil)
5 Tbsp Grapeseed oil

Combine ingredients. Apply lightly onto face every morning and night for healthy, glowing skin. Works well for dry, aging, and mature skin.

Turmeric
Curcuma Longa

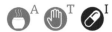

Scan Here To Experience More

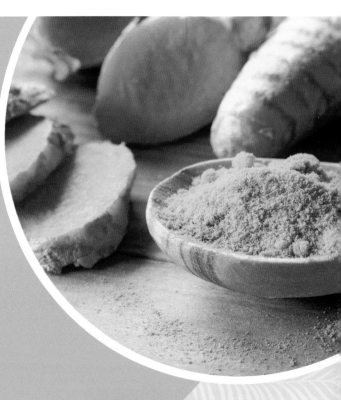

Top Uses

Chronic Pain & Inflammation
Take 2-4 drops under the tongue or in a veggie capsule. Or rub directly onto location.

Heart Palpitations
Rub 2-4 drops over chest; ingest 1-3 drops in a capsule.

Tumors
Take 5 drops in a capsule for assistance with tumorous conditions.

Brain Function
Take 5 drops in a capsule; rub a drop on the bottoms of big toes.

Detoxification
Apply 2 drops to lower back and rib cage.

Anxiety & Depression
Diffuse 5 drops to improve mood and obsessive thoughts.

Main Properties
Analgesic, Anti-inflammatory, Antimutagenic, Anti-parasitic, Anti-rheumatic

Chemical Constituents
α-Phellandrene, Terpinolene, 1,8-Cineole, ρ-Cymene, 2-Octanol

Other Uses
Arthritis, Blood Sugar, Memory Loss, Weight Loss, Wound Healing

Safety
Contraindicated in pregnancy and infants.

Emotional Use
Monoterpenes like α-Phellandrene make Turmeric a restoring oil that helps absorb the seriousness of heavy emotions.

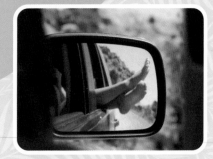

Wrinkle Free Facial Oil

4 drops Turmeric
4 drops Myrrh
4 tsp Argan Oil

Mix the two oils well and massage on your face and neck in an upward motion. Wipe off excess after massaging your face thoroughly. Do this at night to diminish fine lines and wrinkles.

Cracked Heels No More

2 drops Turmeric
1 drop Copaiba
2 Tbsps Castor Oil

Soak feet in warm water for 15 minutes and pat dry. Mix the oils and apply generously to your heels. Do at least once a week to reduce cracked and dry heels.

Vetiver
Vetiveria Zizanioides

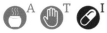

Scan Here To Experience More

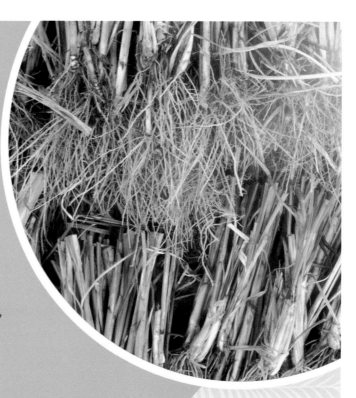

Top *Uses*

ADD/ADHD
Apply 1-2 drops behind ears and on the back of the neck.

Sleep & Insomnia
Apply 1-2 drops along spine.

Skin Irritation
Apply 1-2 drops with carrier oil to affected area.

Neuropathy
Apply 1-2 drops to bottoms of feet, or along spine.

Balance Issues
Apply 1-2 drops behind ears.

Stress-Related Menstrual Issues
Apply 1-2 drops to lower abdomen.

PTSD & Anxiety
Apply 1-2 drops behind ears, or diffuse.

Main Properties
Antimicrobial, Astringent, Cytophylactic, Diuretic, Soporific, Stimulant

Chemical Constituents
Isovalencenol, α & β-Vetivones, Vitivene, Khusimol

Other Uses
Breast Enlargement, Depression, Irritability, Learning Difficulties, Memory Retention, Muscular Pain, Nerve Issues, Nervous Tension, PMS, Postpartum Depression, Restlessness, Termites, Workaholism

Emotional Use
Alcohols like Isovalencenol make Vetiver a stabilizing oil. It centers the mind and makes space for prioritizing and focus.

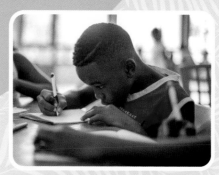

Still and Serene Bath Blend

4 drops Vetiver
2 drops Fennel
1 Tbsp Castile Soap

Mix the oils into castile soap and add to a warm bath for a grounding and nourishing blend.

Kid's Focus Diffuser Blend

2 drops Vetiver
2 drops Lavender
2 drops Rosemary

Diffuse during homework time when your child struggles with focusing.

Wild Orange
Citrus Sinensis

 A T  I

Scan Here To Experience More

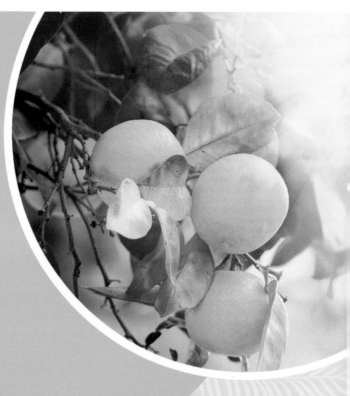

Top *Uses*

Energy
Drink 1-3 drops in water, or inhale from cupped hands.

Cheering & Mood Enhancer
Inhale 1-2 drops from cupped hands, or diffuse.

Anxiety & Depression
Inhale 1-2 drops from cupped hands, or diffuse 5-10 drops.

Immune Support
Gargle 2 drops with water, or apply to bottoms of feet.

Sleep Issues
Put a drop under the tongue before bed.

Smoothies, Dressings, & Sauces
Add according to taste.

Main Properties
Antibacterial, Antiseptic, Depurative, Sedative, Stimulant

Chemical Constituents
δ-Limonene, β-Carotene, Citral

Other Uses
Cellulite, Colds, Creativity, Depression, Detox, Fear, Fluid Retention, Heart Palpitations, Insomnia, Menopause, Nervousness, Scurvy, Sluggish Digestion, Withdrawal Issues

Safety
Avoid sun exposure for 12 hours after topical use.

Emotional Use
Monoterpenes like Limonene make Wild Orange an uplifting oil. Use it to lift a scarcity mindset into an abundance mentality.

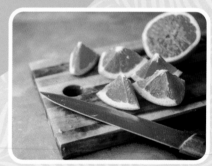

Delightful Zest Sugar Scrub

18 drops Wild Orange
6 drops Madagascar Vanilla
1/2 cup Brown Sugar
1/4 cup FCO

Mix all ingredients together in a small bowl and transfer the mixture to the glass jar. Rub a small amount onto the body and wash off with warm water.

Citrus Slice Roll-on

3 drops Wild Orange
3 drops Bergamot
2 drops Grapefruit
2 tsp FCO

Add all the oils to a small roll-on bottle and shake to blend together. Apply on pulse points to uplift emotions (be aware of photosensitivity).

Wintergreen
Gaultheria Procumbens

 A T I

Scan Here To Experience More

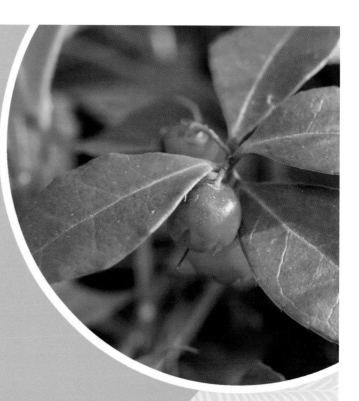

Single Oils

Top *Uses*

Muscle Pain & Inflammation
Massage 1-2 drops with carrier oil into affected areas

Arthritis & Gout
Massage 1-2 drops into inflamed joints, diluting if needed.

Broken Bones
Apply 1-2 drops gently over injury, avoiding open wounds.

Frozen Shoulder & Rotator Cuff
Massage 1-2 drops with carrier oil into affected area.

Teeth Whitening
Brush with a drop of oil and baking soda

Dandruff
Add a drop to shampoo, or massage 1-2 drops directly into scalp before shampooing.

Main Properties
Analgesic, Anti-inflammatory, Antirheumatic, Antiseptic, Stimulant

Chemical Constituents
Methyl salicylate, Salicylic acid

Other Uses
Bone Spurs, Cartilage Injury, Circulation, Muscle Development, Rheumatism

Safety
Potential skin sensitivity.

Emotional Use
Esters like Methyl salicylate make Wintergreen a restoring oil. It transitions control issues and the need to be right into a state of safe surrender.

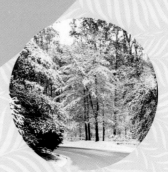

 Sweet Minty Treat Diffuser Blend

2 drops Wintergreen
2 drops Peppermint
2 drops Cassia

Diffuse to enjoy a sweet blend with a burst of mint!

Holiday Vibes Room Spray

2 drops Wintergreen
7 drops Peppermint
5 drops Green Mandarin
1 Tbsp Grain Alcohol
Distilled Water

Add oils and alcohol to a glass spray bottle. Fill the rest with water. Shake again and spray around the room for a holiday vibe.

Yarrow|Pom
Achillea Millefolium

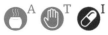 A T I

Scan Here To Experience More

Top *Uses*

High Blood Pressure
Massage 2-4 drops to wrists and bottoms of feet 2x daily.

High Cholesterol
Use 2-4 drops under the tongue or in a veggie capsule 2x daily.

Heart Health
Rub 2-3 drops over heart and wrists.

Insulin Resistance
Rub 2-3 drops onto wrists, and take under tongue or in a veggie capsule.

Varicose Veins
Apply 1-2 drops neat to affected areas.

Hemorrhoids
Apply 1-2 drops heavily diluted to affected area.

Eczema & Skin Irritation
Apply 1-2 drops diluted to affected area.

Main Properties
Antispasmodic, Carminative, Cicatrizing, Circulatory, Expectorant

Chemical Constituents
Azulene, Caryophyllene, Pinene

Other Uses
Congestion, Brain Health, Detox, Excess Sodium, Digestive Discomfort, Flatulence, Gallbladder Pain, Headache, Heart Attack, Inflammation, Metabolism, Muscle Spasms, PMS, Weight Loss

Safety
Contraindicated in pregnancy and with infants.

Emotional Use
Sesquiterpenes like Caryophyllene make Yarrow|Pom a soothing oil, granting protection to the courageous warrior.

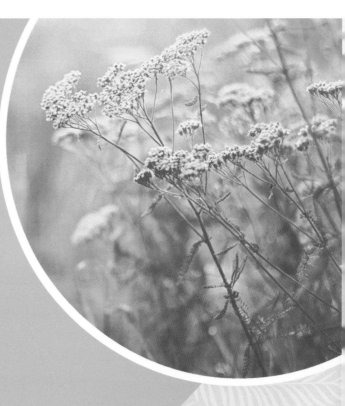

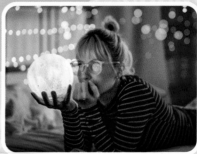

Hair Strengthening Oil

2 drops Yarrow|Pom
1 drop Roman Chamomile
1 tsp Argan oil

Mix the oils and massage on hair from roots to tips. Leave it overnight and rinse in the morning.

Dark Hours Inhaler Blend

5 drops Yarrow|Pom
5 drops Lavender
2 drops Wild Orange

Add all oils to an empty personal inhaler and use at night to help calm the mind when you are feeling restless.

Ylang Ylang
Cananga Odorata

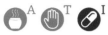

Scan Here To Experience More

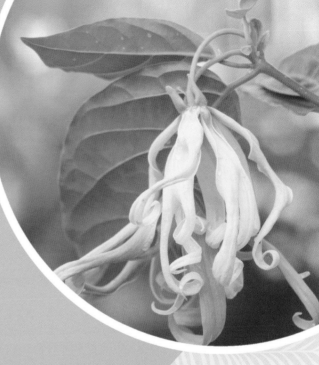

Top *Uses*

Hormone Balance
Apply 1-2 drops to wrists and behind ears.

Low Libido
Apply 1-2 drops to pulse points and reproductive reflex points. Diffuse 4-8 drops during intimacy, or use in massage.

High Blood Pressure
Apply 2 drops to bottoms of feet, and take in a capsule daily.

Infertility
Massage 1-2 drops over abdomen and reproductive reflex points.

Heart Palpitations
Apply 1-2 drops over heart, and diffuse.

Oily Skin
Add a drop to toner or facial moisturizer, or take 1-2 drops in a capsule daily.

Main Properties
Antidepressant, Antiphlogistic, Antispasmodic, Nervine, Sedative

Chemical Constituents
β-Caryophylle, Benzyl acetate & benzoate, Linalool

Other Uses
Anxiety, Arterial Hypertension, Balance Issues, Chronic Fatigue, Circulation, Depression, Diabetes, Exhaustion, Hair Loss, Hypertension, Insomnia, Intestinal Spasms, Tachycardia

Safety
Dilute for highly sensitive skin.

Emotional Use
Sesquiterpenes like Germacrene D make Ylang Ylang a soothing oil that brings out the simplicity and joy of your inner child.

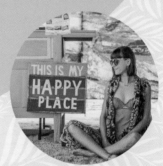

Sensual Massage Blend

5 drops Ylang Ylang
3 drops Sandalwood
3 drops Wild Orange
1 tsp FCO

Mix the oils and massage onto the inner thighs before bed for its aphrodisiac properties.

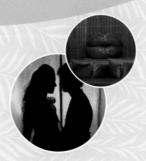

Happy Place Diffuser Blend

2 drops Ylang Ylang
2 drops Grapefruit
1 drop Bergamot

Diffuse to promote a joyful ambiance and overall positivity.

125

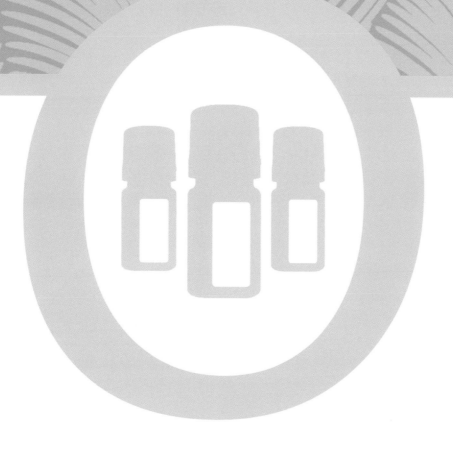

Section 4

Oil Blends

Abōde™
Refreshing Blend

  A T I

Scan Here To Experience More

Top *Uses*

Surface Cleaner Boost
Add several drops to your favorite natural surface cleaner.

Air Freshener
Add 20 drops to a 12 oz. glass spray bottle with water. Spray as needed.

Disinfectant
Add 20 drops to an 8 oz. glass spray bottle with water, along with 1 Tbsp rubbing alcohol.

Bathroom Odors
Drop a couple drops into the toilet bowl before use.

Gloominess
Inhale 1-2 drops from cupped hands or diffuse several drops for a brighter mood.

Main Ingredients
Distilled Lime, Litsea, Cassia, Lemon Eucalyptus, Tea Tree, Arborvitae, Eucalyptus Kochii, Lavandin, and Lemon Myrtle

Safety
May cause skin sensitivity. Use with caution during pregnancy.

Other Uses
Air Polution, Airborne Bacteria, Airborne Viruses, Athlete's Foot, Cold, Cold Sores, Depression, Flu, Respiratory Issues, Staph Infection, Strep Throat

Did You Know?
Distilled Lime doesn't have the same photosensitivity-causing effects as cold pressed Lime. This means you don't have to worry about sun exposure after putting this blend on your skin!

Emotional Use
A fresh environment can reflect a refreshed internal state. Use this blend to tune into a sense of rejuvenation and refreshment from the inside out.

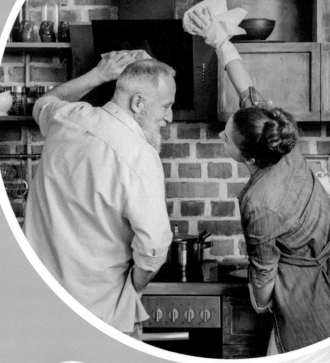

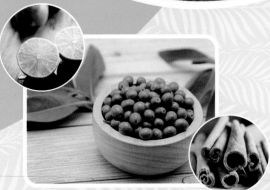

 ## *Spotless Surface Cleaner*

20 drops Abōde™
20 drops Lemon
1 cup Distilled Water
¼ cup White Vinegar

Combine all ingredients into a 12 oz. glass spray bottle. Shake well. Spray on surfaces and wipe clean.

 ## *Clean & Fragrant Toilet Spray*

10 drops Abōde™
5 drops Bergamot
5 drops Grapefruit
1 tsp Witch Hazel
2 oz. Distilled Water

Mix all ingredients in a 4 oz. glass spray bottle. Shake well. Spray directly into toilet bowl before use or into the air after use.

Oil Blends

Adaptiv™
Calming Blend

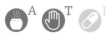 A T I

Scan Here To Experience More

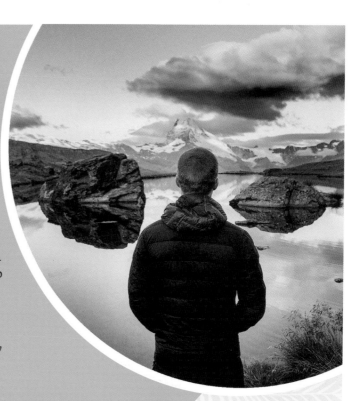

Top Uses

Anxiety
Apply 2 drops onto webs of hands and base of skull. Diffuse throughout the day.

Depression
Massage 1-3 drops onto the base of skull and over solar plexus.

PTSD
Rub 1-2 drops onto insides of arms and onto base of skull.

Hyperactivity
Diffuse several drops. Also rub 2 drops onto bottoms of feet.

Bipolar
Apply 2-4 drops to temples and inner thighs 2x daily.

Adjustment Neuropathy
Apply 1-2 drops to child's stuffed toy or take-along comfort item.

Main Ingredients
Wild Orange, Lavender, Copaiba, Spearmint, Magnolia, Rosemary, Neroli, Sweetgum

Other Uses
Behavioral Issues, Mood Disorders, Postpartum Depression, Seasonal Depression, Sleep Issues, Social Anxiety

Did You Know?
Adaptiv™ oil blend is made to work synergistically with the Adaptiv™ Complex. Together they work systemically to improve neurotransmitter activity.

Emotional Use
The gentle floral and fruity tones of this blend create a sense of safety in the present moment. Take in the feeling and awareness of everything being alright as it is right now.

Oil Blends

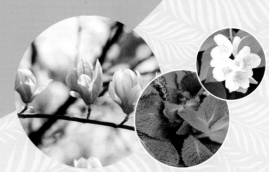

Stress Relief Roller Blend

8 drops Adaptiv™
8 drops Balance
8 drops Copaiba
FCO

Combine oils in a 10ml roller bottle and top with FCO. Apply to pulse points, over heart and behind ears.

Pure Bliss Diffuser Blend

3 drops Adaptiv™
3 drops Lemon
2 drops Green Mandarin

Diffuse to enjoy a joyful ambiance.

129

Air-X™

Air Blend | Air Repair | Clearify™

 A T 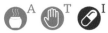 I

Scan Here To Experience More

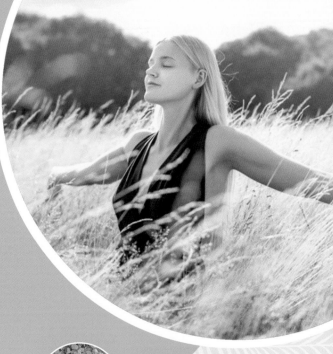

Top *Uses*

Air Polution
Diffuse several drops during times of poor air quality (during forest fires, winter inversions, high traffic seasons, etc.).

Airborne Viruses
Diffuse several drops throughout the day to combat viruses in the air.

Fatigue & Low Energy
Apply a drop to the bottoms of feet and diffuse to arouse the senses and spark energy.

Boredom
Diffuse several drops to ignite creativity and excitement for day-to-day life.

Asthma
Rub a drop diluted with FCO over the chest at the onset of an asthma attack. Also apply a drop to the lung reflex points on the bottoms of the feet.

Main Ingredients
Litsea, Tangerine, Grapefruit, Frankincense, Cardamom

Safety
Can irritate sensitive skin. May cause photosensitivity where applied topically.

Other Uses
Bacterial Infections (Internal), Cellulite, Cold (Common), Congestion, Depression, E. Coli, Flu, Stress-Induced Insomnia, Winter Depression

Did You Know?
This special blend was formulated for areas of China with high air pollution. Breathing it through diffusion introduces valuable detoxifying agents to help the body expel toxicity obtained from breathing poor air quality.

Emotional Use
The chemistry of this blend highlights the release of self doubt. It's a blend for the repairing of self-assurance.

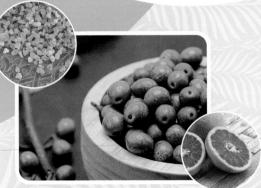

 Purifying Floral Diffuser Blend

4 drops Air-X™
2 drops Lavender
2 drops Ylang Ylang

Diffuse inside your home daily to purify the air from contaminants and to minimize viruses and bacteria

 Clean Breathing Roller Blend

16 drops Air-X™
8 drops Eucalyptus
8 drops Tea Tree
FCO

Place the oils in a 10ml roller bottle and top with FCO. Apply as needed on temples, wrists, and back of neck when exposed to air pollution.

Align
Centering Blend | Affirm

 T I

Scan Here To Experience More

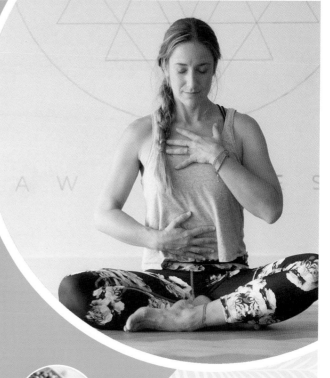

Oil Blends

Top Uses

Warrior II, Triangle, & Gate Yoga Poses
Apply 2 drops over heart, turning your attention within. Reach inside for power, identity, and assurance.

Completeness, Calmness, Courage
Apply 1-3 drops over heart, pulse points, and naval area.

Hyperactivity
Apply a drop to temples; diffuse several drops.

Addictions
Apply 2-4 drops to bottoms of feet, focusing on big toes; diffuse several drops.

Hormone Balancing
Apply 2-4 drops to wrists and inner thighs 2x daily.

Neuropathy
Apply 2-4 drops to bottoms of feet 3x daily.

Main Ingredients
Bergamot, Coriander, Marjoram, Peppermint, Geranium, Basil, Rose, Jasmine

Safety
May cause photosensitivity. Use with caution during pregnancy.

Other Uses
Body Odors, Dizziness, Mood Disorders, Muscle Injury, Nausea, Neuralgia, Vertigo

Did You Know?
The prominent herbaceous notes of this blend stimulate a sense of alignment with the centered way nature caries itself. It smells like a flourishing field of wild herbs and flowers.

Emotional Use
This yoga blend encourages a sense of harmony and calm progress. Release feelings of hastiness and know that growth happens most often in a subtle, ongoing process.

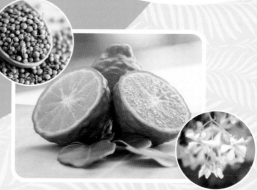

 ## Moving Forward Diffuser Blend

2 drops Align
2 drops Frankincense
1 drop Blue Tansy

Diffuse this blend when you need to let go of past mistakes and move forward positively.

 ## Painful Period Soothing Blend

10 drops Align
5 drops Cinnamon
5 drops Clary Sage
5 drops Chamomile
30ml Jojoba oil

Combine the oils together in a roller bottle and shake gently. Rub onto lower abdomen in a clockwise direction.

Anchor
Steadying Blend

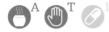

Scan Here To Experience More

Top Uses

Seated Meditation, Seated Twist, & Bhu Mudra yoga poses
Apply a couple drops to heels, over ears, and the base of skull.

Circulation Issues
Apply 2-4 drops to the bottoms of feet morning and evening.

Muscle Spasms
Massage 2-4 drops into the bottoms of feet and into affected muscles.

Energetic Focus
Apply a drop to temples and inhale from cupped hands to center your attention.

Emotional Numbness
Massage 2-4 drops into sacral area and lower spine.

Cracked or Chapped Skin
Massage 2-4 drops with extra FCO into affected areas.

Main Ingredients
Lavender, Cedarwood, Frankincense, Cinnamon, Sandalwood, Black Pepper, Patchouli

Safety
Can irritate sensitive skin. Use with caution during pregnancy.

Other Uses
Agitation, Bipolar Disorder, Calming, Courage, Muscle Fatigue, Sleep Issues

Did You Know?
Sandalwood has a historic reputation for deepening meditation and mindfulness, which makes it fitting for this anchoring meditation and yoga blend.

Emotional Use
This is the oil of anchoring to truth. Use this blend to connect to your inner wisdom and what is true to you, independent of social or cultural expectations or changes.

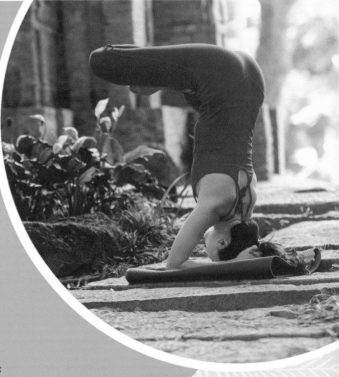

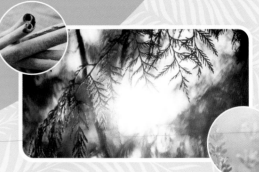

Whole-ly Feelings Diffuser Blend

4 drops Anchor
2 drops Tangerine
1 drop Helichrysum

Diffuse this blend to encourage feelings of wholeness and satisfaction within yourself.

Anchor Foot Soak

4 drops Anchor
2 drops Frankincense
3 drops Clary Sage
2 cups Epsom salt

Mix the oils with the Epsom salt and pour into a foot basin. Add enough warm water to cover feet and stir the mixture with your feet until the salt dissolves. Soak for 20 minutes.

Arise
Enlightening Blend | Ascend

 A T I

Scan Here To Experience More

Top Uses

Standing Arms High, Standing Side Stretch, & Half Moon Yoga Poses
Apply 2-4 drops to inside of arms and wrists. Feel light entering the crown of your head as your own energy rises to meet it.

Lacking Motivation
Apply 1-3 drops to temples and back of neck.

Mental Clarity & Illumination
Apply 1-3 drops to temples and forehead.

Cold & Flu
Massage 2-4 drops into bottoms of feet and spine; diffuse several drops.

Overeating
Massage 2-4 drops over stomach; diffuse several drops.

Cold Sores
Apply a drop to affected area 5x daily.

Main Ingredients
Lemon, Grapefruit, Siberian Fir, Osmanthus, Melissa

Safety
Avoid sun exposure for 12 hours after topical application.

Other Uses
Depression, Fear, Respiratory Infection, Sinus Infection, Toxicity, Viral Infection

Did You Know?
The candy-like aroma in this blend is largely due to the combination of citrus oils with Osmanthus, creating a smell that is sweet and fruity.

Emotional Use
Arise inspires a sense of freedom. It reminds the user that stability and freedom are the paradoxical duo that allows creativity and inspiration to abound.

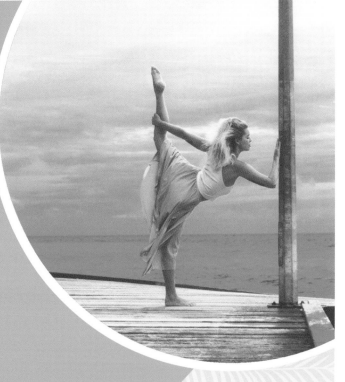

Oil Blends

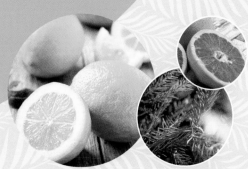

Crystal Clarity Diffuser Blend

6 drops Arise
4 drops Sandalwood

Start diffusing for about 20-30 minutes before you meditate to elevate your state of being.

Happy Homestead Room Spray

10 drops Arise
10 drops Madagascar Vanilla
5 drops Lemon
3/4 cup water

Combine all ingredients to a glass spray bottle and shake well. Spray within your home for a bright and sweet scent.

AromaTouch®
Massage Blend

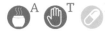 A T ⊘ I

Scan Here To Experience More

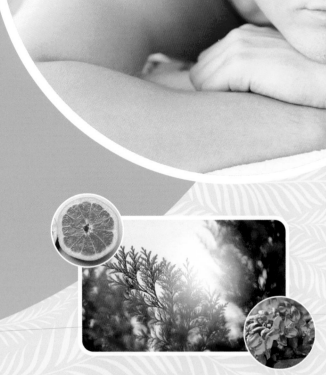

Top *Uses*

Muscle Tension & Aches
Massage 2-4 drops with carrier oil into tight muscles.

Adrenal Fatigue & Lethargy
Apply 1-2 drops to lower back.

Back, Neck, & Shoulder Pain
Massage 2-4 drops with carrier oil into affected muscles, or add to hot bath.

Post-Work Stress
Massage 2 drops into back of neck to relieve stress from work.

Neuropathy
Apply 1-2 drops to bottoms of feet.

High Blood Pressure
Apply 1-2 drops to bottoms of feet.

Headache
Apply 1-2 drops to temples, avoiding eyes.

Main Ingredients
Cypress, Peppermint, Marjoram, Basil, Grapefruit, Lavender

Safety
Can irritate sensitive skin. Use with caution during pregnancy.

Other Uses
Arthritis, Circulation, Ligament Damage, Muscular Dystrophy, Relaxation, Tension

Did You Know?
Marjoram and Cypress are a power duo for muscle-mend. They increase circulation and promote faster muscle repair.

Emotional Use
This blend assists in releasing the tension of the day and shifting into a state of well-deserved relaxation. It opens the mind and heart to the possibility of releasing unnecessary stress.

Soothing Sensation Massage Oil

2 drops AromaTouch®
2 drops Helichrysum
2 drops Siberian Fir

Combine essential oils and massage over shoulders and neck for a relaxing and soothing effect after a long day.

Simply Tranquil Diffuser Blend

3 drops AromaTouch®
2 drops Lime
2 drops Balance
1 drop Citrus Bliss®

Diffuse to create a peaceful atmosphere to help wind down into a space of tranquility.

Oil Blends

Balance
Grounding Blend

 A T I

Top Uses

Emotional Grounding
Inhale 1-3 drops from cupped hands, or apply to bottoms of feet daily.

Focus & Concentration
Apply 1-3 drops to temples and pulse points, or diffuse.

Stress & Anxiety
Apply 1-3 drops to pulse points and temples, or to bottoms of feet.

Meditation
Apply 1-2 drops to wrists and temples.

Neurological Issues
Apply 2-4 drops to bottoms of feet.

Stress-Induced Inflammation
Inhale 2-4 drops from cupped hands, apply to bottoms of feet, or diffuse.

Balance
Apply 1-2 drops behind ears.

Main Ingredients
Spruce, Ho Wood, Frankincense, Blue Tansy, Blue Chamomile, Osmanthus

Other Uses
Anger, Back Pain, Brain Integration, Bursitis, Comas, Confusion, Convulsions, Diabetic Sores, Grief, Herniated Discs, Hyperactivity, Lou Gehrig's Disease, Parkinson's Disease, Tranquility

Did You Know?
Many popular balancing blends have used Rosewood, a now-endangered species. That's why this blend instead leverages the benefits of Blue Tansy and Blue Chamomile in tandem.

Emotional Use
The earthy character of this blend help bring scattered energy and emotions into a space of stability, consistency, and safety.

Scan Here To Experience More

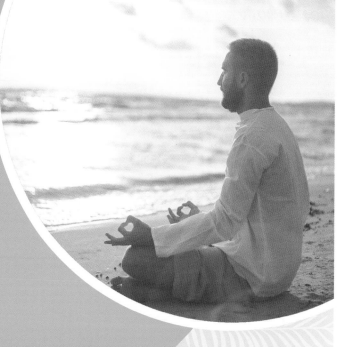

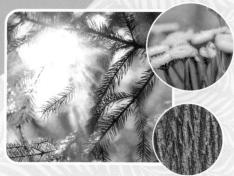

Oil Blends

Strain Away Diffuser Blend

4 drops Balance
2 drops Frankincense
2 drops Vetiver

Diffuse in your office to minimize feelings of stress and pressure.

Joyful Trip Car Diffuser

5 drops Balance
5 drops Citrus Bliss®

Drop the oils to a scent pad and place into a diffuser car clip and close lid.

Breathe

Respiratory Blend | Air | Easy Air®

Scan Here To Experience More

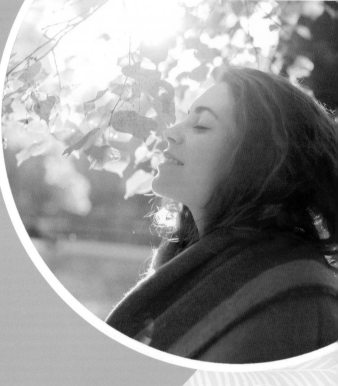

Oil Blends

Top Uses

Cough, Bronchitis, Pneumonia
Inhale 2-4 drops from cupped hands, and apply diluted over chest.

Asthma
Inhale 2-4 drops from cupped hands, and apply to lung reflex points.

Cold & Flu
Diffuse 5-10 drops, or apply with carrier oil over chest.

Allergies
Apply 1-2 drops over bridge of nose and sinuses, avoiding eyes.

Snoring
Apply 1-2 drops over throat and bridge of nose, avoiding eyes.

Closed off from Love
Rub a few drops over heart.

Main Ingredients
Laurel, Eucalyptus, Peppermint, Tea Tree, Lemon, Cardamom, Ravintsara, Ravensara

Safety
Can irritate sensitive skin. Use with caution during pregnancy.

Other Uses
Constricted Breathing, Emphysema, Exercise-Induced Asthma, Nasal Polyps, Respiratory Infections, Sinusitis, Tuberculosis

Did You Know?
The chemistry of this blend produces the properties of expectorant, antitussive, anti-spasmodic, and decongestant.

Emotional Use
Rather than being suffocated by sadness or other constricting emotions, this blend helps one exhale that which no longer serves and inhale the support and embrace to make life rich.

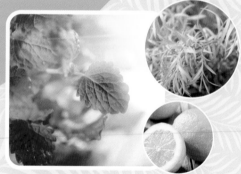

Kick the Cough Massage Roller

12 drops Breathe
15 drops Lime
10 drops Rosemary
FCO

Combine oils in a 10ml roller bottle and then top with FCO. Apply to chest, throat, and lung reflex points 3-5x daily.

Breathe & Rest Diffuser Blend

3 drops Breathe
3 drops Geranium
2 drops Lavender

Diffuse before and during bedtime to promote easy breathing during sleep.

Cheer
Uplifting Blend

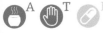 A T I

Scan Here To Experience More

Top *Uses*

Gloominess
Inhale 1-2 drops from cupped hands

Self-Sabotage
Apply 1-2 drops over naval, and diffuse.

Low Energy
Apply 1-2 drops over adrenals on lower back, and diffuse.

Pessimism
Apply 1-2 drops to pulse points, and diffuse.

Detoxification
Apply 2-4 drops to bottoms of feet.

Emotional Disconnect
Apply 1-2 drops to temples or over heart.

Moodiness
Apply 1-2 drops to pulse points, or diffuse.

Main Ingredients
Orange, Clove, Star Anise, Lemon Myrtle, Nutmeg, Ginger, Cinnamon, Zdravetz

Safety
Can irritate sensitive skin. Use with caution during pregnancy.

Other Uses
Digestive Discomfort, Food Addiction, Jaw Pain, Lock Jaw, Low Energy

Did You Know?
Spice essential oils are typically high in antioxidants. Application to the bottom of the feet is a great way to eliminate free radicals.

Emotional Use
This oil of cheer and hope is magnetic for optimistic thoughts and laughter. It reminds the soul that fun can happen for no reason other than that life is meant to be cheerful.

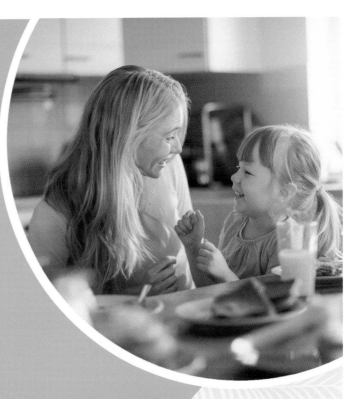

Oil Blends

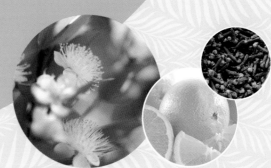

 Feel the Fun Roll-on

15 drops Cheer
20 drops Lemon
15 drops Green Mandarin
FCO

Combine oils in a 10ml roller and top with FCO. Roll onto wrists and neck to promote happy thoughts and laughter.

 Cheerify Diffuser Blend

3 drops Cheer
3 drops Tangerine
2 drops Douglas Fir

Diffuse to transform grumpiness into ease and cheer in everyday life.

137

Citrus Bliss®
Invigorating Blend

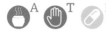 A T I

Scan Here To Experience More

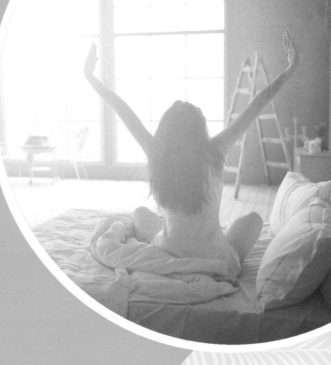

Top Uses

Lack of Creativity & Inspiration
Inhale 2 drops from cupped hands, or diffuse.

Low Energy
Apply 2 drops to pulse points, or diffuse.

Morning Moodiness
Diffuse 5-10 drops next to bedside in the morning, or inhale from cupped hands.

Lymphatic Drainage
Apply 3-4 drops to bottoms of feet.

Stress & Anxiety
Inhale 2 drops from cupped hands, or apply to pulse points.

Depression & Gloom
Inhale 2 drops from cupped hands, or diffuse 5-10 drops.

Main Ingredients
Orange, Lemon, Grapefruit, Mandarin, Bergamot, Clementine, Vanilla

Safety
Avoid sun exposure for 24 hours after topical use.

Other Uses
Air Freshener, Household Cleaning, Eating Disorders, Laundry Freshener, Low Appetite, Mastitis

Did You Know?
Citrus oils are comprised primarily of d-Limonene, a natural dopaminergic. You feel happy with this oil blend because it stimulates your happy neurotransmitters.

Emotional Use
The blissful aromas of this blend inspire creativity. They help bring out artistic expression and daringness to be bold in what you create.

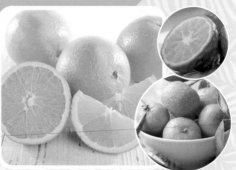

Oil Blends

Soft & Scented Hand Cream

15 drops Citrus Bliss®
¼ cup Argan oil
3 Tbsp beeswax
2 Tbsp coconut oil

Heat the beeswax and coconut oil until it becomes liquid. Add the other oils and mix well. Pour into a glass jar. Let it cool to become solid. Use to massage hands and keep them soft.

Citrus Scented Surface Cleanser

15 drops Citrus Bliss®
10 drops Tea Tree
¼ cup White Vinegar
12 oz. Water

Combine oils and vinegar in a 16 oz. glass spray bottle and shake. Add the white vinegar. Use on countertops and other household surfaces.

Citrus Bloom®
Springtime Blend

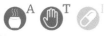

Scan Here To Experience More

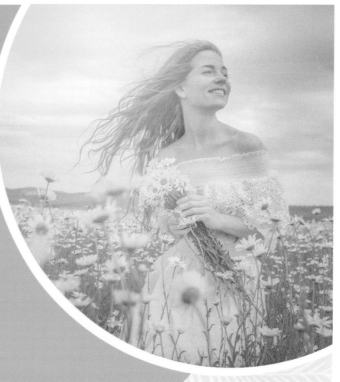

Oil Blends

Top Uses

Calm Energy
Rub 1-2 drops onto the bottoms of feet and massage into the back of neck.

Emotional Stability
Apply 1-2 drops to palms and breathe deeply from cupped hands.

Pleasant Sleep
Rub 1-2 drops into the bottoms of feet and diffuse several drops near bedside.

Anxiety
Massage 1-2 drops into temples and the base of skull. Also diffuse several drops.

Bedtime Wind-down
Begin diffusing several drops in family areas an hour before bed.

PMS & Cramps
Massage 1-2 drops with FCO over lower abdomen as needed.

Main Ingredients
Wild Orange, Grapefruit, Lavender, Roman Chamomile, Magnolia

Safety
Citrus oils can cause photosensitivity where applied topically for up to 24 hours.

Other Uses
Bee Stings, Crying, Diaper Rash, Hyperactivity, Muscle Spasms, Nervous Disorders, Parasites, Sleep Disorders, Spider Bites, Worms

Did You Know?
The chemistry of this blend is a unique balance between calming agents and energizing constituents. Citrus oils are adaptogenic - meaning that this blend can serve as an energizer or a relaxant based on when it is used.

Emotional Use
This blend represents the balance of collected energy and graceful calm. It shows the user feelings of being fully charged and ignited, rooted in pure presence and peace of mind.

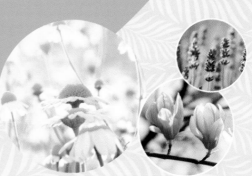

Woodsy Bloom Perfume Roller

20 drops Citrus Bloom
11 drops Sandalwood
FCO

Combine essential oils in a 10ml roller bottle and top with FCO. Apply this perfume blend over pulse points for a fragrant balance of deep, woodsy, bright, and floral.

Bright Dreams Diffuser Blend

4 drops Citrus Bloom
1 drop Ylang Ylang
1 drop Basil

Use this diffuser blend by your bedside to incite happy dreams while giving the body rejuvenating sleep.

139

ClaryCalm®
Women's Monthly Blend

  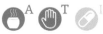

Scan Here To Experience More

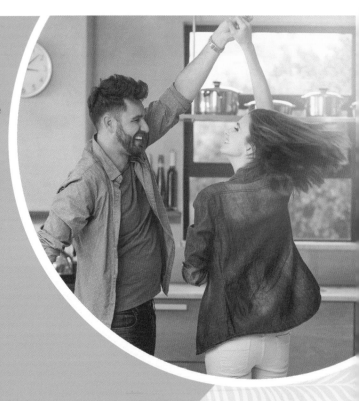

Oil Blends

Top Uses

PMS
Apply to wrists and over lower abdomen.

Cramping
Apply to lower abdomen.

Hormone Balance
Apply to wrists and over lower abdomen.

Hot Flashes
Apply to wrists and back of neck.

Mood Swings
Inhale from cupped hands, and apply to pulse points.

Self-Confidence
Inhale from cupped hands, and apply to pulse points.

Heavy Menstruation
Apply to lower abdomen.

Main Ingredients
Clary Sage, Lavender, Bergamot, Chamomile, Cedarwood, Ylang Ylang, Geranium, Fennel, Carrot Seed, Palmarosa, Vitex

Safety
Avoid sun exposure to application site for 24 hours after topical use.

Other Uses
Aphrodisiac, Sedative, Sleep Issues

Did You Know?
Vitex is distilled from Monk's Pepper and has been used to treat menstrual health since the days of ancient Greece.

Emotional Use
This oil of vulnerability helps ease fear of rejection and need to constantly meet expectations. It opens a space to feel accepted, nurtured, and enough at any given moment.

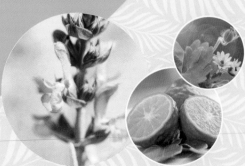

Calm the Cramps Blend

3 drops ClaryCalm®
1 drop Pink Pepper
1 drop Rose
FCO

Combine the oils with several drops of FCO and gently massage onto the lower abdomen to ease the pain of monthly periods.

Nurtured Emotions Inhaler

8 drops ClaryCalm®
2 drops Rose
5 drops Green Mandarin
Empty essential oil inhaler

Add essential oils onto the cotton wick and assemble the inhaler. Breathe in deeply as needed to help calm and balance emotions.

140

Console
Comforting Blend

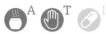

Scan Here To Experience More

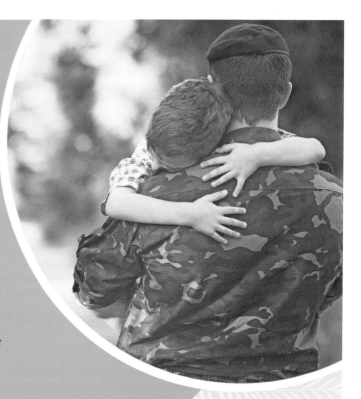

Top Uses

Grief, Sorrow, Despair
Apply 1-2 drops over heart, or diffuse.

Hormone Balance
Apply 1-3 drops to pulse points before bed.

Self-Esteem
Inhale from cupped hands, or diffuse during meditation.

Perfume
Wear on pulse points for a floral aroma.

Anti-Aging
Apply 1-3 drops with carrier oil to wrinkles, sun spots, and fine lines.

Nightmares
Diffuse 3-6 drops next to bedside.

Rheumatoid Arthritis
*Massage diluted into affected area.***i**

Main Ingredients
Frankincense, Ylang Ylang, Patchouli, Labdanum, Sandalwood, Rose, Osmanthus

Other Uses
Anger, Brain Health, Bladder Infection, Emotional Processing, Heart Health, Resentment

Did You Know?
The floral oils in this blend all provide a unique way of calming heavy emotions while balancing hormones. That's why this blend is a powerful aid in processing sadness or grief.

Emotional Use
The soothing qualities of this blend assist in processing grief, loss, and trauma. It facilitates a sense of being whole and knowing that the greater good is unfolding.

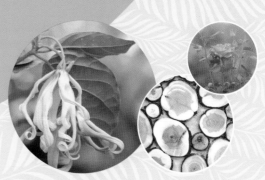

Sweet Comforting Necklace

2 drops Console
Diffuser necklace

Simply drop the oil to your aromatherapy necklace and enjoy a comforting aroma on the go!

Hopeful Massage Oil

3 drops Console
3 drops Wild Orange
2 drops Rosemary
1 oz. FCO

Blend oils together and use for an uplifting massage when you need emotional healing.

DDR Prime®
Cellular Complex Blend

Scan Here To Experience More

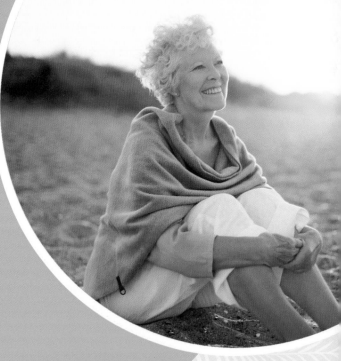

Top Uses

Damaged DNA Repair
Apply 2-4 drops to bottoms of feet and spine morning and night.

Thyroid (hypo, Hashimoto's)
Apply diluted over thyroid or to thyroid reflex point, or take 1-2 drops in capsule.

Smoking Addiction
Rub onto bottom of big toe.

Immune Support
Take 1-2 drops in a capsule.

Antioxidant
Take 1-2 drops in a capsule, or use in cooking.

Liver Detox
Rub over liver, or on liver reflex point.

Rheumatoid Arthritis
Massage diluted into affected area.

Main Ingredients
Frankincense, Wild Orange, Lemongrass, Thyme, Summer Savory, Clove, Niaouli

Safety
Can irritate sensitive skin. Use with caution during pregnancy.

Other Uses
Addictions, Blood Clots, Candida, Cataracts, Fever, Herpes Simplex, Hodgkin's Disease, Glaucoma, Gingivitis, Lipoma, Lupus, Lyme

Did You Know?
This blend helps the body repair damaged systems and functions by utilizing oils that are known regeneratives and tonics.

Emotional Use
Just as this blend helps transform health at a cellular and DNA level, it is also useful in emotional transformation. Use it to turn toxicity into a rebirth.

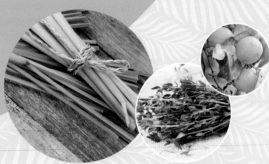

 ## Healthy Cells Citrus Juice

1-2 drops DDR Prime®
8oz fresh squeezed orange juice

Mix the oil into the juice and consume daily to protect the body from free radicals.

 ## Daily Shield Roller Blend

4 drops DDR Prime®
2 drops Eucalyptus
2 drops Cinnamon
FCO

Combine oils in a 10ml roller bottle and top with FCO. Apply to temples, wrists, and back of neck for a daily immune booster.

Deep Blue®
Soothing Blend | Ice Blue®

Scan Here To Experience More

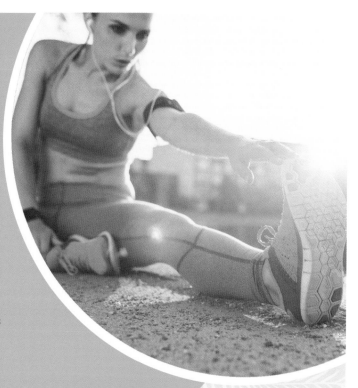

Oil Blends

Top Uses

Muscle Pain & Inflammation
Massage 2-4 drops with carrier oil or lotion into affected areas.

Joint Pain & Arthritis
Apply 1-2 drops to affected areas.

Lupus & Fibromyalgia
Apply 1-2 drops with carrier oil when experiencing flare-ups.

Whiplash
Apply 2-4 drops to affected areas.

Bruises
Gently apply 1-2 drops to bruising.

Headache
Apply 1-2 drops to temples and back of neck.

Bone Pain
Apply 2-4 drops directly over pain.

Main Ingredients
Wintergreen, Camphor, Peppermint, Blue Tansy, Helichrysum, Blue Chamomile

Safety
Can irritate sensitive skin. Use with caution during pregnancy.

Other Uses
Back Pain, Bursitis, Frozen Shoulder, Growing Pains, Injured Joints, Tendinitis, Tennis Elbow, Workout (Pre and Post)

Did You Know?
This blend combines anti-inflammatory minty oils with the tissue-healing power of floral oils, making it perfect for quick pain relief and long-term healing.

Emotional Use
Sometimes growth is restricted because pain must first be surrendered. This blend encourages the individual to embrace and move through difficulties in order to find the joy that lies beyond pain.

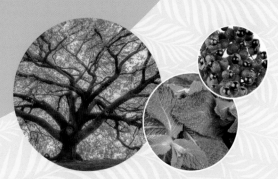

Super Cool Muscle Rub

15 drops Deep Blue®
15 drops Frankincense
15 drops Copaiba
FCO

Combine oils in a 10ml roller bottle and top with FCO. Use when undiluted Deep Blue® is too intense for sensitive tissues.

Head Tension Buster

15 drops Deep Blue®
15 drops Lavender
15 drops Frankincense
FCO

Combine oils in a 10ml roller bottle and top with FCO. Apply on temples, back of neck, and shoulders to help minimize head and neck tension.

DigestZen®
Digestive Blend | ZenGest®

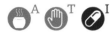

Scan Here To Experience More

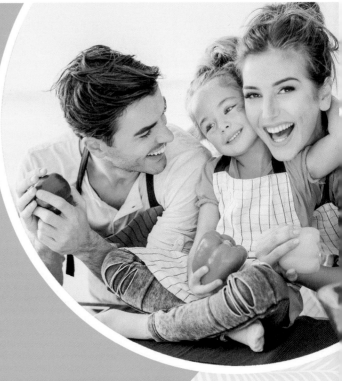

Oil Blends

Top *Uses*

Stomach Upset
Drink 1-3 drops in water, or take in a capsule.

Gas & Bloating
Massage 2-4 drops over stomach, or take in a capsule.

Diarrhea & Constipation
Massage 2-4 drops over stomach, or take in a capsule.

Irritable Bowel Syndrome
Massage 2-4 drops over stomach, or take in a capsule.

Food Poisoning
Drink 3-5 drops in water, or take in a capsule.

Nausea
Put a drop under the tongue, or rub over stomach.

Main Ingredients
Peppermint, Ginger, Caraway, Coriander, Anise, Tarragon

Safety
Can irritate sensitive skin. Use with caution during pregnancy.

Other Uses
Abdominal Cramps, Acid Reflux, Colitis, Crohn's Disease, Gastritis, Heartburn, Morning Sickness, Motion Sickness, Parasites, Sinusitis

Did You Know?
This blend works by combining oils that have exceptional carminative (gas-reducing) and digestive stimulant properties.

Emotional Use
The digestion oils in this blend make it useful for digesting difficult emotions, assimilating new information, and achieving a state of feeling nourished.

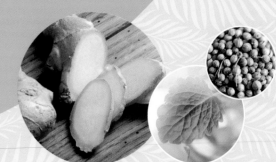

 ## Tame a Tummy Baby Rub

1 drop DigestZen®
1 drop Grapefruit
2 Tbsp
FCO

Add oils to fractionated coconut oil and massage onto the baby's tummy when upset.

After Taste Remedy

1 drop of DigestZen®
1 drop Lemon
1 oz. Water

Gargle oils in an ounce of water as a mouth rinse at night or if you have eaten a meal with strong smells such as garlic or onion.

Elevation
Joyful Blend

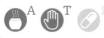

Scan Here To Experience More

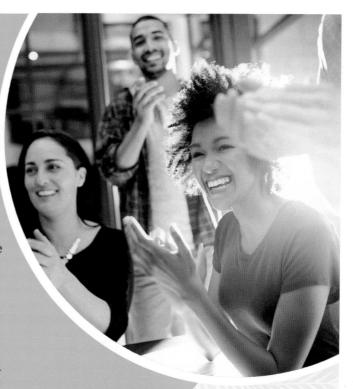

Top Uses

Depression
Carry on your person, and inhale 1-2 drops from cupped hands as needed.

Stress & Anxiety
Diffuse 4-8 drops, or inhale 1-2 drops from cupped hands.

Abuse Recovery
Apply 1-2 drops to back of neck and over heart.

Grief & Sorrow
Apply 1-2 drops to pulse points, or diffuse.

Poison Oak/Ivy
Apply 1-2 drops with carrier oil to affected areas.

Lupus & Fibromyalgia
Inhale 1-2 drops from cupped hands, and apply diluted to inflamed areas.

Main Ingredients
Lavandin, Lavender, Sandalwood, Tangerine, Melissa, Ylang Ylang, Osmanthus, Lemon Myrtle

Safety
Can irritate sensitive skin. Avoid sun exposure for 12 hours after topical use.

Other Uses
Cushing's Syndrome, Lethargy, Postpartum Depression, Sadness, Shock, Weight Loss

Did You Know?
Melissa oil in this blend has been shown to inhibit GABA-induced currents, making it a valuable antidepressant.

Emotional Use
This floral-citrussy aroma brings with it true joy. It elevates the heavy-hearted into an optimistic and care-free state of being.

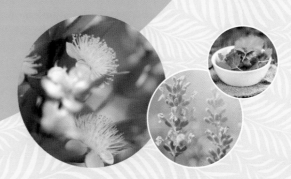

Weekend Vibe Diffuser Blend

4 drops Elevation
2 drops Lemon
2 drops Lime

Diffuse to create a positive and energized mood on a weekend staycation.

Glee and Free Roller Blend

5 drops Elevation
10 drops Citrus Bliss®
5 drops Balance
FCO

Combine essential oils to a 10ml roller bottle and then fill the remainder of the bottle with FCO. Apply to wrists and back of neck to elevate your spirits.

Forgive
Renewing Blend

   A T I

Scan Here To Experience More

Oil Blends

Top *Uses*

Anger, Resentment, Guilt
Apply 1-2 drops to pulse points, and inhale from cupped hands.

Attachment Issues
Apply 1-2 drops to pulse points, and diffuse.

Critical Thinking
Apply 1-2 drops to temples and back of neck, and diffuse.

Circulation
Apply 2-4 drops to bottoms of feet.

Insect Repellent
Apply with carrier oil over exposed skin.

Prostate Issues
Apply 1-2 drops over lower abdomen.

Irritability
Inhale 1-2 drops from cupped hands.

Main Ingredients
Spruce, Bergamot, Juniper Berry, Myrrh, Arborvitae, Nootka, Thyme, Citronella

Safety
Can irritate sensitive skin. Avoid sun exposure for 12 hours after topical use.

Other Uses
Bitterness, Emotional Stagnation, Kidney Stones, Liver Issues, Muscle Pain, Sadness, Shame, Skin Infection

Did You Know?
Arborvitae and Nootka oils come from sustainable harvesting in British Columbia. The oils are procured from sawdust residue so that not one extra tree is cut down. Even the pulp is recycled into paper.

Emotional Use
This oil blend brings the promise of peace that comes with forgiving others and self. It turns resentment and judgment into allowing and acceptance, the two ingredients critical for growth.

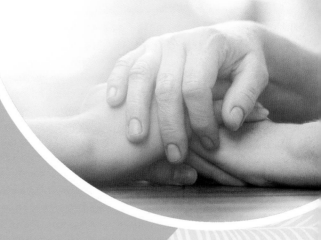

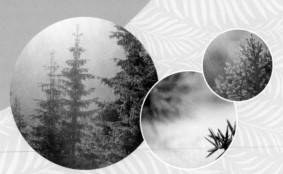

 Sweet Surrender Diffuser Blend

3 drops Forgive
1 drop Geranium
1 drop Lime

Diffuse throughout the day to let go of anger and frustrations.

 Positive Heart Roller blend

15 drops Forgive
10 drops Melissa
FCO

Combine oils in a 10ml roller bottle and top with FCO. Apply over heart to avoid negative emotions throughout the day.

Hope
Hopeful Blend

 A T I

**Scan Here To
Experience More**

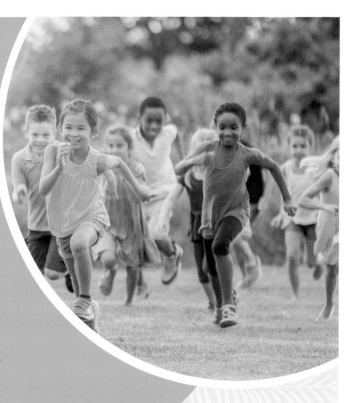

Top Uses

Emotional Trauma
Apply to pulse points, and inhale from cupped hands.

Grief & Trust Issues
Apply to pulse points, and inhale from cupped hands.

Hormone Balance
Apply to wrists and bottoms of feet.

Perfume
Apply 1-2 drops to pulse points.

Adrenal Fatigue
Apply to neck and lower back.

Stress
Apply to temples, and inhale from cupped hands.

Focus & Concentration
Apply to temples.

Main Ingredients
Bergamot, Ylang Ylang, Frankincense, Vanilla

Safety
Use with caution during pregnancy

Other Uses
Addictions, Alzheimer's, Appetite Loss, Autism, Discouragement, Parkinson's, Self-Worth Issues

Did You Know?
FCF Bergamot is distilled with steam distillation, rather than the usual cold pressing of citrus oils. It does not cause photosensitivity.

Emotional Use
This blend facilitates renewing trust in people and self after experiencing abuse or trauma. It helps regenerate the ability to connect in safe, healthy, and consensual ways.

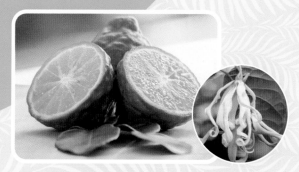

Drawer Fragrance Balls

1-3 drops Hope
1 drop Cedarwood
Cotton balls

Add a few drops onto a plain cotton ball and place into drawers or closets to give clothes a fresh scent.

Light and Dreamy Diffuser Blend

4 drops Hope
1 drop Jasmine

Diffuse when you need to just lay down and enjoy the sunset while thinking about your hopes and dreams.

HD Clear®
Skin Clearing Blend

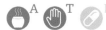

Scan Here To Experience More

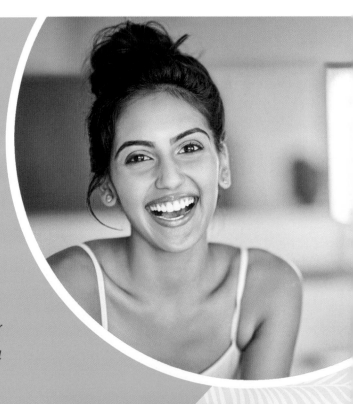

Oil Blends

Top Uses

Acne & Blemishes
Apply directly to areas of concern.

Skin Impurities
Rub into skin before washing.

Oily Skin
Apply to areas of concern.

Eczema & Dermatitis
Apply with carrier oil to affected areas.

Bacterial Infection
Apply to affected areas.

Main Ingredients
Black Cumin, Ho Wood, Tea Tree, Geranium, Eucalyptus, Litsea

Safety
May irritate sensitive skin with continued use

Did You Know?
The oils chosen for this blend are dominant in antibacterial constituents. While many of them have similar chemical foundations, their individual methods of addressing bacteria create a synergistic effect for fighting acne and breakouts.

Emotional Use
This topical blend helps suppressed feelings of anger and blame resolve before they boil to the surface. It's all about understanding the gift of imperfections.

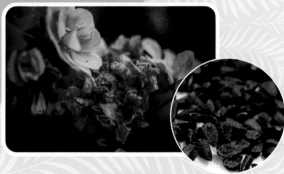

Acne Be gone

HD Clear®
Frankincense

Apply a dab of Frankincense to acne blemishes and pat until the oil is absorbed. Then apply a dab of HD Clear®, allowing to air dry.

Youthful Un-Chemical Peel

HD Clear®
1 oz. Lemon Juice

Combine several drops of lemon juice with a swipe of HD Clear® on your face and massage in a circular motion for 30 seconds. Wash face immediately after.

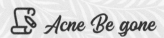

Immortelle
Anti-Aging Blend | Salubelle®

A T I

Scan Here To Experience More

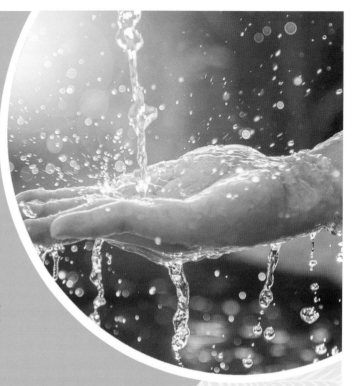

Top Uses

Wrinkles & Fine Lines
Apply to desired areas morning and night.

Age Spots
Apply to affected areas 3x daily.

Scarring
Massage for 30 seconds into scar tissue 2-3x daily until desired appearance.

Skin Cancer
Apply neat to affected area 3x daily.

Skin Discoloration
Apply to affected areas 3x daily.

Meditation
Apply to pulse points during meditation.

Bleeding
Apply neat to stop minor bleeding.

Main Ingredients
Frankincense, Sandalwood, Lavender, Myrrh, Helichrysum, Rose

Other Uses
Aging, Blisters, Chapped Skin, Cuts, Dry Skin, Eczema, Hyper-pigmentation, Psoriasis, Sunburns

Did You Know?
This blend helps skin remain youthful by restoring tissue integrity (Curzerene in Myrrh), regenerating cells (β-Caryophyllene in Frankincense), and inhibiting the degradation of collagen and elastin (Neryl Acetate in Helichrysum), among other properties.

Emotional Use
Sacred trees and woodsy oils in this blend make it ideal for inviting spiritual insight during prayer and meditation.

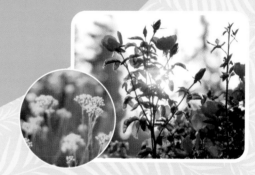

 ## Smooth & Glowing Facial Oil

5 drops Immortelle
4 tsp Jojoba oil

Mix the two oils well and massage on your face, neck, and decolletage in an upward motion. Do this in the morning followed by your moisturizer.

Radiantly Youthful Massage Blend

5 drops Immortelle
3 drops Helichrysum
2 drops Tulsi
1 tsp Argan Oil

Mix the oils and massage onto skin before bed for smoother, more radiant, and youthful-looking skin.

Oil Blends

InTune®
Focus Blend

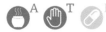 A T I

Scan Here To Experience More

Oil Blends

Top Uses

ADD & ADHD
Apply to back of neck and behind ears.

Focus & Concentration
Apply to back of neck and behind ears.

Anxiety
Apply to pulse points, or inhale from cupped hands.

Hyperactivity
Apply to pulse points, or inhale from cupped hands.

Seizures
Apply to bottoms of feet and back of neck.

Skin Irritations
Apply with carrier oil to affected areas.

Sedative
Apply to pulse points or bottoms of feet.

Main Ingredients
Amyris, Patchouli, Frankincense, Lime, Ylang Ylang, Sandalwood, Chamomile

Safety
Repeated use can irritate highly sensitive skin.

Other Uses
Alzheimer's, Emotional Balance, Hormone Balance, Memory, Parkinson's, Relaxation, Sleep

Did You Know?
Essential oils with base notes are common enhancers of focus. That's why this blend contains four of them (Amyris, Patchouli, Frankincense, & Sandalwood).

Emotional Use
The bright citrus and deep woodsy fragrance combo in this blend facilitates happily living in the present moment. It promotes indulging in the goodness of the here and now.

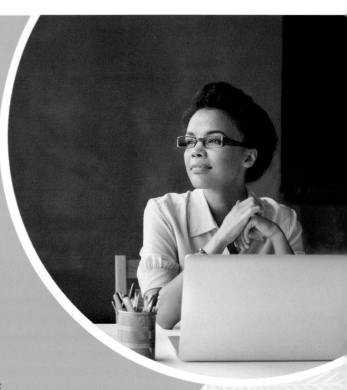

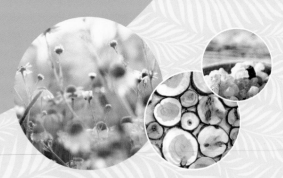

Prep & Plan Diffuser Blend

5 drops InTune®
5 drops Spearmint
4 drops Wild Orange

Diffuse this blend to help inspire healthy study and planning patterns.

Attention Booster Bracelet Diffuser

7 drops InTune®
4 drops Rosemary
7 drops Wild Orange
3 drops Cedarwood
30 drops FCO

Mix oils in a glass dropper bottle. Apply 1-2 drops onto clay beads of a diffuser bracelet and let your child wear to school.

Kid's Brave
Kid's Courage Blend

 A T I

Scan Here To Experience More

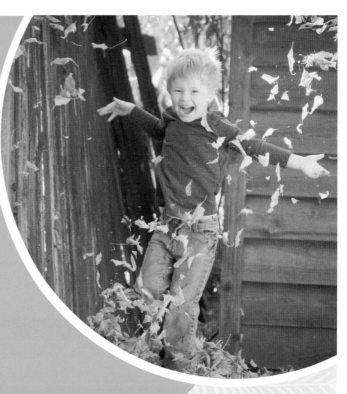

Oil Blends

Top Uses

Making New Friends
Apply to wrists and inhale from cupped hands. Speak out loud a few reasons you make a great friend for others!

Team Sports
Apply over chest to bring the courage to do your best and be a team player.

Potty Training
Apply over lower back and back of neck to feel excited about being a big kid.

Electronics Addiction
Apply to wrists and temples to find ambition to experience new adventures.

Imagination Sparks
Apply to the back of neck and temples to spur creativity and new ideas.

Trying New Things
Apply to the naval and chest to feel brave when trying new things.

Main Ingredients
Wild Orange, Amyris, Osmanthus, Cinnamon

Safety
Avoid sun exposure for 12 hours after topical use.

Other Uses
Anxiety, Fear, Immune Support, Motivation, Nervousness, Reassurance, Self-Doubt

Did You Know?
Osmanthus oil is extracted from a beautiful asian flower. It is associated with feelings of happiness and joy, making it an emotional match to the bravery-enhancing properties of this blend.

Emotional Use
This blend brings out the bravery in every kid. It reminds kids the value of self-expression, and what it means to be yourself and hold strong to values.

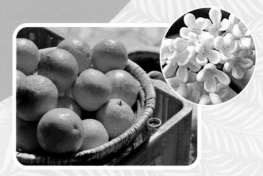

Artwork Inspiring Ritual

Kids's Brave
Kid's art supplies

Encourage your child's creativity by applying the oil to the back of the neck, wrists, and temples during art time.

Play Protection Blend

Kids's Brave
1 drop Frankincense

Apply Kid's Courage Blend over the chest and back of neck followed by Frankincense before playing outdoors.

Kid's Calmer
Kid's Restful Blend

 A 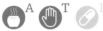 T I

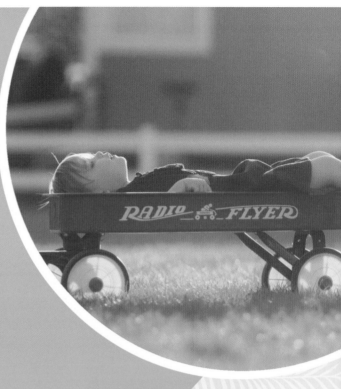

Top Uses

Easy Sleeping
Apply to bottoms of feet and back of neck 30 minutes before bedtime for an easier time falling asleep.

Monsters in the Closet
Apply over chest and wrists to ease nighttime fears.

Argument Diffuser
Apply to temples and back of neck to ease contention.

Tornado Thoughts
Apply to temples, wrists, and back of neck to soothe runaway and irrational thoughts.

Grown-Up Relaxation
Apply liberally to temples and chest before getting into a warm bath to let go of a stressful day of kid's duties.

Main Ingredients
Lavender, Cananga, Buddha Wood, Roman Chamomile

Other Uses
Behavioral Disorders, Bee Sting, Crying, Diaper Rash, Hyperactivity, Hyper-pigmentation, Neuralgia, Shock, Spider Bite, Sunburn, Worms

Did You Know?
Buddha Wood is an Australian tree known for its soporific (sleep-inducing) and sedative benefits.

Emotional Use
The gentle floral aromas of this blend invite purposeful communication. It reminds the wearer to choose words that uplift and edify over words that make you right.

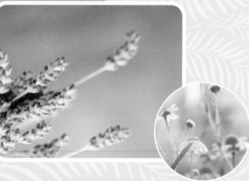

Unruffled Nap Time

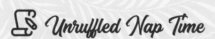

Kids's Calmer
1 drop Wild Orange
1 drop Ylang Ylang

Apply oils to the bottom of feet and back of neck 20 minutes before your kid's nap time to encourage peaceful rest.

Tantrum-Buster Blend

Kids's Calmer
1 drop Clary Sage

Apply over temples and back of neck to discourage outbursts.

Kid's Rescuer
Kid's Soothing Blend

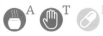 A T I

Scan Here To Experience More

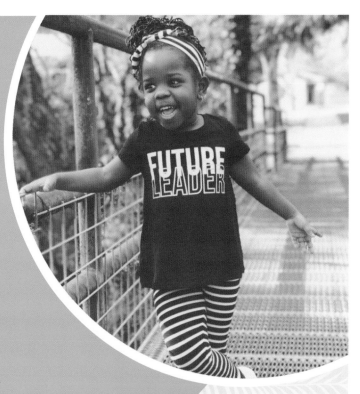

Top *Uses*

Battle Wounds
Apply liberally to ease pain and injury that happen with the dangers of being an active kid.

Sports Injury
Apply to injured muscles, joints, and connective tissue 5x daily.

Bumps & Bruises
Apply every couple hours to reduce the appearance of bruises or bumps.

Self-Trust
Apply to the back of neck and temples to remember the power of trusting your good instincts.

Stinky Feet
Apply to feet before and after school.

Mighty Muscles
Apply to legs, arms, and shoulders as a pre-workout before sports and exercise.

Main Ingredients
Copaiba, Lavender, Spearmint, Zanthoxylum

Safety
Can irritate sensitive skin. Use with caution during pregnancy

Other Uses
Charley Horse, Growing Pains, Headache, Lethargy, Joint Pain, Muscle Pain, Muscle Tension

Did You Know?
Zanthoxylum helps with pain management and recovery by calming nerves and stress that prolong pain.

Emotional Use
This blend provides the refresh and reprieve needed for soul-soothing. It turns trouble into a pathway to move forward better and wiser.

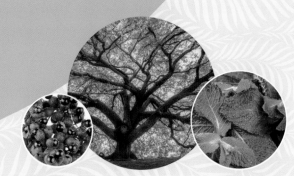

Oil Blends

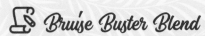 **Bruise Buster Blend**

Kids's Rescuer
Dab of Wintergreen

Roll Kid's Soothing Blend onto bruises followed by a dab of Wintergreen to help minimize the appearance of bruises or bumps.

Active Kid Cooling Blend

Kids's Rescuer
1 drop Peppermint

Use this blend to provide comfort to tired muscles after a physical activity. Also pat a bit onto the back of child's neck on a hot play day.

153

Kid's Steady
Kid's Grounding Blend

 A T I

Scan Here To Experience More

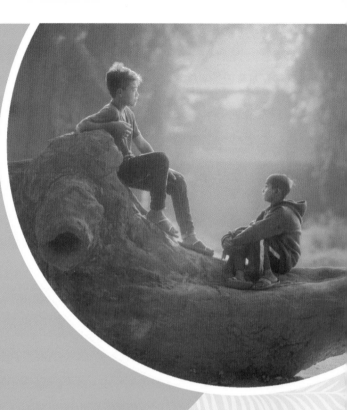

Oil Blends

Top Uses

Social Anxiety
Apply to wrists and lower back to add a feeling of steadiness to social situations.

Frazzled School Mornings
Start the morning right by applying to bottoms of feet and the back of the neck.

Useful Time-Outs
Turn time-outs from unhelpful punishment to a time of valuable reflection on the importance of keeping your word and being true to who you are.

Superhero Confidence
Apply over chest and the back of neck.

Waaaah-Baby
Apply to temples and wrists to calm temper tantrums.

Bad News Buster
Apply over chest to help ease disappointment or discouragement.

Main Ingredients
Amyris, Balsam Fir, Coriander, Magnolia

Other Uses
Chronic Pain, Circulation Issues, Cough, Cramps, Depression, Procrastination, Scrapes, Stress

Did You Know?
Amyris is a base note with fixative properties, meaning that the aroma will stay for longer as it compliments lighter notes like Magnolia. It's a significant part of how this blend provides a long-lasting steadying effect.

Emotional Use
This blend brings a sense of steadiness to every day. It fosters feelings of safety in the present moment, reminding the user everything can eventually work out.

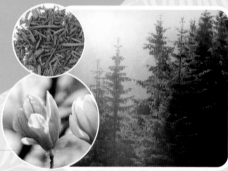

Pick Me Up Blend

Kids's Steady
1 drop Vetiver
1 drop Cypress

Apply to child's bottoms of feet and back of neck after an active day outdoors.

Tame That Temper Blend

Kids's Steady
1 drop Lavender
1 drop Melissa

Apply Kid's Grounding Blend to bottoms of feet followed by Lavender and Melissa to help pacify cranky kids.

Kid's Stronger

Kid's Protective Blend

 A T I

Scan Here To Experience More

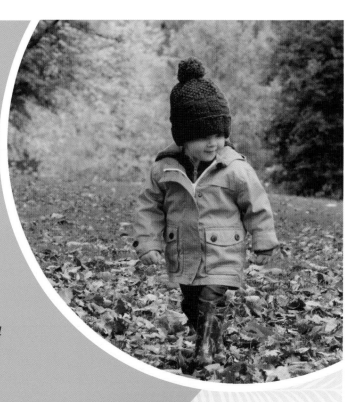

Top Uses

Playtime-Ready
Rub on hands, back of neck, and under nose to ward off germs during play with other kids.

Cold & Flu
Apply to chest, spine, and bottoms of feet 5x daily.

Super Hero Immunity
Apply to bottoms of feet each morning for immune system boost.

Zombie Attacks (Bacteria, Virus, Fungus)
Apply 3-5x daily to infected areas.

Fatigue
Apply over kidneys and adrenals 2x daily to improve stamina.

Inner Circle Friends
Inhale from cupped hands to remember maintaining healthy boundaries and respect in friendships.

Main Ingredients
Cedarwood, Litsea, Frankincense, Rose

Safety
Can irritate highly sensitive skin.

Other Uses
Athlete's Foot, Dandruff, Fungal Infection, Heartache, Ingrown Toenail

Did You Know?
Rose is the unanticipated plant with a profound ability to combat serious types of bacteria like MRSA. Yet it's also gentle enough for even the most sensitive skin.

Emotional Use
This blend brings strong heart into social interactions. It helps fortify boundaries of love, promoting a sense of true community.

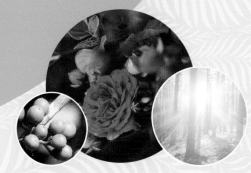

 Baby Pacifier Blend

Kids's Stronger
1 drop Roman Chamomile

Apply the blend on the bottoms of feet to comfort irritable emotions.

 Summer Skin Soother

Kids's Stronger
1 drop Tea Tree

Use this combination to help soothe skin irritations, scrapes, or cuts.

Kid's Tamer
Kid's Digestive Blend

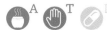 A T I

Scan Here To Experience More

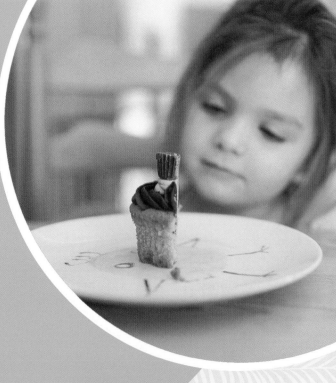

Top Uses

Tummy Bugs
Rub a few drops worth clockwise over stomach several times throughout the day.

Car Sick-Speedster
1-2 drops to bottoms of feet or temples for car sickness.

Food Allergies
Massage 1-2 drops over lower back after exposure to allergens.

Grown-Up Food Envy
Rub over stomach with a drop of Ginger after eating foods that cause stomach upset.

Theme Park Junkie
Rub clockwise onto stomach and wrists before activities that cause motion sickness.

Summer Burn-up
Rub over back of neck to cool overheated skin.

Main Ingredients
Spearmint, Japanese Peppermint, Ginger, Parsley Seed, Black Pepper

Safety
Can irritate highly sensitive skin.

Other Uses
Acid Reflux, Colic, Croup, Flu, Food Poisoning, Heart Burn, Loss of Apetite, Nausea, Sour Stomach, Sunburn

Did You Know?
Japanese Ginger is especially useful for uplifting mood. Because emotions and hormones are housed in the gut, a cheerful mood is an important part of healthy digestion.

Emotional Use
Rich in oils with 1,8-cineole, this blend is full of dopaminergics and quickly invites a sense of cheerfuly digesting life and all its adventures with ease.

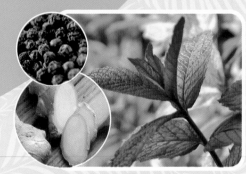

Kids Belly Roll-on Relief

Kids's Tamer
Dab of Peppermint

Gently roll Kid's Digestive Blend clockwise onto your kid's upset stomach followed by a small dab of Peppermint.

Motion Sickness Buster

Kids's Tamer
1 drop Lavender

Apply this blend on the back of the neck or bottoms of feet to reduce dizziness associated with motion.

Kid's Thinker
Kid's Focus Blend

 A T I

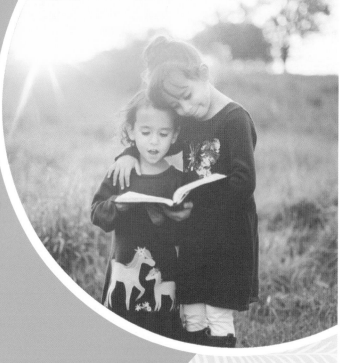

Scan Here To Experience More

Top Uses

Homework Booster
Apply to back of neck at the beginning of homework time to boost concentration.

ADD/ADHD
Apply to the back of neck 3x daily or as needed.

Creative Writing
Apply to temples to incite new ideas during writing projects.

Household Chores
Apply to naval and wrists to stay focused during chore time so that playtime can come sooner.

Test Taking
Apply to temples while studying for a test, and again while taking the test.

Confusion & Distractions
Apply to temples and inhale from cupped hands to promote mental clarity.

Main Ingredients
Vetiver, Peppermint, Clementine, Rosemary

Safety
Can irritate sensitive skin. Avoid sun exposure for 12 hours after topical use.

Other Uses
Autism, Asperger's, Hyperactivity, Mental Handicaps, Nervous Disorders

Did You Know?
Peppermint and Rosemary enhance memory retention. They make it easier to recall information when they're used first during study time and then during test-taking.

Emotional Use
This blend is the oil for peaceful thoughts. It helps turn agitation and frustration into centered thinking that is both realistic and useful.

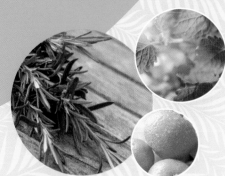

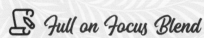 **Full on Focus Blend**

Kids's Thinker
2 drops Ylang Ylang

Apply on temples, wrists, and the back of the neck to help kids stay alert and focused.

 Chillax and Relax Blend

Kids's Thinker
2 drops Frankincense

Apply on temples while studying for a test to prevent feeling overwhelmed and pressured.

Oil Blends

Motivate
Encouraging Blend

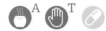 A T I

Scan Here To Experience More

Top *Uses*

Discouragement, Low Confidence, Low Motivation
Inhale 1-2 drops from cupped hands, or diffuse.

Detox
Apply 1-2 drops to bottoms of feet, or massage over endocrine organs.

Adrenal Fatigue
Massage 1-2 drops with carrier oil over lower back.

Flatulence
Rub 1-2 drops with carrier oil over stomach.

Depression
Diffuse 5-10 drops, or rub 1-2 drops onto temples.

Respiratory Issues
Apply 1-2 drops over chest, or diffuse.

Main Ingredients
Clementine, Peppermint, Coriander, Basil, Melissa, Rosemary

Safety
Can irritate sensitive skin. Use with caution during pregnancy

Other Uses
Asthma, Confusion, Creativity, Fatigue, Loneliness, Overwhelm, Uncertainty

Did You Know?
The energizing properties of Clementine (powered by Limonene) with the dopaminergic properties of Peppermint (powered by 1,8-Cineole) create the perfect motivating aroma.

Emotional Use
The combination of citrus and herbs in this blend make it a powerful motivator. It turns lethargic energy into enthusiasm and a sense of "I can do this!"

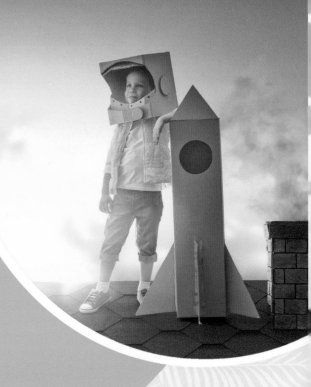

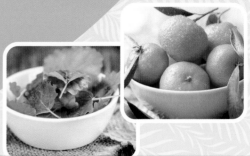

Morning Go-Go Foot Massage

2 drops Motivate
2 drops Melissa
2 drops Siberian Fir

Combine essential oils and apply to the bottom of feet in the morning before going out to work.

Get It Done Diffuser Blend

3 drops Motivate
3 drops Lemon
3 drops Grapefruit

Diffuse in the office to inspire motivation to finish all your tasks at hand.

Oil Blends

Northern Escape
Woodland Blend

 A T I

Scan Here To Experience More

Top *Uses*

Mental Clarity
Apply a drop to the temples or diffuse several drops during focus time.

Respiratory Issues
Massage 1-2 drops with FCO over chest and upper back; Diffuse several drops.

Airborne Pathogens
Diffuse several drops.

Muscle Aches & Pain
Massage 3-4 drops with FCO into affected areas. Also add 6 drops to 1 cup Epsom salt and add to hot bath.

Workout Recovery
Massage 2-3 drops with FCO over muscles and joints.

Nervous Disorders
Massage 2-3 drops with FCO into the spine, bottoms of feet, and directly over affected areas 2-3x daily.

Main Ingredients
Black Spruce, Siberian Fir, Balsam Fir, Lavandin (Sweet Lavender), Cedarwood, Cypress, Hinoki, Frankincense, Nootka, Cananga, Clove Bud

Safety
Can irritate sensitive skin. Dilute if needed. Use with caution when pregnant.

Other Uses
Anger Issues, Cabin Fever, Cold, Congestion, Cough, Disinfectant, Flu, Headache, High Blood Pressure, Migraine, Muscle Tension

Did You Know?
The woodsy oils in this blend are complimented by two floral aromas: Lavendin and Cananga. Both of these florals are also unique and harder to find as individual oils.

Emotional Use
This blend represents the feeling of effortless stability. The energy of effortless stability comes through this blend, reminding the user that life is always balancing itself out and moving in the flow of prosperity.

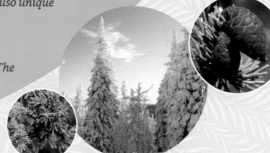

 ## Ever Fresh Muscle Salve

15-20 drops Northern Escape
3 drops Peppermint
½ cup Unrefined Coconut Oil
1 oz Beeswax

Melt the coconut oil and beeswax in a double boiler. Remove from heat and stir in the essential oils. Pour into a small glass jar before mixture cools. Massage a generous amount into muscles and joints as needed.

Vibrant Woods Diffuser Blend

3 drops Northern Escape
3 drops Lemon
2 drops Green Mandarin

Diffuse this blend in the morning or during the workday to arouse the senses and stimulate free, creative thinking.

On Guard
Protective Blend

 A 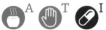 T I

Scan Here To Experience More

Top *Uses*

Immune Support
Take 1-2 drops in capsule as daily supplement, or apply to bottoms of feet.

Colds & Flu
Apply 1-2 drops to bottoms of feet, and take with water or in a capsule.

Airborne Viruses
Diffuse 5-10 drops.

Mouthwash
Rinse mouth with 2 drops and water.

Cold Sores
Apply a drop with carrier oil to needed areas.

MRSA
Apply 1-2 drops diluted to affected areas.

Gum Disease & Cavities
Rinse mouth with 2 drops and water.

Main Ingredients
Orange, Clove, Cinnamon, Rosemary, Eucalyptus

Safety
Can irritate sensitive skin. Use with caution during pregnancy.

Other Uses
Autoimmune Disorders, Cough, Germs, Household Cleaning, Hypoglycemia, Laundry Booster, Mold, Pneumonia, Staph Infection, Strep Throat, Warts

Did You Know?
This bend contains many natural antibiotics, but does not injure the immune system by harming healthy flora in the gut.

Emotional Use
The protective properties of this blend extend from harmful pathogens to harmful energy. It promotes feelings of being independently capable and strong.

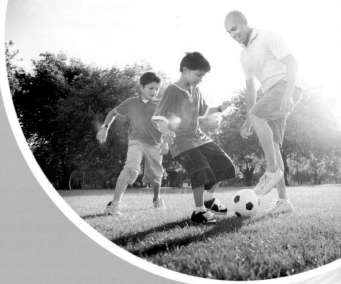

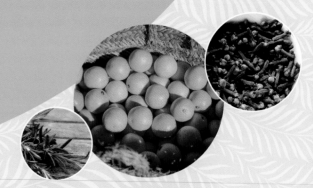

Oil Blends

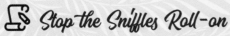 **Stop the Sniffles Roll-on**

10 drops On Guard
10 drops Black Pepper
10 drops Tea Tree
5 drops Frankincense
5 drop Siberian Fir

Mix all oils in a 10ml roller bottle and top with FCO. Apply to neck, throat, chest, and back to help reduce cold symptoms.

 Immunity Support Diffuser Blend

5 drops On Guard
5 drops Tea Tree
3 drops Oregano

Diffuse daily to help boost the immune system.

160

Passion
Inspiring Blend

  A T I

Scan Here To Experience More

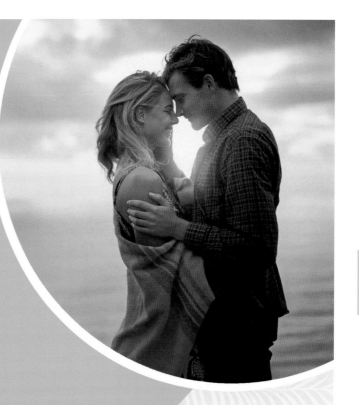

Top Uses

Apathy & Boredom
Inhale 1-2 drops from cupped hands, or diffuse.

Low Sex Drive
Apply 1-2 drops with carrier oil to pulse points, or use diluted in massage.

Digestive Issues
Apply 1-2 drops to stomach reflex points, or apply diluted over stomach.

Aphrodisiac
Apply 1-2 drops to pulse points.

Slow Digestion
Apply 1-2 drops with carrier oil over stomach.

Lack of Creativity
Diffuse 5-10 drops.

Main Ingredients
Cardamom, Cinnamon, Ginger, Sandalwood, Jasmine, Damiana

Safety
Can irritate sensitive skin. Avoid topical use during pregnancy.

Other Uses
Depression, Hormone Balance, Menopause, PMS Discomfort, Slow Bowel Movements

Did You Know?
Cinnamon, Ginger, Sandalwood, Jasmine, and Damiana are all natural aphrodisiacs. This blend can really turn up the heat.

Emotional Use
The passion-inspiring oils in this blend are all about coming out of self-denial and finding the vitality and love of taking risks and being more playful with life.

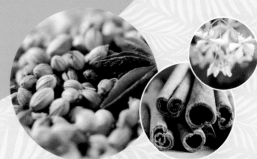

Be Inspired Diffuser Blend

1 drop Passion
2 drops Bergamot
3 drops Lime

Combine and diffuse in the morning to start the day feeling energized and enthusiastic.

In the flow Roller Blend

10 drops of Passion
7 drops of Ylang Ylang
12 drops Frankincense
15 drops Tangerine

Combine oils in a 10ml roller bottle and top with FCO.

Oil Blends

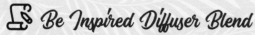

PastTense®
Tension Blend

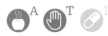 A T I

Scan Here To Experience More

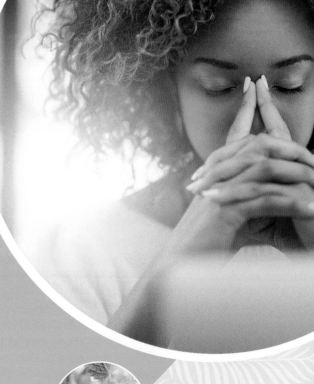

Top Uses

Headache & Migraine
Massage into temples and forehead, avoiding eyes.

Muscle Tension
Massage into areas of concern.

Hot Flashes
Apply to back of neck.

Fevers
Apply to back of neck.

Bruises
Apply gently over bruises.

Hangover
Apply to temples and over stomach.

Arthritis
Massage into aching joints.

Main Ingredients
Wintergreen, Lavender, Peppermint, Frankincense, Cilantro, Marjoram, Chamomile, Rosemary

Safety
Can irritate sensitive skin. Use with caution during pregnancy.

Other Uses
Alertness, Calming, Inflammation, Muscle Cramps, Swelling

Did You Know?
The dominant chemical makeup of this blend is Methyl Salicylate (anti-inflammatory), Linalool (calming), and β-Caryophyllene (analgesic).

Emotional Use
This blend of relief brings equilibrium and calm where there was nervousness and burnout. It helps relieve stress before it becomes a setback.

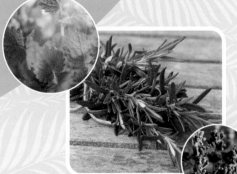

Tense No More Massage Blend

PastTense®
1-2 drops Frankincense

Apply Tension Blend to shoulders, neck, and back followed by Frankincense. Massage gently for a cooling and soothing sensation.

Mellow Me Night Blend

PastTense®
1-2 drops Lavender
1-2 drops Cedarwood

Roll Tension blend on bottoms of feet followed by Lavender and Cedarwood. Massage gently and wear socks. Do this before bedtime for peaceful sleep.

Peace
Reassuring Blend

 A T I

Scan Here To Experience More

Top Uses

Fear & Insecurity
Apply 1-2 drops over temples or chest.

Worry
Inhale 1-2 drops from cupped hands.

Restlessness & Irritability
Apply 1-2 drops to temples or bottoms of feet, or diffuse.

Sleep Issues
Diffuse 4-8 drops near bedside, or apply 1-2 drops to temples.

Focus Issues
Apply 1-2 drops to back of neck or temples

Social Disorders
Inhale 1-2 drops from cupped hands, or rub onto back of neck.

Main Ingredients
Vetiver, Lavender, Ylang Ylang, Frankincense, Marjoram, Spearmint, Labdanum

Safety
Use with caution during beginning of pregnancy.

Other Uses
Addictive Personality, Postpartum Recovery, Social Anxiety

Did You Know?
Labdanum (AKA Cistus) is used in this blend for its stress-reducing properties, but it is also known for combating many types of infections.

Emotional Use
The peaceful oils in this blend help one move from feeling attacked or controlled by people or life to a place of understanding, lightness, and freedom.

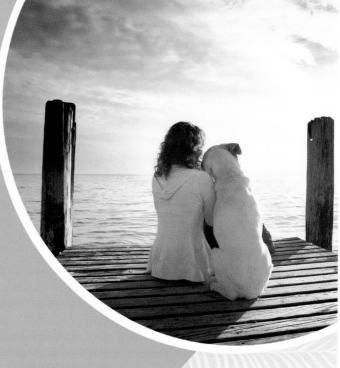

Oil Blends

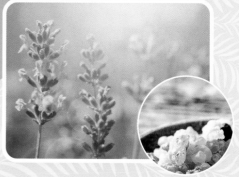

Still Silence Roller Blend

10 drops Peace
5 drops Bergamot
2 drops Clary Sage
FCO

Combine oils in a 10ml roller bottle and top with FCO. Apply to the back of neck, chest, and along spine to help re-balance and calm emotions.

Hushed Lullaby

4 drops Peace
3 drops Cedarwood
3 drops Juniper Berry

Apply to the chest, wrists, and bottoms of feet to assist with falling asleep and to enjoy a deeper night's sleep.

Purify
Cleansing Blend

 A T I

Scan Here To Experience More

Oil Blends

Top *Uses*

Air Freshener
Add 10 drops to glass spray bottle with water. Spray as needed.

Foot Odors
Apply neat to feet. Spray inside shoes.

Laundry
Add 4-5 drops to detergent.

Disinfectant
Add 20 drops to glass spray bottle with water and 1 Tbsp rubbing alcohol.

Deodorant
Apply 1-2 drops with carrier oil to armpits.

Mildew
Use several drops with a clean sponge.

Bites & Stings
Apply 1 drop neat to bite or sting.

Main Ingredients
Lime, Lemon, Siberian Fir, Citronella, Tea Tree, Cilantro

Safety
Can irritate sensitive skin. Avoid direct sun exposure 12 hours after application.

Other Uses
Airborne Bacteria & Viruses, Boils, Household Cleaning, Insect Repellent, Mice Repellent, Skin Ulcers

Did You Know?
The prominent levels of λ-terpinene in this blend enhance its deodorizing properties.

Emotional *Use*
The purifying effects of this blend assist in releasing trapped, unhealthy emotions. It can clear negative energy from a room so that goodness can be noticed and felt.

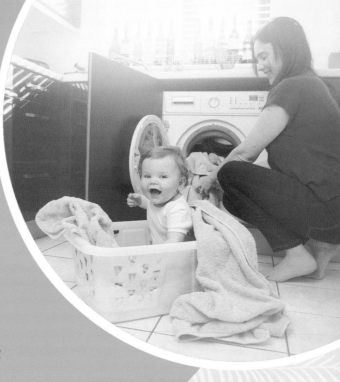

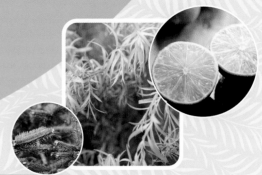

Flu-Away Diffuser Blend

2 drops Purify
2 drops Lemongrass
2 drops Green Mandarin
2 drops Melissa

Diffuse during the flu season to help protect against environmental threats.

Purifying Room Spray

10-15 drops Purify
1 tsp salt
Distilled water

Add the oils and salt in a 2 oz glass spray bottle and shake well. Fill the rest with water and shake again. Use to freshen up the air in any room.

Serenity
Restful Blend | Lavender Peace®

Scan Here To Experience More

Top Uses

Sleep Issues
Apply 1-2 drops to temples and bottoms of feet, and diffuse near bedside.

Stress & Anxiety
Apply 1-2 drops to pulse points, and inhale from cupped hands

ADD & ADHD
Apply 1-2 drops to back of neck, and diffuse.

Itchy Skin
Apply 1-2 drops with carrier oil to affected areas.

Anger & Restlessness
Massage 1-2 drops into back of neck.

Hormone Balance & Mood Swings
Apply 1-2 drops to pulse points, or diffuse.

Main Ingredients
Lavender, Sweet Marjoram, Chamomile, Ylang Ylang, Sandalwood, Cedarwood, Vetiver, Vanilla

Safety
Use with caution during pregnancy.

Other Uses
Addictions, Hyperactivity, Insomnia, Lock Jaw, Mental Fatigue, Temporomandibular Joint Disorder (TMJ), Tension

Did You Know?
The dominant chemistry in this blend is Linalool and an array of esters, all powerful sedatives and calming agents.

Emotional Use
This oil of tranquility has incredible sedative properties for the mind and heart. It soothes agitation and restlessness to make room for peace, compassion, and connection.

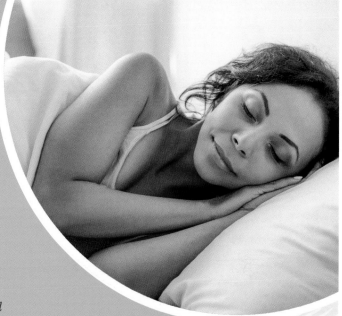

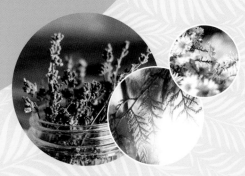

Quiet Solitude Bath

12 drops Serenity
6 drops Rosemary
2 drops Thyme
2 cups Epsom salt

Add oils to salt in an airtight container and mix well. Put 1/2 cup of the mixture in a warm bath and soak for up to 30 minutes.

Sleep Tight Diffuser Blend

4 drops Serenity
3 drops Frankincense
3 drops Vetiver

Use this diffuser blend to calm your mind and body and slowly drift to dreamland.

TerraShield®
Outdoor Blend | TerraArmour®

 A T I

Scan Here To Experience More

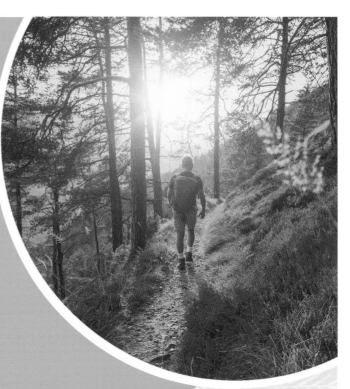

Oil Blends

Top Uses

Insect Repellent
Apply directly to exposed skin, and diffuse if possible.

Fly Infestation
Diffuse 10 drops, or apply lightly over clothing.

Energetic Toxicity
Use 1-3 drops during meditation, journaling, or prayer.

Main Ingredients
Ylang Ylang Flower, Tamanu Seed, Nootka, Cedarwood, Catnip, Lemon Eucalyptus, Litsea, Vanilla Bean, Arborvitae

Other Uses
Ants, Flies, Mites, Mosquitoes, Termites, Tics

Did You Know?
Tamanu seed oil is added to this blend to help soothe and nourish skin. It's harvested in tandem with humanitarian and fair farming & sourcing programs in Madagascar.

Emotional Use
Just as TerraShield® shields you from pests, so can it shield you from relationships or situations where your boundaries may be breached. It lets others be responsible for their energy, and you for yours.

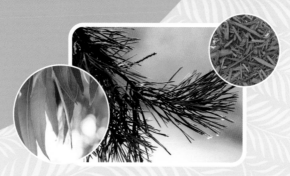

Supercharged Repellent Spray

40 drops TerraShield®
10 drops Arborvitae
10 drops Citronella
2 ounces Witch Hazel
2 ounces distilled water

Mix the witch hazel and distilled water with the oils. Shake well before use. Use as often as needed.

Bugs Adieu Diffuser Blend

6 drops TerraShield®
2 drops Citronella

Diffuse to keep bugs and insects away from your home.

Whisper
Women's Perfume Blend

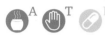

Scan Here To Experience More

Top Uses

Perfume
Apply 1-2 drops to pulse points.

Hormone Balance
Apply 1-2 drops to pulse points and back of neck.

Aphrodisiac
Apply 1-2 drops to neck and wrists.

Sedative & Calming
Inhale 1-2 drops from cupped hands.

Low Sex Drive
Apply 1-2 drops to pulse points.

Menopause
Apply 1-2 drops to pulse points.

Main Ingredients
Bergamot, Ylang Ylang, Patchouli, Jasmine, Vanilla, Cinnamon, Labdanum, Vetiver, Cocoa, Rose

Other Uses
Loss of Vision, Skin Irritation

Did You Know?
Cocoa absolute oil is a well-known aphrodisiac. Besides being good for feelings of contentment and well-being, it has always been associated with indulgence, love, and sensuality.

Emotional Use
This blend brings out the best of femininity. Where unexpressed feminine or overtly masculine energy may be a pattern, this blend brings balance to embracing your sexuality.

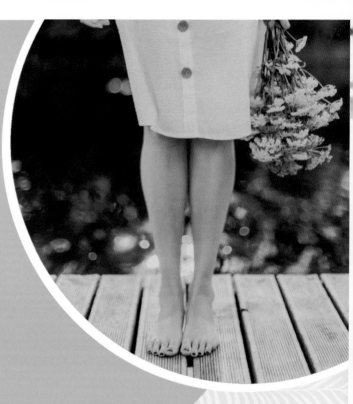

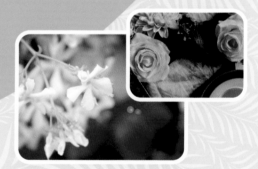

Night Out Perfume Roll-on

20 drops Whisper
15 drops Tangerine
3 drops Rose
FCO

Combine oils in a 10ml roller bottle and top with FCO. Apply to wrists, back of neck, and pulse points on a ladies' night out.

Perfumed Beddings Spray

10 drops Whisper
1 ounce Witch Hazel
3 oz. water

Place the oil and witch hazel first in a glass spray bottle and shake well. Add the water and shake again to blend the mixture well. Spray on beddings for a graceful fragrance.

Zendocrine®
Detoxification Blend

A T I

Scan Here To Experience More

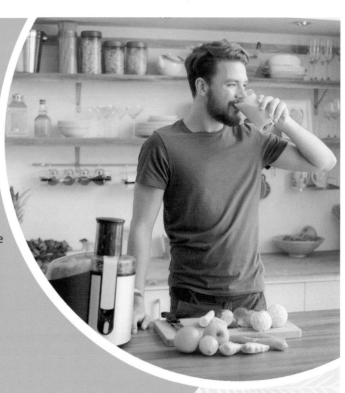

Top Uses

Detoxification
Take 2-4 drops in a capsule, or apply to bottoms of feet.

Allergies
Apply 2-4 drops to bottoms of feet, or diffuse.

Smoking Cravings
Rub onto bottom of big toe, or drink 1-3 drops in water after meals.

Liver & Kidney Support
Massage 1-3 drops over liver or kidneys.

Antioxidant
Take 1-2 drops in a capsule.

Heavy Metal Detox
Apply 2-4 drops to bottoms of feet.

Adrenal Fatigue
Massage 1-3 drops over lower back.

Main Ingredients
Tangerine, Geranium, Rosemary, Juniper Berry, Cilantro

Safety
Can irritate sensitive skin. Avoid sun exposure for 12 hours after topical use.

Other Uses
Hangover, Hormone Balance, Gallbladder Detox, Urinary Infection, Weight Loss

Did You Know?
This blend is designed to help the body purge chemical, imbalanced hormones, and even heavy metal toxicity.

Emotional Use
Purging physical toxins also sets the stage for emotional detox. Use this blend to purge self-sabotage and apathy, and transition to vitality.

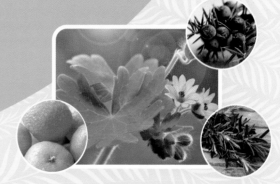

Clean Up Toxins Bath Soak

6 drops Zendocrine®
1 Tbsp Jojoba oil
1/4 cup Pink Himalayan Salt

Combine oils together then mix in pink salt. Add into warm bath water and soak for at least 20 minutes.

Detoxifying Herbal Tea

1 drop Zendocrine®
1 drop Lemon
8 oz. Herbal tea

Swirl the oils into the tea and drink in the morning to help cleanse and support the body's systems.

Oil Blends

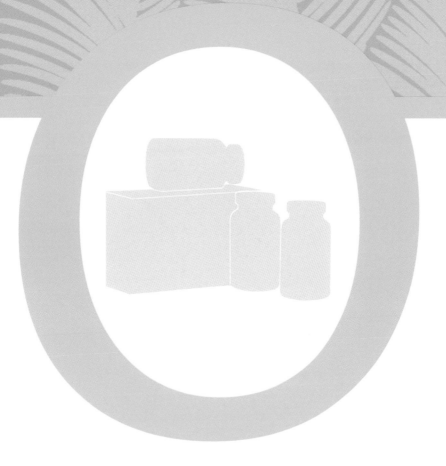

Section 5

Supplements & Softgels

Lifelong Vitality *Pack*®

Components
- Microplex VMz®
- xEO Mega®
- Alpha CRS®

Key Uses
- Vitality & Wellness
- Immune System Support
- Pain & Inflammation
- Sleep
- Mood, Depression, Anxiety
- Energy
- Hormone Balance
- Provides bioavailable crucial nutrients to cells for building healthy organs, tissues, and body systems.

Every protocol starts with Lifelong Vitality!

Every ailment and disease has roots in inflammation, and every real solution happens at the cellular level. Essential oil protocols should always include Lifelong Vitality Pack®.

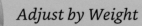

Adjust by Weight

A full dose of the trio is intended for an average-size adult. Try increasing or decreasing dosage for bigger or small body sizes!

a2z Chewable™

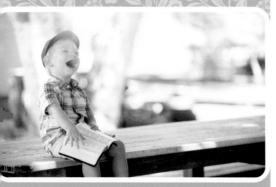

Main Ingredients
Vitamins A, C, D, E, B1, B2, B3, B6, B12, B5, Folic Acid, Biotin, Calcium, Iron, Iodine, Magnesium, Zinc, Copper, Manganese, Superfood Blend, Cellular Vitality Blend

Key Uses
• Complete daily nutrient for children
• Food-derived nutrients
• Easy to ingest
• Pairs perfectly with other supplements

Take twice daily for:

• Supplementing imperfect diet
• Supporting proper development

Adaptiv™ Complex

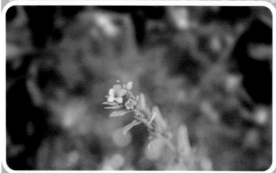

Main Ingredients
Lavender oil, Coriander oil, Wild Orange oil, Fennel oil, Ahiflower® oil, Gamma aminobutyric acid, Sceletium extract

Key Uses
• Provides neurotransmitter support
• Provides fatty acids to the brain
• Provides neurological and bio-chemical improvements through systemic pathways.

Avoid Calming Blend Complex when taking GABA inhibiting medication. Start slowly with your Calming Blend dosage and carefully observe your physical and mental response.

Take 1-2x daily for:

• Anxiety
• Depression
• Stress
• Bipolar Disorder & OCD
• Seizure disorders
• Mood balance

Alpha CRS®

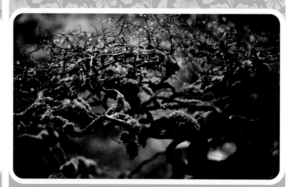

Main Ingredients
Boswellia Serrata, Scuttelaria Root, Milk Thistle, Pineapple Extract, Polygonum Capsudatum, Turmeric Root, Red Raspberry, Grape Seed, Marigold Flower, Tomato Fruit

Key Uses
• Protects body against free radicals
• Maintains proper cellular function
• Improves cellular vitality & energy
• Reduces inflammation

Take 2 twice daily for:

• Food-based nutrition
• Supplementing imperfect diet
• Cellular fuel
• Low energy

Bone Nutrient

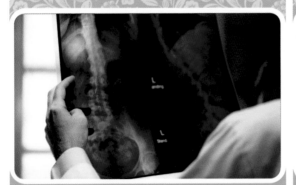

Main Ingredients
Calcium (coral calcium), Vitamin C, Vitamin D-2, Biotin, Magnesium, Zinc, Copper, Manganese, Boron

Key Uses
- Promotes Bone Health
- Prevents age-related calcium loss
- Maintains bone mineralization
- Maximizes calcium utilization

Take 1-2 capsules twice daily for:

- Osteoporosis
- Weak bones
- Fragile hips
- Aggressive sports

Deep Blue® Complex

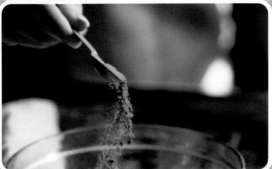

Main Ingredients
Frankincense Extract, Turmeric, Ginger, Green Tea Extract, Pomegranate Extract, Grape Seed Extract, Resveratrol

Key Uses
- Reduces inflammation and pain
- Provides relief to tension headaches, as well as back, neck, and shoulder pain
- Antioxidant support
- Internal complement to Soothing Blend

Take 1-3 daily for:

- Chronic pain (take 2 twice daily)
- Headaches & migraines (take 3)
- Lupus, Fibromyalgia, and other inflammatory issues (take 2 twice daily)
- Post-workout recovery

DigestTab™

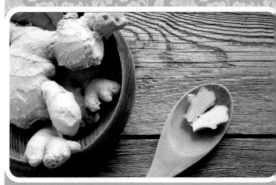

Main Ingredients
Calcium Carbonate, Ginger, Fennel, Coriander, Peppermint, Tarragon, Anise, Caraway

Key Uses
- Soothes GI discomfort
- Relieves heartburn and indigestion
- Relieves sour stomach
- Reduces belching and bloating

Take 1-2 as needed for:

- Excessive gas
- Stinky gas
- Diarrhea
- Gurgling stomach
- Acid reflux

Fiber

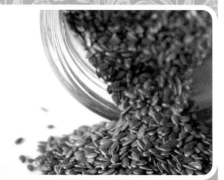

Main Ingredients

Apple, Tapioca, Flaxseed, Jerusalem Artichoke, Chicory Root, Lemon Essential Oil, 200 mg of Vitamin C.

Key Uses
- High source of fiber
- Contains high potency vitamin C
- Helps maintain a healthy microbiome
- Promotes healthy digestive function
- Supports cardiovascular health
- Supports the immune system
- Supports metabolic processes
- Supports weight management goals

Mix one scoop with 10 oz of liquid for:

- Health improvement of your gut microbiome
- Support for a healthy and regular digestive system

Greens

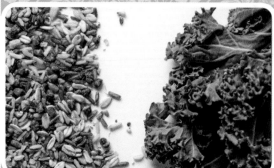

Main Ingredients

Kale, Dandelion, Collard Greens, Wheat Grass, Alfalfa, Barley Grass, Goji Berry, Mangosteen, Lemon & Ginger Oil

Key Uses
- Provides essential nutrients
- Supports Immune Health
- Supports Digestive Health
- Supports Weight Loss
- All natural ingredients

Use 1-2 servings daily for:

- Supplementing low produce consumption
- Higher energy
- Enhancing smoothies & juices
- Better nutrition while traveling

GX Assist®

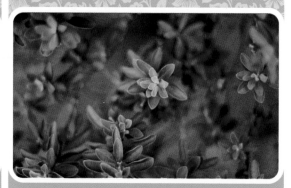

Main Ingredients

Caprylic Acid; Oregano, Melaleuca, Lemon, Lemongrass, and Thyme Oils

Key Uses
- Helps rid gut of parasites, Candida, and other harmful agents
- Supports healthy digestive environment
- Helps improve microbial balance

Take 1 capsule with each meal (no more than 10 days*) for:

- Candida & parasite cleanse
- Removing biofilm in gut

* Begin with 1 capsule/day. Work your way up to 3.

IQ Mega®

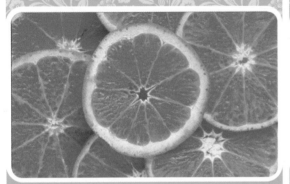

Main Ingredients
Fish Oil (EPA, DHA), Vitamin D, Vitamin E, Vitamin C, Orange Essential Oil

Key Uses
- Provides benefits of fish oil without fishy taste
- Easy to take plain, or add to juice
- Supports brain, joint, and cardiovascular development

Take 1-2 Tbs twice daily for:

- Heart support
- Brain support & development
- Joint support
- Healthy skin
- Use extra for ADD/ADHD, Autism, and developmental issues

Microplex VMz®

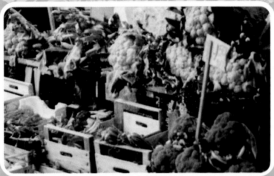

Main Ingredients
Vitamins A, C, D, E, K, B6, B12, Thiamin, Riboflavin, Niacin, Folate, Biotin, Pantothenic Acid, Calcium, Iron, Iodine, Magnesium, Zinc, Selenium, Copper, Manganese

Key Uses
- Whole-food comprehensive vitamin and mineral nutrient
- Provides bioavailable crucial nutrients to body systems, organs, and cells

---

Take 2 twice daily for:

- Sustainable energy
- Fuel for your cells & body systems
- Supplementing more veggies & fruits into your diet

Mito2Max®

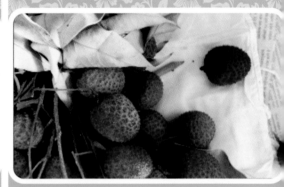

Main Ingredients
Acetyl-L-Carnitine, Alpha-Lipolic Acid, Coenzyme Q10, Lychee Fruit, Green Tea Leaf, Quercetine Dihydrate, Cordyceps Mycelium, Ginseng, Ashwagandha

Key Uses
- Increases cellular energy
- Improves micro-circulation
- Stimulates mitochondria
- Improves stamina

Take 1-2 capsules 1-2x daily for:

- Low energy
- Pre-workout
- Exhaustion
- Cold extremities
- Endurance

Supplements

On Guard® + Softgels

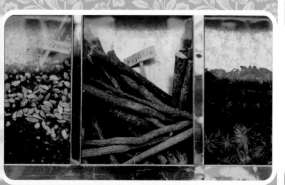

Main Ingredients
Clove, Wild Orange, Black Pepper, Cinnamon, Eucalyptus, Oregano, Rosemary, Melissa

Key Uses
- Supercharged Protective Blend
- Combats viral and bacterial infections
- Supports immune system

Take 1-2 softgels as needed for:

- Combating cold & flu
- Preventing illness
- Immune system boost
- Antioxidant support

PB Assist®

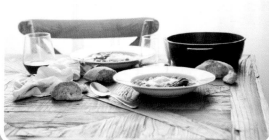

Main Ingredients
L. acidophilus, B. lactis, L. salivarius, L. casei, B. longum, B. bifidum

Key Uses
- 6 billion CFUs
- Supports digestive & immune systems
- Unique double-encapsulated delivery
- Shelf stable with prebiotics to sustain probiotics
- Helps digestion of food nutrients

Take 1-3x daily for:

- Healthy immune system
- Replenishing flora after antibiotics
- Hormone balance
- Proper digestive functions
- Higher absorption rates than other probiotic delivery forms

PB Assist® Jr

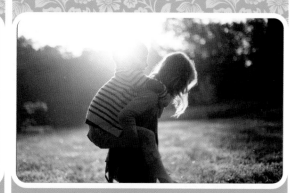

Main Ingredients
Lactobacillus Rhamnosus, Lactobacillus Salivarius, Lactobaccilus Plantarum LP01 & LP02, Bifidobacterium Breve, Bifidobacterium Lactis

Key Uses
- 5 billion live cells of 6 strains of flora
- Supports healthy digestive, neurological, immune, and brain function
- Shelf-stable unique delivery process
- Special micro-encapsulation protects probiotics until they reach the gut

Take twice daily for:

- Healthy immune system
- Proper digestive function
- Healthy mood balance

Supplements

Phytoestrogen Complex

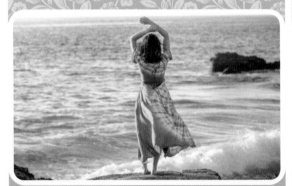

Main Ingredients
Soy Extract (64% isoflavones, 50% Genistein), Flaxseed Extract (40% Lignan), Pomegranate Extract (40% Ellagic Acid)

Key Uses
- Promotes hormone balance by blocking estrogen binding to cells
- Manages harmful metabolite byproducts of hormone metabolism

Take 1-2 capsules daily for:

- Pre-menopausal hormone balance (take 1-2)
- Post-menopausal hormone balance (take 2)

Protein (Whey)*

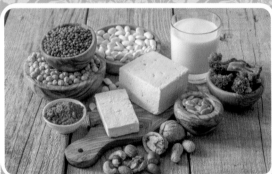

Main Ingredients
Whey Protein Concentrate, Calcium Caseinate, Tapioca Fiber, Flaxseed Powder, Oat Flour, Cream, Maltodextrin, Nonfat Dry Milk, Sunflower Lecithin, Gum Acacia, Sea Salt, Guar Gum, Steviol Glucosides, Xanathan Gum, Natural Flavors, Monk Fruit Extract

Key Uses
- Increase protein intake
- Meal replacement
- Manages appetite and cravings
- Healthy protein-carb-fat ratio

Plant protein also available

Use 1-2 servings daily for:

- Protein supplementation
- Weight training/muscle building
- Weight loss program support
- Smoothie & shake enhancement
- Enhanced appetite control

Serenity Complex

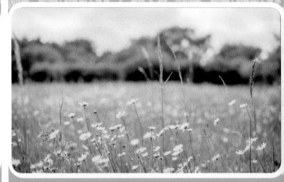

Main Ingredients
Lavender, L-theanine, Lemonbalm, Passion Flower, Chamomile

Key Uses
- Promotes falling asleep faster
- Supports more meaningful sleep
- Promotes waking up feeling refreshed

Take 2 30 minutes before bed for:

- Falling asleep more easily
- Waking feeling more refreshed
- Use in addition to Restful essential oil blend (diffuse & rub 2 drops on bottoms of feet)

TerraZyme®

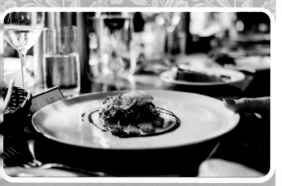

Main Ingredients
Protease, Amylase, Lipase, Alpha Galactosidase, Cellulase, Maltase, Sucrase, Tummy Taming Blend, Enzyme Assimilation Blend

Key Uses
- Facilitates breakdown of food
- Increases nutrient absorption
- Promotes comfortable digestion
- Increases usability of nutrients
- Facilitates proper gut function

Take 1-3x daily with meals for:

- Digestive comfort after eating out
- Increasing nutrient absorption
- Gluten sensitivities
- Lactose sensitivities
- Restoring proper digestive function

TriEase® Softgels

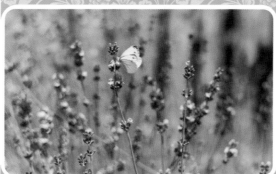

Main Ingredients
Lemon, Lavender, & Peppermint Essential Oils

Key Uses
- Reduces histamine response
- Opens airways
- Relieves itchiness
- Eases sinus congestion
- Useful for seasonal and pet allergies

Take 1-2 as needed:

- Constricted airways
- Hayfever
- Pet allergies

* Let 1 softgel dissolve under the tongue for faster results.

Turmeric Capsules

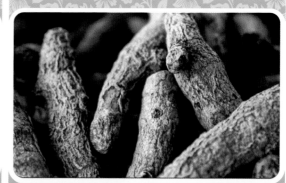

Main Ingredients
Curcuminoids (from Turmeric Root Extract), Turmeric Rhizome Oil

Key Uses
- Unique dual chamber delivery method with botanicals and essential oil
- Disrupts inflammation communication pathways
- Improved bioavailability by combining curcuminoids with turmerones

Take 1-2x daily for:

- Pain & inflammation
- Muscle tension
- Organ & tissue inflammation
- Heart palpitations
- Healthy brain function

Supplements

xEO Mega®

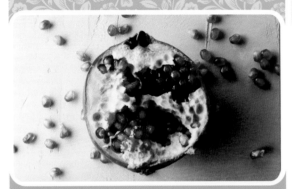

Main Ingredients

Fish Oil (EPA DHA), Astaxanthin, Flaxseed Oil, Borage Seed Oil, Cranberry Seed Oil, Pomegranate Seed Oil, Vitamin D

Key Uses
- Promotes heart, brain, joint, eye, skin, and circulatory health
- Protects against lipid oxidation
- Molecularly filtered fish oil combined with internal dose of 9 essential oils

Take 2 twice daily for:

- Brain support
- Depression, Anxiety, & ADD/ADHD
- Heart support
- Joint support
- Healthier skin

Yarrow|Pom Complex

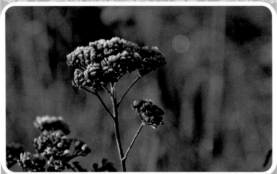

Main Ingredients

Pomegranate Seed Oil, Grape Seed Extract, Yarrow Oil, Frankincense Oil, Celery Seed Oil, Palmarosa Oil, Turmeric Oil, Melon Fruit Concentrate, Melissa Oil

Key Uses
- Promotes healthy tissue remodeling
- Reduces appearance of aging signs
- Supports cellular health
- Combats oxidative stress
- Supports healthy skin from the inside out

Take 2 capsules daily for:

- Youthful looking skin
- Antioxidant support
- Promoting healthy tissues
- Anti-aging

Zendocrine® Complex

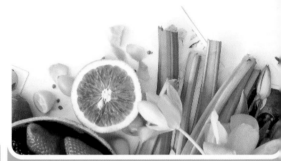

Main Ingredients

Psyllium Seed Husk, Barberry Leaf, Turkish Rhubarb, Kelp, Milk Thistle, Osha Root, Safflower, Acacia Gum, Burdoc Root, Clove, Enzyme Assimilation Complex

Key Uses
- Natural detoxification herbal blend
- Promotes healthy endocrine system
- Promotes toxin filtration
- Complements Detoxification Oil Blend

Take 1-3x daily for:

- Liver & kidney issues
- Fatigue
- Toxicity-related acne & skin issues
- Toxicity from medications
- Toxicity from food, air, or other environmental factors

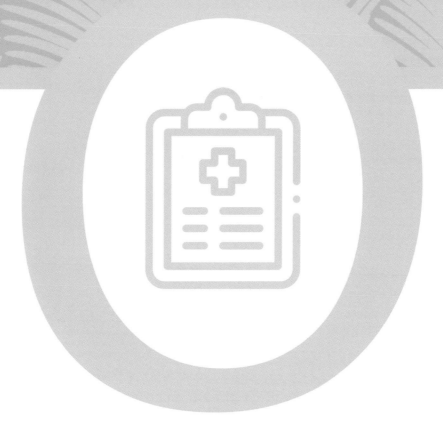

Section 6
Ailment Protocols

How to Use *Ailment Protocols*

While using plant-based medicine to remedy a health challenge is very much an individual process, this chapter offers protocols that provide more specific direction.

Each protocol gives detailed instructions on which essential oils and supplements to use, including dosage, frequency, and duration.

It is recommended that you use the protocols as they are written in order to achieve the best results. Consistency creates greatest impact.

How to Stay Consistent

- Set recurring reminders in your phone
- Place your oils and supplements where you'll see them
- Take products you need when you leave the house
- Commit to fully experiencing the protocol

Safety & Dosage

These protocols are not intended to replace instruction or care from your physician. Consult your physician before changing medications or other prescribed routines.

If the recommended dosage of oils or supplements feels off to you, adjust how much you're using. Refer to the safety and dilution chart at the beginning of this book. Listen to your body.

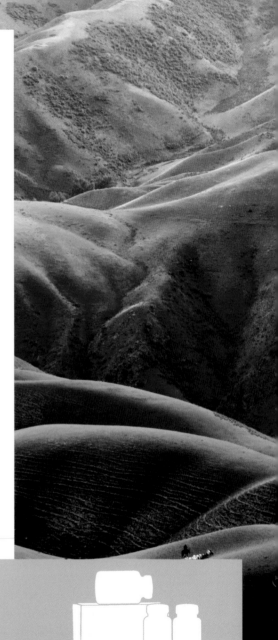

Build from the Lifelong Vitality *Pack*®

Lifelong Vitality is recommended as the basis for all protocols. Every health challenge will involve at least one of the main focuses of Lifelong Vitality: *Inflammation, Immune Response, Energy, and Hormones.*

Protocols

Acid Reflux

Condition in which acidic gastric fluid is regurgitated into the esophagus.

Description
Improves the integrity of gut cell junctions and repairs the intestinal mucosa. Doing so will reduce the symptoms of acid reflux.

Suggested Duration
3-6 months

DigestZen® (1), Turmeric (1), Yarrow|Pom(2)
Combine oils in an empty capsule and take 3x daily on an empty stomach. Also rub over upper abdomen.

Celery Seed & Lemon/Lime
Add 2 drops of each to morning smoothie or juice.

DigestZen® Softgels
Take 2 capsules with food.

DigestTab™
Chew 1-2 tabs as needed.

Additional Support
- PB Assist® (take 2 capsules 2x daily on an empty stomach)
- TerraZyme® (take 1 capsule with each meal)

Acne (bacterial)

Inflamed sebaceous glands and pimples due to bacteria trapped in pores.

Description
Combats bacterial overgrowth that becomes trapped in pores.

Suggested Duration
Ongoing

HD Clear® Facial Cleanser
Cleanse skin morning and night before bed.

HD Clear®
Apply a small amount evenly over clean skin after showering daily.

Citronella & Cedarwood
Apply a dab to blemishes.

Frankincense
Apply a dab to healing blemishes to prevent scarring.

Additional Support
- Eliminate fast food and un healthy fats from diet
- Tea Tree
- Immortelle
- Helichrysum

Acne (hormones)

Inflamed sebaceous glands and pimples due to hormonal imbalance.

Description
Balances hormone production and maintenance throughout the body, including the gut.

Suggested Duration
Until desired appearance is achieved, then as needed.

Phytoestrogen Complex
Take 1 capsule 2x daily (for men and women).

Clary Sage
Rub 1 drop on pulse points before bed.

HD Clear®
Apply a small amount to blemishes daily as needed.

Lifelong Vitality Pack® Necessary

Additional Support
- Tea Tree
- Helichrysum
- Zendocrine®

Acne (toxicity)

Outbreak occurring when the skin is used to eliminate toxins from the body.

Description
Alleviates toxicity overload by detoxing organs and skin.

Suggested Duration
3-5 weeks

Zendocrine® Softgels
Take 1 softgel with each meal.

Zendocrine® Complex
Take 1 capsule with breakfast and dinner.

DDR Prime® Softgels
Take 1 softgel with each meal.

HD Clear®
Apply small amount to blemishes daily as needed.

Additional Support
- Eliminate fast food and un healthy fats from diet
- GX Assist®
- Helichrysum
- Zendocrine® (use on bottoms of feet)

Lifelong Vitality Pack® should be the base of every protocol. Use as directed.

ADD/ADHD

Behavioral disorder with symptoms of poor concentration and hyperactivity.

Description
Activates the parasympathetic nervous system and induces a more calm and focused mental state.

Suggested Duration
6 months, then as needed

PB Assist® (or PB Assist® Jr)
Take 2 capsules in the morning on an empty stomach.

Vetiver, Frankincense, Rose, Copaiba
Combine 10 drops each in a 10 ml roller and top with FCO. Apply to spine and bottoms of feet 2x daily.

InTune®
Carry in your pocket and roll a small amount on back of neck as needed for focus.

Additional Support
- Ylang Ylang
- Sandalwood
- Siberian Fir
- Roman Chamomile
- Black Spruce

Adrenal Fatigue

Stress-related deterioration of adrenal glands' ability to produce hormones.

Description
Supports healthy adrenal function.

Suggested Duration
4-8 weeks

Lemon (22), Rosemary (9), Frankincense (9), Basil (9)
Combine in roller bottle. Fill the rest with carrier oil. Massage into neck and kidneys 2-3x daily.

Rosemary & Peppermint
Breathe a drop of each from cupped hands, or diffuse for energy as needed.

Mito2Max®
Take 2 capsules 2x daily.

Lifelong Vitality Pack® Necessary

Additional Support
- Citrus Bliss®
- Zendocrine®

AIDS/HIV

Sexually transmitted retrovirus that can become autoimmune dysfunction.

Description
Provides emotional support, promotes a properly functioning immune system.

Suggested Duration
6 months, then as needed

DDR Prime®
Rub 3-5 drops onto spine morning & night.

DDR Prime® Softgels
Take 2 softgels 3x daily.

On Guard & Melissa
Rub 2 drops each on bottoms of feet 2x daily.

Elevation
Carry with you, and inhale from hands for emotional support throughout the day.

Lifelong Vitality Pack® Necessary

Additional Support
- Helichrysum
- Pink Pepper
- Zendocrine®

Allergies (food)

Abnormal immune response to certain foods.

Description
Lowers histamine response triggered by food allergies and creates calm in the gut.

Suggested Duration
4 weeks to begin, then as needed

PB Assist®
Take 1 capsule 3x daily on an empty stomach.

Deep Blue® Complex
Take 1 capsule 3x daily

TerraZyme®
Take 1 with each meal.

Lavender
Put 1 drop under tongue. Drink water after 30 seconds.

Additional Support
- Do a 14-day bone broth cleanse
- Zendocrine® Complex
- Zendocrine®

Lifelong Vitality Pack® should be the base of every protocol. Use as directed.

Allergies (seasonal/pet)

Overreaction of the immune system to ordinarily harmless substances.

Description
Reduces histamine response and boosts immune response.

Suggested Duration
4-8 weeks, then as needed

PB Assist®
Take 1 capsule 3x daily on an empty stomach.

Lemon, Lavender, Peppermint
Put 1 drop each under tongue. Drink water after 30 seconds.

Breathe
Inhale from cupped hands when experiencing attack.

On Guard
Gargle 2 drops with water nightly, then swallow.

Additional Support
- TriEase® Softgels
- Siberian Fir

Allergies (skin)

Hypersensitivity to typically harmless substances that come in contact with skin.

Description
Calms irritation due to skin contact with allergens.

Suggested Duration
As needed

Lavender, Helichrysum, Frankincense, Lemon
Combine 10 drops of each in a roller bottle. Fill the rest with carrier oil. Roll onto affected area often.

Lavender
Put a drop under tongue. Drink water after 30 seconds.

PB Assist®
Take 1 capsule 3x daily on an empty stomach.

Additional Support
- Zendocrine® Complex
- Zendocrine®
- Yarrow|Pom

Alzheimer's

Progressive mental deterioration due to degeneration of the brain.

Description
Supports healthy mental activity, boosts alertness.

Suggested Duration
Ongoing

DDR Prime®
Rub 3-5 drops along spine and bottoms of feet 3x daily.

DDR Prime® Softgels
Take 1 softgel 3x daily.

Peppermint & Rosemary
Massage a drop each into scalp and diffuse several drops daily to increase alertness & memory.

Vitality Supplement Trio Necessary

Additional Support
- Cilantro
- Frankincense
- Extra xEO Mega®
- Balance

Anxiety

Condition of worry, nervousness, or unease.

Description
Systemically addresses GABA receptors, neurotransmitters, & emotions.

Suggested Duration
3 months, then as needed

PB Assist®
Take 2 capsules in the morning on an empty stomach.

Adaptiv™ Complex*
Take 2 capsules daily.

Adaptiv™
Apply to web of hands and base of skull. Diffuse throughout the day.

Magnolia & Copaiba
Apply 1-2 drops each to the back of neck and bottoms of feet 2x daily, especially before bed.

*Start slowly with Adaptiv™ Complex and observe yourself closely.

Vitality Supplement Trio Necessary

Additional Support
- Frankincense
- Rose
- Sandalwood
- Vetiver

Protocols

Lifelong Vitality Pack® should be the base of every protocol. Use as directed.

Arthritis

Painful inflammation and stiffness of the joints.

Description
Decreases the inflammatory response within joint tissues.

Suggested Duration
6 months, then as needed

Turmeric Capsules
Take 2 capsules in the morning.

Turmeric & Copaiba
Massage 1-2 drops each into affected area in the morning.

Deep Blue® Rub
Massage into affected areas as needed throughout the day.

Copaiba Softgels
Take 2 capsules in the evening before bed.

Additional Support
- Deep Blue® Complex
- Marjoram
- Lemongrass
- Oregano
- Myrrh

Asperger's

Developmental disorder impacting social interactions and communication.

Description
Increases the integrity of the gut lining and promotes brain health.

Suggested Duration
1 to 3 years

PB Assist® or PB Assist® Jr
Take 2 capsules in the morning on an empty stomach.

Vetiver & Clary Sage
Apply a drop of each to bottoms of feet 3x daily.

DDR Prime®
Apply 2 drops to spine 3x daily.

InTune®
Apply to temples and sides of neck 3x daily.

Additional Support
- DigestZen® Softgels (2x daily)
- Serenity Complex (2 at bedtime)
- Yarrow|Pom (under the tongue)
- Lavender
- Sandalwood

Asthma

Respiratory condition marked by spasms in the bronchi of the lungs.

Description
Promotes open airways and easy breathing.

Suggested Duration
As needed

Breathe
Rub 2 drops on chest and inhale from cupped hands during attacks.

Lavender
Massage a drop behind and over ears to promote calm.

Cardamom
Gargle a drop for 30 seconds, then swallow as needed.

PB Assist®
Take 1 capsule 2x daily.

Additional Support
- Rosemary
- Siberian Fir
- Eucalyptus

Autism

Developmental disorder impacting social interactions and communication.

Description
Increases the integrity of the gut lining and promotes brain health.

Suggested Duration
1 to 3 years

PB Assist® or PB Assist® Jr
Take 2 capsules in the morning on an empty stomach.

TerraZyme®
Take 1 capsule with each meal.

DDR Prime® & Rose
Apply 2 drops each diluted to spine 2x daily.

Vetiver, Turmeric, Clary Sage
Apply a drop of each diluted to back of neck and bottoms of feet 3x daily.

Lavender, Tea Tree, Copaiba, Frankincense, DigestZen®
Combine 10 drops each with FCO in roller bottle. Roll clockwise over stomach 2x daily.

Additional Support
- DigestZen® Softgels (2x daily)
- Serenity Complex (2 at bed time)
- Yarrow|Pom (under the tongue)

Protocols

Lifelong Vitality Pack® should be the base of every protocol. Use as directed.

Auto-Immune

Condition in which the immune system turns on healthy cells.

Description
Induces the parasympathetic nervous system, eliminates antigens and latent infections, and reduces the immune response.

Suggested Duration
1 to 3 years

PB Assist®
Take 2 capsules in the morning on an empty stomach.

Frankincense, Yarrow|Pom, Turmeric, Clary Sage
Apply a drop of each to back of neck and bottoms of feet 2x daily.

DDR Prime® Softgels
Apply 2-4 drops to spine 2x daily. Also take 2 softgels 2x daily.

Zendocrine®
Apply 2 drops to sides of neck 2x daily.

Vitality Supplement Trio Necessary

Additional Support
- Copaiba
- Sandalwood
- Zendocrine® Herbal Complex
- Serenity Complex
- PB Assist® Jr

Back Pain

Inflammation and pain in the back due to injury, aging, or other issues.

Description
Increases circulation, reduces scar tissue, promotes healing.

Suggested Duration
6-12 months

Turmeric Capsules
Take 2 capsules in the morning.

Turmeric & Copaiba
Massage 1-2 drops each into affected area in the morning.

Marjoram, Siberian Fir, Deep Blue®
Apply a drop of each onto spine and painful areas 3x daily.

Copaiba Softgels
Take 2 capsules in the evening before bed.

Additional Support
- Frankincense
- Lemongrass
- Wintergreen
- Deep Blue® Rub

Bipolar Disorder

Mood disorder resulting in mania, depression, and psychotic issues.

Description
Normalizes brain activity and regulates the nervous system.

Suggested Duration
12 months

PB Assist®
Take 2 capsules in the morning on an empty stomach.

Adaptiv™ Complex*
Take 2 capsules daily.

DDR Prime®
Apply 2-4 drops to spine 2x daily.

Adaptiv™ & Vetiver
Apply to web of hands and base of skull. Diffuse throughout the day.

Start slowly with Adaptiv™ Complex and observe yourself closely.

Lifelong Vitality Pack® Necessary

Additional Support
- Balance
- Clary Sage
- Rosemary
- Sandalwood
- Lavender

Blood Pressure (high)

Hypertension resulting unhealthy pressure on artery walls.

Description
Regulates blood pressure by dilation of blood vessels and reducing the viscosity of the blood.

Suggested Duration
6-12 months

Cypress, Marjoram, Ylang Ylang, Lemon
Apply a drop of each over the chest and bottom of feet 2x daily.

Marjoram, Ylang Ylang, Lemon, Yarrow|Pom
Take 2 drops each in a capsule 2x daily.

Additional Support
- Clary Sage
- Lavender
- DDR Prime®

Lifelong Vitality Pack® should be the base of every protocol. Use as directed.

Bone Spurs

New bone material that develops along the edges of existing bones.

Description
Alleviates agitation of surrounding tissue and decreased functionality by decreasing pain and inflammation.

Suggested Duration
2-3 months

Frankincense & Turmeric
Massage a drop of each into affected area in the morning.

Deep Blue® Rub
Massage into affected area as needed throughout the day.

Copaiba Softgels
Take 2 softgels 3x daily.

Additional Support
• Turmeric Capsules
• Wintergreen
• Rosemary
• Yarrow|Pom

Bronchitis

Inflammation of the mucous membrane in the bronchial tubes.

Description
Increases immune response to address possible infections and open the airways for symptomatic relief.

Suggested Duration
1-2 weeks

Cardamom, Black Pepper, Rosemary, Lime
Apply drop of each to chest and bottoms of feet 3-5x daily.

Breathe
Diffuse several drops; inhale 2 drops from cupped hands as needed.

On Guard+ Softgels
Take 2 softgels 2x daily until symptoms subside.

Additional Support
• Pink Pepper
• Oregano
• Melissa
• Lemon Eucalyptus

Calluses

Thickened or hardened part of the skin due to excess friction.

Description
Softens thickened skin for easy removal.

Suggested Duration
1-2 weeks

Tea Tree, Peppermint, Roman Chamomile
Apply a drop each to callused area 3x daily for 3 days.

After 3 days, place feet in a cold water soak with 10 drops of each and use a pumice stone to remove the calluses.

Additional Support
• Oregano
• Basil
• Rosemary
• Lavender

Cancer

Neoplastic mass composed of abnormal cell growth resulting in a complex disease.

Description
Increases the immune response and slows the growth of abnormal cell proliferation.

Suggested Duration
1-3 years

PB Assist®
Take 2 capsules in the morning on an empty stomach.

Adaptiv™ Complex*
Apply 2-4 drops to back of neck, spine, and bottoms of feet 4x daily.

Frankincense, Sandalwood, Turmeric, Lemongrass
Take a drop of each in a capsule 4x daily.

Zendocrine®
Apply 2 drops diluted to sides of neck 3x daily

Lifelong Vitality Pack® Necessary

Additional Support
• Zendocrine® Softgels
• Zendocrine® Complex
• DigestZen® Softgels
• Pink Pepper

Lifelong Vitality Pack® should be the base of every protocol. Use as directed.

Cancer (Leukemia)

Malfunction of white blood cells in the body's blood. Often affects the bone marrow and lymphatic system.

Description
Improves the immune response and reduces a hyperactive immune system.

Suggested Duration
1-3 years

PB Assist®
Take 2 capsules in the morning on an empty stomach.

DDR Prime®
Apply 2-4 drops to back of neck, spine, and bottoms of feet 4x daily.

Frankincense, Sandalwood, Turmeric, Lemongrass
Take a drop of each in a capsule 4x daily.

Zendocrine®
Apply 2 drops diluted to sides of neck 3x daily.

Lifelong Vitality Pack® Necessary

Additional Support
• Zendocrine® Softgels
• Zendocrine® Complex
• DigestZen® Softgels
• Pink Pepper

Candida

Fungal infection often caused by the overuse of antibiotics. Occurs frequently as vaginal yeast infections skin infections and oral thrush.

Description
Combats fungus overgrowth, restores healthy flora.

Suggested Duration
2-3 months

GX Assist®
Take 1 softgel 3x daily with meals for 10 days (start with 1 daily and work your way up).

PB Assist®
Take 2 capsules in the morning and evening on an empty stomach.

Lemon Eucalyptus, Clove, Tea Tree
Carry in your pocket and roll a Apply a drop of each diluted over lower abdomen or affected area 6x daily.

Zendocrine® Softgels
2 softgels 2x daily after food.

Additional Support
• Arborvitae
• Thyme
• Green Mandarin

Canker Sores

Iritation that often occurs in the mouth but can also affect the lips.

Description
Decreases iritation and maintains a preventative regimen.

Suggested Duration
5-10 days

PB Assist®
Take 2 capsules in the morning and evening on an empty stomach.

Tea Tree, Oregano, Clove
Apply a dab of each with FCO directly to canker sore. Hold in mouth for 3 minutes. Apply 6x daily.

Combine 3 drops each to 20 drops of carrier oil and swish for 2 minutes daily for ongoing prevention.

On Guard+ Softgel
Take 2 softgels 2x daily.

Additional Support
• Tulsi
• Frankincense
• Myrrh
• Thyme

Celiac's

Autoimmune disorder affecting the small intestine.

Description
Promotes nutrient absorption, calms digestive system.

Suggested Duration
Ongoing

PB Assist®
Take 2 capsules morning and evening on an empty stomach.

TerraZyme®
Take 2-3 capsules with meals.

DigestZen®
Rub on outside of stomach at onset of pain.

Slim & Sassy® Softgels
Take 1-2 softgels 2-3x daily.

Additional Support
• Cinnamon
• Grapefruit
• Frankincense

Lifelong Vitality Pack® should be the base of every protocol. Use as directed.

Cholesterol (high)

Excess lipid molecules found in the blood, often the contributing cause of heart disease and heart attacks.

Description
Reduces the amount of cholesterol in the blood to prevent the formation of dangerous clots.

Suggested Duration
6-12 months

PB Assist®
Take 2 capsules morning and evening on an empty stomach.

Yarrow|Pom, Frankincense, Rosemary
Take 2 drops each in a capsule 2x daily.

DDR Prime®
Apply 2-4 drops to bottoms of feet 2x daily.

Additional Support
- Citronella
- Turmeric
- Lavender

Cold Sores

Inflamed blister in or near the mouth caused by herpes simplex virus.

Description
Combats viral infection, promotes skin healing and pain relief.

Suggested Duration
5-10 days

Tea Tree & Melissa
Apply a dab of each diluted 3-5x daily.

PB Assist®
Take 2 capsules in the morning on an empty stomach.

On Guard+ Softgels
Take 2 softgels 2x daily.

Helichrysum
Apply a dab diluted at night to help tissue heal.

Additional Support
- Arborvitae
- Black Pepper
- Frankincense

Colds (common)

Respiratory infection resulting in excess mucus, cough, and sinus issues.

Description
Provides antiviral and respiratory support.

Suggested Duration
5-10 days

Celery Seed & Lime
Add 2 drops each to morning juice or smoothie.

On Guard+ Softgels
Take 2 softgels 2-3x daily.

On Guard, Black Pepper, Tea Tree
Rub a drop each on bottoms of feet 3x daily.

Breathe
Rub 2 drops onto chest and diffuse several drops as needed.

Additional Support
- Rosemary
- Cardamom
- Lemon Eucalyptus
- Litsea
- Mito2Max®

Constipation

Difficulty emptying bowels, usually associated with hardened feces.

Description
Stimulates proper digestive function and elimination.

Suggested Duration
2-3 months, then as needed

PB Assist®
Take 2 capsules morning and evening on an empty stomach.

TerraZyme®
Take 2-3 capsules with meals.

DigestZen® Softgels
Take 1 softgel after meals.

Clary Sage & Petitgrain
Rub 1-2 drops each over stomach in a clockwise motion 3x daily.

Additional Support
- Bergamot
- DigestZen®
- Cassia

Lifelong Vitality Pack® should be the base of every protocol. Use as directed.

Cough (chronic)

Chronic and involuntary respiratory expulsion.

Description
Increases immune response to address possible infections; opens the airways for symptomatic relief.

Suggested Duration
1-2 weeks

Cardamom & Lime
Gargle a drop each with water for 30 seconds, then swallow 3x daily.

Breathe, Rosemary, Black Pepper
Apply 1-2 drops each to chest and bottoms of feet 2x daily. Also diffuse several drops throughout the day.

On Guard+ Softgels
Take 2 softgels 2x daily until symptoms subside.

Additional Support
- Oregano
- Melissa
- Arborvitae
- Eucalyptus
- Madagascar Vanilla

Crohn's Disease

Inflammatory disease of intestines, colon, and ileum.

Description
Reduces inflammation and swelling in the bowels.

Suggested Duration
6 months

GX Assist®
Take 1 softgel 1-2x daily with food for 2 weeks.

Peppermint, Frankincense, Basil
Take 1-2 drops each in capsule daily for 2 weeks after GX Assist®.

PB Assist®
Take 1 capsule w/each meal.

DigestZen® Softgels
Take 1 softgel to ease discomfort 3-5x daily.

Additional Support
- Ginger
- Marjoram
- Copaiba Softgels
- Turmeric Capsules

Cysts (ganglion)

Non-cancerous lumps that most commonly develop along the tendons or joints of your wrists or hands.

Description
Reduces the size or eliminates the cyst by softening the cyst and allowing the fluid to be absorbed and dispersed into the surrounding tissue.

Suggested Duration
2-4 weeks

Lemongrass & Oregano
Massage a drop of each diluted into the cyst 2x daily.

Then apply a small cloth soaked in caster oil over the cyst. Wrap tightly with tape or muslin fabric overnight.

Additional Support
- DDR Prime®
- Thyme
- Cypress

Deodorant (body)

Unpleasant smell from pheromones or bacterial or mildew development.

Description
Helps manage bacteria and odor-causing toxicity

Suggested Duration
4 weeks, then as needed

Zendocrine®
Apply 2 drops to bottoms of feet 30 minutes before showering daily.

Cilantro
Take 2 drops in a capsule daily 2x daily.

Purify
Use diluted with carrier oil under arms after showering.

Additional Support
- Abōde™
- Tea Tree
- Arborvitae
- Petitgrain
- Zendocrine® Softgels

Lifelong Vitality Pack® should be the base of every protocol. Use as directed.

Depression

Experience of a more depressed mood and loss of interest in previously interesting activities.

Description
Increases mood by stimulation through senses.

Suggested Duration
3 months, then as needed

Adaptiv™
Apply to web of hands and base of skull. Diffuse throughout the day.

Adaptiv™ Complex*
Take 2 capsules daily.

PB Assist®
Take 2 capsules in the morning on an empty stomach.

Melissa or Frankincense
Use a drop under the tongue 2x daily.

Copaiba
Apply 2 drops to back of neck and spine before bed.

*Start slowly with Adaptiv™ Complex and observe yourself closely.

Lifelong Vitality Pack® Necessary

Additional Support
• Cheer
• Arise
• Tangerine
• Hawaiian Sandalwood

Detox (full body)

Elimination of toxic substances accumulated in organs and tissues.

Description
Helps the body eliminate toxicity and free up filtering organs.

Suggested Duration
30 days (in 10 day segments)

GX Assist®
Take 1 softgel w/each meal for 10 days (start with 1 a day, and work up to 3).

Zendocrine® Softgels & Zendocrine® Complex
Take 1 w/each meal.

TerraZyme®
Take 1 capsule w/each meal.

DDR Prime® Softgels
Take 1 softgel 2x daily.

PB Assist®
Take 1 capsule w/each meal during last 10 days.

Lifelong Vitality Pack® Necessary

Additional Support
• Lemon (in water)
• Cilantro
• Lemon Eucalyptus
• Grapefruit

Diabetes (type 1)

Autoimmune condition in which little or no insulin is produced by the pancreas.

Description
Stimulates cellular maintenance, helps balance blood sugar.

Suggested Duration
3-6 months, then as needed

Rosemary, Siberian Fir, Cassia
Take 1 drop each in capsule daily. Also rub diluted onto pancreas reflex points.

Geranium & Rosemary
Add 3 drops of each to a hot bath nightly.

Additional Support
• DDR Prime®
• Coriander
• Juniper Berry
• Bergamot

Diabetes (type 2)

Condition in which the body becomes resistant to insulin.

Description
Helps balance blood sugar, supports pancreas.

Suggested Duration
3-6 months, then as needed

Coriander, Cinnamon, Juniper Berry
Take 1-2 drops each in capsule daily.

DDR Prime® Softgels
Take 2 softgels 2x daily.

Zendocrine®
Rub 2 drops onto pancreas reflex point or over pancreas daily.

Lifelong Vitality Pack® Necessary

Additional Support
• Cassia
• Slim & Sassy®

Lifelong Vitality Pack® should be the base of every protocol. Use as directed.

Digestive Issues

Symptoms of gas, stomach ache, bloating, indigestion, and cramping.

Description
Relieves inflammation, gas, and discomfort in digestive system.

Suggested Duration
4 weeks, then as needed

PB Assist®
Take 2 capsules in the morning on an empty stomach.

Frankincense & Cardamom
Rub a drop of each onto stomach reflex points in the morning.

DigestZen®
Drink 1-2 drops with water, or rub over stomach to ease discomfort.

TerraZyme®
Take 1 capsule w/each meal.

Additional Support
- Ginger
- Fennel
- Peppermint Softgels
- Celery Seed

Ear Ache

Inflammation or infection of the middle ear usually caused by bacteria or virus.

Description
Provides assistance in dispersing the infection and draining the surrounding tissue.

Suggested Duration
2 weeks

Lavender & Basil
Apply a dab of each diluted around ear (do not place oils inside ear).

On Guard+ Softgels
Take 2 softgels 3x daily with food.

PB Assist®
Take 2 capsules in the morning on an empty stomach.

Additional Support
- Ginger
- Tea Tree
- Frankincense
- Helichrysum

Eczema/Dermatitis

A condition of the skin causing patches of scales and dryness, often caused by bacterial infection.

Description
Reduces the infection, increases moisture, and promotes new skin cell growth.

Suggested Duration
3 months, then as needed

Arborvitae, Tea Tree, Frankincense
Combine 1-2 drops each with FCO and apply to the affected area 5x daily.

Apply a warm towel compress over the area after oils are applied in the evening

On Guard+ Softgels
Take 2 softgels 3x daily with food.

PB Assist®
Take 2 capsules in the morning on an empty stomach.

Additional Support
- Myrrh
- Hawaiian Sandalwood
- Helichrysum

Endometriosis

A condition where uterine lining grows outside the uterus.

Description
Provides relief from pain and discomfort by increasing blood flow and circulation to the area.

Suggested Duration
1 year, then as needed

Clary Sage, Frankincense, Eucalyptus
Apply a drop of each to lower abdomen 3x daily.

Cover with a hot compress towel after application in the evening.

DDR Prime®
Apply to abdomen 2x daily.

Additional Support
- Yarrow|Pom
- Hawaiian Sandalwood
- Myrrh
- Patchouli

Lifelong Vitality Pack® should be the base of every protocol. Use as directed.

Slim & Sassy®
Metabolic Blend / Smart & Sassy®

 A 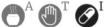 T I

Scan Here To Experience More

Top Uses

Weight Loss
Take 2-4 drops in capsule or drink in water 3-5x daily.

Appetite Control
Drink 2-4 drops in water throughout the day, or diffuse.

Blood Sugar Regulation
Take 1-2 drops in water or in a capsule.

Cellulite & Visceral Fat
Massage several drops with carrier oil into needed areas.

Antioxidant
Take 1-2 drops in a capsule.

Eating Disorders
Take a drop under the tongue, or diffuse 4-8 drops.

Main Ingredients
Grapefruit, Lemon, Ginger, Peppermint, Cinnamon

Safety
Can irritate sensitive skin. Use with caution during pregnancy. May cause photosensitivity.

Other Uses
Colds, Congestion, Detox, Energy, Food Addiction, Gallbladder Stones, High Cholesterol, Lymphatic Stimulation, Obesity, Over-Eating

Did You Know?
This blend combines the power of balancing blood sugar (Cinnamon), detoxification (citrus oils), and appetite suppressing (Peppermint) to assist with weight loss.

Emotional Use
The Metabolic Blend invites the user to release self-criticism, judgment and shame. It turns focus inward where true beauty originates from.

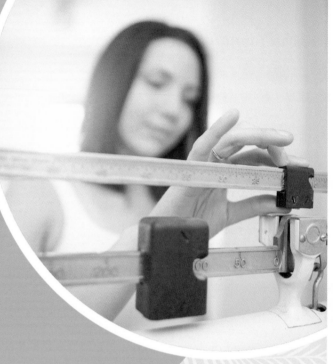

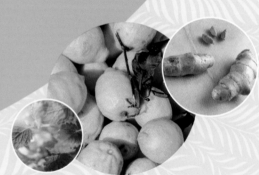

Cellulite Buster Massage Blend

7 drops Slim & Sassy®
5 drops Juniper Berry
4 tsp Argan oil

Massage well onto the thighs, buttocks, and any other regions affected by cellulite and leave on for 60 minutes before washing.

Kick the Cravings Diffuser Blend

5 drops Slim & Sassy®
1 drop Coriander

Diffuse this blend to help kick cravings and feel satiated.

Energy (low)
Fatigue caused by lack of sleep, toxicity, nervous issues, or regenerative issues.

Description
Increases energy by stimulation of the sympathetic nervous system, eliminating toxins, and inducing cellular pruning and regeneration.

Suggested Duration
6 months, then as needed

Peppermint, Bergamot, Lemongrass
Apply a drop of each to back of neck and bottoms of feet 2-3x daily.

Mito2Max®
Take 2 capsules 2x daily.

PB Assist®
Take 2 capsules in the morning on an empty stomach.

xEO Mega®
Take 2 capsules 2x daily.

Lifelong Vitality Pack® Necessary

Additional Support
- Frankincense
- Peppermint
- Tangerine
- Elevation

Fibromyalgia
Condition where one experiences widespread muscle pain and tenderness.

Description
Decreases inflammation, promotes healthy cellular function.

Suggested Duration
1-3 years

Frankincense, Yarrow|Pom, Copaiba, Turmeric
Apply a drop of each to back of neck and bottoms of feet 2x daily.

DDR Prime® & Softgels
Apply 2-4 drops to spine 2x daily. Also take 2 softgels 2x daily.

Deep Blue® Rub
Massage into inflamed areas 3x daily or as needed.

PB Assist®
Take 2 capsules in the morning on an empty stomach.

Melissa
Use 1 drop under tongue daily.

Lifelong Vitality Pack® Necessary

Additional Support
- Copaiba Softgels
- Turmeric Capsules
- Mito2Max®
- Zendocrine®

Flu/Influenza
Viral infection of the respiratory passages.

Description
Combats viruses, boosts immune system, supports respiratory system.

Suggested Duration
5-10 days

On Guard, Tea Tree, Black Pepper
Rub 2 drops each on bottoms of feet 3x daily.

On Guard+ Softgels
Take 2 softgels 3x daily.

DigestZen®
Drink 1-3 drops in water, or rub over stomach to ease nausea & vomiting.

Breathe
Diffuse 8-10 drops. Sit/sleep near the diffuser. Also rub 2 drops over chest as needed.

Additional Support
- Melissa
- Cardamom
- GX Assist®
- Pink Pepper

Focus & Concentration
Need for improved ability to remain on-task and mentally centered.

Description
Actives the parasympathetic nervous system and induces a more calm and focused mental state.

Suggested Duration
6 months

Vetiver, Frankincense, Wild Orange, Peppermint
Diffuse 2 drops each during focus times. Also apply a drop of each to back of neck and brain reflex point (the bottom of the big toe).

InTune®
Apply to forehead and temples 2x daily and as needed.

PB Assist®
Take 2 capsules in the morning on an empty stomach.

Additional Support
- Sandalwood
- Ylang Ylang
- Roman Chamomile
- Siberian Fir

Lifelong Vitality Pack® should be the base of every protocol. Use as directed.

Gout

Excess buildup of uric acid in the blood, often caused by poor dietary habits.

Description
Relieves pain, disperses and dilutes excess uric acid.

Suggested Duration
1 week

Frankincense, Turmeric, Lavender
Apply a drop of each to painful areas 3x daily.

Deep Blue®
Massage into affected areas after above oils 3x daily.

Deep Blue® Complex
Take 2 capsules 2x daily on an empty stomach.

DDR Prime®
Apply 2 drops to painful areas before bed each night.

Additional Support
- Yarrow|Pom
- Copaiba
- Fennel
- Wintergreen

Headache

Continuous pain in the head or sinuses.

Description
Increases circulation and relieves pain.

Suggested Duration
As needed

PastTense®
Apply roller regularly to forehead, neck and temples. Add a drop of Helichrysum if needed.

Deep Blue® Complex
Take 2 capsules 2x daily on an empty stomach.

DDR Prime®
Rub 1-2 drops into bottoms of feet and spine 3x daily.

Additional Support
- Peppermint
- Frankincense
- Lavender
- Copaiba

Heartburn

Indigestion felt as a burning sensation in the chest.

Description
Balances stomach acid, eases pain of indigestion.

Suggested Duration
As needed

DigestTab™
Chew 2 tablets as needed.

DigestZen®
Drink 1-2 drops in water.

TerraZyme®
Take 1-3 capsules with each meal.

Cardamom
Rub 1-2 drops over stomach.

Additional Support
- Ginger
- Fennel
- Coriander

Hemorrhoids

Swollen veins that often lead to the formation of a small blood clot inside or outside the anus.

Description
Reduces the inflammatory response to the veins, shrinks the size of the clot, reduces pain.

Suggested Duration
8 weeks to 12 months

Geranium & Cypress
Apply a drop of each diluted to the location of the hemorrhoid 3x daily.

DDR Prime®
Apply 2-4 drops with carrier oil to inside of legs from ankles to inner thighs 2x daily.

Additional Support
- Cypress
- Myrrh
- Sandalwood
- Juniper Berry

Lifelong Vitality Pack® should be the base of every protocol. Use as directed.

Hepatitis C

Viral infection that attacks the liver over several years.

Description
Combats bacterial overgrowth that becomes trapped in pores.

Suggested Duration
2-3 months

Helichrysum, Oregano, Frankincense
Apply a drop of each diluted to the sides of the lower back 6x daily. (If infection is on the face or body, follow the same protocol.)

PB Assist®
Take 2 capsules in the morning and evening on an empty stomach.

DigestZen® Softgels
Take 2 softgels 2x daily after food.

Additional Support
- Neroli
- Thyme
- Greenland Moss
- Carrot Seed

Herniated Disc

Bulging of the central portion of a disc beyond the damaged outer rings.

Description
Increases circulation, reduces scar tissue, promotes healing.

Suggested Duration
6-12 months

Frankincense, Turmeric, Copaiba
Apply 1 drop of each to painful areas 3x daily.

Deep Blue® Rub
Massage into affected area after above oils 3x daily.

Deep Blue® Complex
Take 2 capsules 2x daily on an empty stomach.

DDR Prime®
Apply 2-4 drops to affected area before bed each night.

Additional Support
- Turmeric Capsules
- Lavender
- Coriander
- Wintergreen

Herpes Simplex

Viral infection that often occurs in the mouth but can also affect the lips.

Description
Decreases the expression of the virus and maintains a preventative regimen.

Suggested Duration
1 week to 3 months

Cardamom, Tea Tree, Melissa
Apply a dab of each diluted directly to blister sore 6x daily.

PB Assist®
Take 2 capsules in the morning and evening on an empty stomach.

xEO Mega®
2 softgels 2x daily.

Helichrysums
Apply a dab at night to help tissues heal.

Additional Support
- Clary Sage
- Geranium
- Lemon Myrtle

Immune Boost

Need for improved immune response to combat bacteria, viruses, and pathogens.

Description
Provides bacteria and virus-fighting agents, boosts immune system.

Suggested Duration
4 weeks

On Guard, Black Pepper, Tea Tree
Rub 2-4 drops each on bottoms of feet daily.

Celery Seed & Lime
Add 2 drops each to morning juice or smoothie.

PB Assist®
Take 2 capsules in the morning on an empty stomach.

Vitality Supplement Trio Necessary

Additional Support
- Frankincense
- Melissa
- Thyme
- On Guard+ Softgels

Lifelong Vitality Pack® should be the base of every protocol. Use as directed.

Infertility

Inability to conceive children.

Description
Supports the reproductive system and proper hormone balance.

Suggested Duration
2-6 months

Full Body Detox
Follow protocol for Detox (full body).

AromaTouch® Technique
Receive from a certified practitioner weekly.

Clary Sage & Geranium
Apply a drop each to reproductive reflex points 2x daily.

Yarrow|Pom
Take 2 drops under tongue 2x daily.

DDR Prime® Softgels
Take 2 softgels 2x daily.

Lifelong Vitality Pack® Necessary

Additional Support
- Zendocrine®
- Rose
- Thyme
- AromaTouch®

Irritable Bowels

A collection of symptoms relating to the GI tract often attributed to possible infection or damage to the intestinal mucosa.

Description
Relieves symptoms of gas, bloating, constipation, diarrhea, and belching.

Suggested Duration
3-6 months

Peppermint Softgels
Take 2 softgels with meals.

TerraZyme®
Take 1-3 capsules w/each meal.

PB Assist®
Take 2 capsules in the morning and evening.

Cardamom & Turmeric
Drink a drop each in water to soothe discomfort as needed.

Lavender, Tea Tree, Frankincense, DigestZen®
Combine 10 drops each w/ FCO in 10ml roller. Apply over stomach 3x daily.

Additional Support
- Fennel
- Coriander
- Basil
- Lemongrass
- Caraway

Libido (low)

Decreased sex drive or sexual desire.

Description
Inspires an uninhibited sex drive.

Suggested Duration
2 weeks, then as needed

Passion®
Diffuse several drops and use a few drops diluted in intimate massage.

Ylang Ylang
Rub 1-2 drops on pulse points.

Clary Sage
Take 1-2 drops in capsule daily.

Lifelong Vitality Pack® Necessary

Additional Support
- Mito2Max®
- Whisper
- Cinnamon

Lupus

Autoimmune disease marked by inflammation of the skin and organs.

Description
Induces the parasympathetic nervous system, eliminates antigens and latent infections, and reduces the immune response.

Suggested Duration
1-3 years

Frankincense, Yarrow|Pom, Copaiba, Turmeric
Apply a drop of each to back of neck and bottoms of feet 2x daily.

DDR Prime®
Apply 2-4 drops to spine 2x daily. Also take 2 softgels 2x daily.

Deep Blue®
Massage into inflamed areas 3x daily or as needed.

PB Assist®
Take 2 capsules in the morning on an empty stomach.

Lifelong Vitality Pack® Necessary

Additional Support
- Turmeric Capsules
- Serenity Complex
- Zendocrine® Complex
- Yarrow|Pom
- DigestZen® Softgels

Protocols

Lifelong Vitality Pack® should be the base of every protocol. Use as directed.

Lyme Disease

Inflammatory disease caused by bacteria transmitted by ticks.

Description
Induces the parasympathetic nervous system, eliminates antigens and latent infections, and reduces the immune response

Suggested Duration
1-3 years

DDR Prime® & Copaiba
Apply 1-2 drops each to spine, back of neck, and bottoms of feet 3x daily.

Cinnamon, Sandalwood, Turmeric, Clary Sage
Take a drop of each in a capsule 2x daily.

Zendocrine®
Apply 2 drops to sides of neck 2x daily.

PB Assist®
Take 2 capsules in the morning on an empty stomach.

Copaiba Softgels
Take 1 softgel 3x daily.

Lifelong Vitality Pack® Necessary

Additional Support
- Yarrow|Pom
- Zendocrine® Complex
- Serenity Complex

Memory Issues

Difficulty recalling thoughts, names, events, and experiences.

Description
Increases the integrity of the gut lining and promotes brain health.

Suggested Duration
1-3 years

Rosemary, Vetiver, Black Spruce, Rose
Diffuse 2 drops each throughout the day. Apply a drop of each to back of neck 3x daily.

PB Assist®
Take 2 capsules in the morning on an empty stomach.

DDR Prime®
Apply 2-4 drops to spine and bottoms of feet 3x daily.

Copaiba Softgels
Take 1 softgel daily.

Additional Support
- Clary Sage
- Frankincense
- Sandalwood
- Yarrow|Pom

Menopause

The ceasing of menstruation, typically between 45 and 50 years of age.

Description
Aids in hormone and mood balance, calms hot flashes.

Suggested Duration
4 months, then as needed

ClaryCalm®
Rub onto pulse points 2x daily (avoid sun exposure for 12 hours after application).

Phytoestrogen Complex
Take 1 capsule 3x daily.

Peppermint
Apply a drop to back of neck to ease hot flashes.

Whisper
Wear as perfume daily

Lifelong Vitality Pack® Necessary

Additional Support
- Ylang Ylang
- Rose
- Geranium

Menstruation (PMS)

The discharge of blood and other materials from the lining of the uterus.

Description
Balances mood and hormones during menstruation.

Suggested Duration
2 weeks as needed

ClaryCalm®
Rub onto pulse points and over ovaries. Apply to calm cramping as needed (avoid sun exposure for 12 hours after application).

Balance
Rub behind ears to balance mood.

Phytoestrogen
Take 1 capsule 3x daily.

Lifelong Vitality Pack® Necessary

Additional Support
- Clary Sage
- Serenity
- PastTense®
- Madagascar Vanilla

Lifelong Vitality Pack® should be the base of every protocol. Use as directed.

Migraine

Recurrent throbbing headache accompanied by nausea and disturbed vision.

Description
Increases circulation and relieves pain.

Suggested Duration
1 day to 3 months

PastTense® & Helichrysum
Apply roller and a drop of Helichrysum to forehead, neck, and temples at the early onset of tension.

Deep Blue® Complex
Take 2 capsules 2x daily on an empty stomach.

DDR Prime®
Rub 2 drops onto bottoms of feet and spine 2x daily.

Copaiba Softgels
Take 2 softgels nightly.

Additional Support
- Copaiba
- Turmeric Capsules
- Frankincense
- Roman Chamomile
- Wintergreen

Mononucleosis

Viral disease with swelling of the lymph glands and prolonged lassitude

Description
Provides antiviral support.

Suggested Duration
8-16 weeks

Oregano, On Guard, Thyme
Take 1-2 drops each in a capsule 3x daily.

Frankincense, Black Pepper
Rub 2 drops each to bottoms of feet.

Mito2Max®
Take 1-2 capsules 2x daily.

Lifelong Vitality Pack® Necessary

Additional Support
- Melissa
- Cassia

Mood Balance

Need for stabilized emotional state, often related to stress or hormone levels.

Description
Activates the parasympathetic nervous system, induces a more calm and focused mental state.

Suggested Duration
6 months

Adaptiv™
Apply to web of hands and base of skull. Diffuse throughout the day.

Adaptiv™ Complex*
Take 1-2 capsules daily.

PB Assist®
Take 2 capsules in the morning on an empty stomach.

Serenity Complex
Take 2 softgels before bed.

Start slowly with Adaptiv™ Complex and observe yourself closely.

Additional Support
- Balance
- Ylang Ylang
- Roman Chamomile
- Frankincense
- Black Spruce
- Tulsi

Multiple Sclerosis

Nerve degeneration including the breakdown of the myelin sheath.

Description
Reduces symptoms of muscle weakness, muscle spasm, and chronic pain.

Suggested Duration
1-3 years

Frankincense, Sandalwood, Turmeric, Clary Sage
Take a drop of each in a capsule 3x daily.

Zendocrine®
Apply 2 drops to sides of neck 2x daily.

PB Assist®
Take 2 capsules in the morning on an empty stomach.

DDR Prime®
Apply 2-4 drops to spine, back of neck, and bottoms of feet 3x daily.

Lifelong Vitality Pack® Necessary

Additional Support
- Yarrow|Pom
- Lavender
- Serenity Complex
- Zendocrine® Complex

Lifelong Vitality Pack® should be the base of every protocol. Use as directed.

Muscle Aches

Inflammation and pain in one or more muscle region.

Description
Reduces inflammation, spasms, and pain in muscles.

Suggested Duration
2 weeks, then as needed

AromaTouch®
Massage 2-4 drops into aching muscles 3x daily.

Deep Blue® Complex
Take 1 capsule 3x daily

Frankincense, Lemon
Take 1-2 drops each in capsule 2x daily.

Magnolia
Apply to affected muscles as needed throughout the day.

Additional Support
- Deep Blue®
- Cypress
- Douglas Fir
- Black Pepper

Neuropathy

Condition of weakness, numbness and tingling due to nerve damage.

Description
Increases blood flow, reduces pain and assists in repair of damaged nerves.

Suggested Duration
1-3 years

DDR Prime® & Vetiver
Apply 2-4 drops each to spine and bottoms of feet 4x daily.

Deep Blue® Rub
Massage into affected area after above oils 4x daily.

Frankincense, Copaiba, Turmeric, Black Pepper
Take a drop of each in a capsule 2x daily.

PB Assist®
Take 2 capsules in the morning on an empty stomach.

Lifelong Vitality Pack® Necessary

Additional Support
- Zendocrine® Complex
- Deep Blue® Complex
- Rosemary
- Lavender

Nerve Damage

Dysfunction or breakdown of isolated nerves or the nervous system.

Description
Increases blood flow, reduces pain and assists in repair of damaged nerves.

Suggested Duration
3-6 months

DDR Prime® & Copaiba
Apply 1-2 drops each to spine and affected areas 4x daily.

Vetiver & Frankincense
Apply 2 drops of each to bottoms of feet 2x daily.

Yarrow|Pom
Use 3-6 drops under the tongue 3x daily.

Lifelong Vitality Pack® Necessary

Additional Support
- Copaiba
- Wintergreen

Obsessive Compulsive Disorder

Excessive or obsessive thoughts that lead to compulsive behaviors.

Description
Increases a general calming state due to the interaction of oils with neurotransmitters.

Suggested Duration
12 months

Roman Chamomile, Rose, Vetiver
Apply a drop of each to bottoms of feet 3x daily.

Adaptiv™
Apply to web of hands and base of skull. Diffuse throughout the day

Adaptiv™ Complex*
Take 1-2 capsules daily.

PB Assist®
Take 2 capsules in the morning on an empty stomach.

Lifelong Vitality Pack® Necessary

Additional Support
- Melissa
- Black Spruce
- Sandalwood
- Lavender

Lifelong Vitality Pack® should be the base of every protocol. Use as directed.

Pets (anxiety)

Excessive uneasiness due to a variety of causes.

Description
Induces a general calming state and promotes proper neurotransmitters.

Suggested Duration
3 weeks, then as needed

Roman Chamomile, Lavender, OR Vetiver
Dilute 1 drop to 1 Tbs FCO and apply to coat of animal 2x daily (dilute more for sensitie animals).

Balance
Diffuse a few drops during the day.

Serenity
Diffuse a few drops at night.

Additional Support
- Frankincense
- Siberian Fir
- Sandalwood
- Black Spruce

Pets (fleas & bugs)

Fleas, ticks, and other pests.

Description
Prevents, removes, and repels fleas and various insects.

Suggested Duration
3 months, then as needed

Rosemary, Peppermint, Eucalyptus, Tea Tree
Add 10 drops of each to 20 oz spray bottle of water. Shake and spray the solution on the coat of pet 3x daily.

TerraShield®
Combine 15 drops with carrier oil and apply to coat of pet 2x daily.

Additional Support
- Citronella

Plantar Fasciitis

Inflammation of the fascia attached to the from the heel to the metatarsal bones of the foot.

Description
Reduces pain and inflammation.

Suggested Duration
Ongoing

Turmeric Capsules
Take 2 capsules in the morning.

DDR Prime® & Turmeric
Apply 2 each to affected area 3x daily

Deep Blue® Rub
Massage into affected area as needed.

Copaiba Softgels
Take 2 softgels before bed.

Additional Support
- Frankincense
- Rosemary
- Yarrow|Pom
- Wintergreen

Pneumonia

Infection that inflames air sacs in lungs, accompanied by cough, phlegm, fever, and chills.

Description
Increases immune response to address possible infections and open the airways for symptomatic relief.

Suggested Duration
1-2 weeks

Cardamom, Black Pepper, Rosemary, Lime
Apply drop of each to chest and bottoms of feet 3-5x daily.

Breathe
Diffuse several drops; inhale 2 drops from cupped hands as needed.

On Guard+ Softgels
Take 2 softgels 2x daily until symptoms subside.

Lifelong Vitality Pack® Necessary

Additional Support
- Pink Pepper
- Oregano
- Melissa
- Lemon Eucalyptus

Lifelong Vitality Pack® should be the base of every protocol. Use as directed.

Pregnancy (postnatal)

Care for mother after giving birth.

Description
Promotes pain relief, tissue healing, and emotional support after giving birth.

Suggested Duration
4-8 weeks

Helichrysum, Myrrh, Frankincense, Lavender
Apply a drop each diluted to areas with tearing and over stretch marks 3x daily.

Ylang Ylang or Adaptiv™
Diffuse for mood balancing.

Phytoestrogen
Take 1 capsule 3x daily.

Adaptiv™ Complex*
Take 1 capsule 2x daily

ClaryCalm®
Apply over lower abdomen.

Start slow with Adaptiv™ Complex and observe yourself closely.

Lifelong Vitality Pack® Necessary

Additional Support
- Geranium
- Clary Sage

Pregnancy (prenatal)

Care for mother during pregnancy.

Description
Relieves pregnancy sickness, provides vital nutrients, provides emotional support.

Suggested Duration
9 months

DigestZen® or Ginger
Drink 2 drops to ease nausea.

Bone Nutrient Complex
Take 1 capsule w/meals.

TerraZyme®
Take 1 capsule w/meals.

Black Spruce
Rub a drop diluted over lower abdomen daily to improve immunity at the placenta

Lavender & Lemon
Add a drop each to a glass of water daily to minimize pregnancy complications.

Lifelong Vitality Pack® Necessary

Additional Support
- Ylang Ylang
- Balance
- Elevation
- Rose

Psoriasis

Skin disease marked by red, itchy, scaly patches.

Description
Relieves itchy, swollen skin, and promotes proper immune system function.

Suggested Duration
4-8 weeks

Helichrysum, Lavender, Frankincense, Tea Tree
Combine 10 drops each with carrier oil in roller bottle. Apply 3x daily

PB Assist®
Take 2 capsules in the morning on an empty stomach.

TerraZyme®
Take 1-3 w/each meal.

DDR Prime®
Take 1-2 softgels 3x daily.

Additional Support
- Copaiba
- Immortelle
- Cedarwood
- Yarrow|Pom

Rash

Patches of scales, dryness, pustules or redness of the skin.

Description
Reduces infection, calms inflammatory response, promotes new skin cell growth.

Suggested Duration
2-4 weeks, then as needed

Arborvitae, Tea Tree, Frankincense
Combine a drop of each with carrier oil and apply 3-5x daily.

Apply a warm towel compress over the area after oils are applied in the evening.

PB Assist®
Take 2 capsules in the morning on an empty stomach.

On Guard+ Softgels
Take 2 softgels 2x daily.

Additional Support
- Myrrh
- Sandalwood
- Yarrow|Pom

Lifelong Vitality Pack® should be the base of every protocol. Use as directed.

Rheumatoid Arthritis

Often hereditary condition causing nodules on the fingers, pain, and stiffness.

Description
Relieves pain and discomfort by increasing blood flow and circulation to the area.

Suggested Duration
Ongoing

Copaiba, Turmeric, Frankincense
Apply a drop of each to affected areas 3x daily.

Deep Blue® Rub
Massage into affected areas after above oils 3x daily.

Deep Blue® Complex
Take 2 capsules in the evening with food.

DDR Prime® Softgels
Take 2 softgels 3x daily.

Copaiba Softgels
Take 1 softgel daily

Lifelong Vitality Pack® Necessary

Additional Support
- Marjoram
- Lemongrass

Scarring (uterine)

Trauma to the uterine lining resulting in excess scar tissue.

Description
Increases circulation, reduces scar tissue, promotes healing.

Suggested Duration
1 year, then as needed

Clary Sage, Frankincense, Ylang Ylang
Apply a drop of each to lower abdomen 2x daily. Cover with a hot compress towel with evening application.

DDR Prime®
Apply 2-4 drops to abdomen 2x daily.

PB Assist®
Take 2 capsules in the morning on an empty stomach.

Additional Support
- Yarrow|Pom
- Sandalwood
- Myrrh
- Patchouli

Sciatica

Condition often caused by injury, overuse, or general degradation to the sciatic nerve.

Description
Reduces pain, increases circulation, and promotes healing.

Suggested Duration
6-12 months

DDR Prime®
Apply 2-4 drops to bottoms of feet 2x daily.

Frankincense, Turmeric, Lavender
Massage a drop each into painful areas 2x daily.

Deep Blue® Rub
Massage into painful areas throughout the day as needed.

Deep Blue® Complex
Take 2 capsules 2x daily on an empty stomach.

Lifelong Vitality Pack® Necessary

Additional Support
- Yarrow|Pom
- Copaiba
- AromaTouch®
- Turmeric Capsules

Seizures (myoclonic)

Disease where nerve cell activity is disturbed in the brain.

Description
Reduces the duration and frequency of seizures.

Suggested Duration
6-12 months, then as needed

DDR Prime®
Take 2 capsules in the morning on an empty stomach.

Frankincense & Copaiba
Take a drop of each in a capsule or hold to the roof of mouth for 30 seconds 2x daily.

PB Assist®
Take 2 capsules in the morning on an empty stomach.

Immediately apply 4 drops of Frankincense to back of neck and bottoms of feet during seizure.

Lifelong Vitality Pack® Necessary

Additional Support
- Yarrow|Pom
- Turmeric

Lifelong Vitality Pack® should be the base of every protocol. Use as directed.

Shingles
Viral infection that often occurs on the face or intercostal region.

Description
Decreases the expression of the viral infection, alleviates pain, and maintains a preventative regiment.

Suggested Duration
1 week to 3 months

PB Assist®
Take 2 capsules morning and evening on an empty stomach.

Melissa & Tea Tree
Apply a drop of each with carrier oil to blisters 6x daily.

On Guard+ Softgels
Take 2 softgels 2x daily after food.

xEO Mega®
Take 2 softgels 2x daily.

Lifelong Vitality Pack® Necessary

Additional Support
· On Guard
· Siberian Fir
· Lemon Myrtle

Sinusitis
Bacterial infection resulting in pressure in the face, mucus discharge, and fatigue.

Description
Clears the bacterial infections and assists in the remediation of the symptoms.

Suggested Duration
1–4 weeks

PB Assist®
Take 2 capsules morning and evening on an empty stomach.

Myrrh & Melissa
Apply a drop of each with carrier oil over the maxillary sinus region 6x daily.

On Guard+ Softgels
Take 2 softgels 2x daily after food.

xEO Mega®
Take 2 softgels 2x daily.

Additional Support
· Cardamom
· Rosemary
· Oregano
· Helichrysum

Sleep (insomnia)
Inability to fall or stay asleep.

Description
Induces a calming state that allows one to fall and stay asleep.

Suggested Duration
3 months, then as needed.

PB Assist®
Take 2 capsules in the morning on an empty stomach.

Serenity Complex
Take 2 softgels 30 minutes before bed.

Serenity
Apply 2 drops to temples and bottoms of feet. Diffuse 4-8 drops near bedside.

Vetiver & Wild Orange
Take a drop of each under the tongue before bed.

Additional Support
· Frankincense
· Sandalwood
· Balance
· Peace

Sleep Apnea
Disorder with pauses in or periods of shallow breathing during sleep.

Description
Promotes open airways and more meaningful sleep.

Suggested Duration
Ongoing

Breathe
Diffuse 5-10 drops next to bedside at night. Also apply over bridge of nose and to sinus reflex points.

On Guard
Gargle 2 drops with water for 30 seconds, then swallow right before bed.

Serenity Complex
Take 2 softgels 30 minutes before bed.

Lifelong Vitality Pack® Necessary

Additional Support
· Peppermint
· Rosemary
· Wintergreen

Lifelong Vitality Pack® should be the base of every protocol. Use as directed.

Smoking (stop)

Addiction to smoking cigarettes, vape pens, or other forms of nicotine.

Description
Helps curb cravings and smoking addiction, aids in detox.

Suggested Duration
6-12 weeks

Grapefruit
Drink 1-3 drops in water throughout the day.

On Guard
Swish 2 drops with water when cravings arise, especially after eating.

Black Pepper
Apply 1 drop to big toes 2x daily. Also inhale or diffuse throughout the day.

Zendocrine®
Apply 2-4 drops to bottoms of feet 30 minutes before showering.

Additional Support
- Clove
- Zendocrine® Complex

Snoring

Disturbed vibrating or grunting sound in a person's breathing during sleep.

Description
Promotes open airways during sleep.

Suggested Duration
Ongoing

Breathe
Diffuse 5-10 drops near bedside at night. Also apply to bridge of nose, throat, and lung reflex points.

On Guard
Gargle 2 drops with water for 30 seconds, then swallow.

Lemon
Drink 1-3 drops in water before bed.

Additional Support
- Eucalyptus
- Rosemary
- Peppermint

Sore Throat

Pain in the throat due to inflammation from a virus or bacteria.

Description
Relieves pain and soreness in throat, provides antiviral and antibacterial support.

Suggested Duration
5-10 days

Lemon (20), On Guard (15), Helichrysum (4)
Combine in 15ml glass spray bottle with carrier oil. Spray toward back of throat as needed

Lavender, Arborvitae
Massage 1-2 drops with carrier oil to outside of throat.

Additional Support
- Melissa
- Black Pepper
- Petitgrain

Stress

Emotional upset, physical malfunction, and mental stress.

Description
Increases a general calming state due to the interaction of oils with neurotransmitters.

Suggested Duration
4-8 weeks, then as needed

Adaptiv™
Apply to web of hands and base of skull. Diffuse throughout the day.

Adaptiv™ Complex*
Take 1-2 capsules daily.

Balance
Apply 1-2 drops to temples during 10 minute daily meditation.

Serenity Complex
Take 2 softgels 30 minutes before bed.

Additional Support
- Rose
- Roman Chamomile
- Black Spruce
- Sandalwood
- Citrus Bloom®

Lifelong Vitality Pack® should be the base of every protocol. Use as directed.

Sunburn

Reddening, inflammation, and sometimes blistering from sun overexposure.

Description
Relieves discomfort from sunburn, promotes healing.

Suggested Duration
3-7 days

Lavender, Yarrow|Pom, Helichrysum
Apply 2-4 drops with carrier oil or aloe to sunburnt skin 3-5x daily.

Peppermint
Add 5 drops to small glass spray bottle with water. Spritz to cool skin.

Additional Support
- Cedarwood
- Copaiba
- Roman Chamomile

Thrush

Infection of the mouth and throat from yeast-like fungus causing white patches.

Description
Provides anti-fungal support, eases oral discomfort.

Suggested Duration
1-3 weeks

Lemon, Tea Tree, IQ Mega®-
Combine 2 drops of each essential oil with 1 Tbs of omegas. Apply with clean finger to child's gums and tongue 2-3x daily.

Tea Tree & Lavender
Massage a drop into bottoms of child's feet 1x daily.

Additional Support
- Geranium
- Helichrysum

Thyroid
(Hyper/ Grave's)

Autoimmune disorder resulting in excess of thyroid hormone.

Description
Assists with regulating the metabolism, detoxifying the body, and restoring balance.

Suggested Duration
1-3 years

PB Assist®
Take 2 capsules in the morning on an empty stomach.

Vetiver (10), Turmeric (10), Myrrh (10), Siberian Fir (5)
Combine oils in a 10ml roller with FCO. Apply over thyroid 3-5x daily.

Balance
Apply 2-4 drops to bottoms of feet morning and night.

Zendocrine®
Take 2 softgels 2x daily.

Lifelong Vitality Pack® Necessary

Additional Support
- Sandalwood
- Basil
- Zendocrine® Complex

Thyroid
(Hypo/ Hashimoto's)

Autoimmune disorder resulting in insufficient thyroid hormone.

Description
Assists with regulating the metabolism, detoxifying the body, and restoring balance.

Suggested Duration
1-3 years

Myrrh (10), Turmeric (10), Clove (6), Lemongrass (6), Copaiba (10)
Combine oils in a 10ml roller with FCO. Apply over thyroid 3-5x daily.

Mito2Max®
Take 2 capsules 2x daily.

Zendocrine® Softgels
Take 2 softgels 2x daily.

DDR Prime® & Softgels
Apply 2 drops to bottoms of feet 2x daily. Also take 1-2 softgels 2x daily.

Lifelong Vitality Pack® Necessary

Additional Support
- PB Assist®
- Lemon Myrtle
- Rosemary
- Basil

Lifelong Vitality Pack® should be the base of every protocol. Use as directed.

Tinnitus

The feeling of noise or ringing in the ears.

Description
Soothes auditory canal and neurological auditory triggers.

Suggested Duration
3 months, then as needed

Helichrysum & Balance
Apply a drop of each around outside of ears and back of neck 3x daily.

Mito2Max®
Take 2 capsules 2x daily.

DDR Prime® Softgels
Take 2 softgels 2x daily.

Additional Support
- Frankincense
- Siberian Fir
- Sandalwood

Toenail Fungus

Infection often caused by the overuse of antibiotics.

Description
Combats fungus growth and provides preventative regimen.

Suggested Duration
1-3 months

Citronella & Tea Tree
Apply 1-2 drops each to affected area 3x daily.

On Guard+ Softgels
Take 2 softgels 2x daily.

DDR Prime® Softgels
Take 2 softgels 2x daily.

Additional Support
- Neroli
- Oregano
- Clove
- Arborvitae

Tourette's

Nervous system disorder that leads to repetitive vocalizations, limb or facial movement.

Description
Lessens the severity and occurrence of tics.

Suggested Duration
1-5 years

Rose, Clary Sage, Vetiver
Apply a drop each to back of neck, spine, and bottoms of feet 3x daily.

InTune®
Apply to temples and sides of neck 3x daily.

PB Assist®
Take 2 capsules in the morning on an empty stomach.

DDR Prime® Softgels
Take 2 softgels 2x daily

Lifelong Vitality Pack® Necessary

Additional Support
- Frankincense
- Siberian Fir
- Roman Chamomile

Urinary Tract Infection

Infection of the ureters from the kidneys t the bladder

Description
Aids in combating bacterial infection and restoring regular immune defenses.

Suggested Duration
1-4 weeks

Oregano, Lemongrass, Frankincense, Clove
Take a drop each in a capsule 3-5x daily (discontinue Oregano and Lemongrass if more than 10 days).

DDR Prime® & Cypress
Rub 2 drops each over lower abdomen 2x daily. Dilute for sensitive skin.

PB Assist®
Take 2 capsules in the morning on an empty stomach.

Additional Support
- Arborvitae
- Thyme
- On Guard
- Melissa

Protocols

Lifelong Vitality Pack® should be the base of every protocol. Use as directed.

Weight Loss (skin condition)

Stretch marks and sagging skin after weight loss.

Description
Improves appearance of scar tissue and helps restore skin elasticity.

Suggested Duration
8-12 weeks

Myrrh, Helichrysum, Frankincense, Yarrow|Pom
Massage 2 drops each with carrier oil into stretch marks 2x daily.

Slim & Sassy® & Myrrh
Rub 3-5 drops each with carrier oil onto sagging skin. Cover oils with warm towel compress for 30 minutes before bed.

Additional Support
- Veráge® or Anti-Aging skincare line
- Yarrow|Pom body spray

Weight Loss

Excess weight usually due to the body's inability to access ketosis.

Description
Assists with burning glucose and glycogen supplies at a faster rate in order to access the ketotic fat burning state.

Suggested Duration
3-6 months

Slim & Sassy®
Apply 10-15 drops with carrier oil to abdomen and fatty areas at night.

Also drink 3-5 drops in water throughout the day

DDR Prime®
Apply 2-4 drops of oil to lower abdomen 2x daily. Take 2 softgels 2x daily.

Zendocrine® Softgels
Take 2 softgels 2x daily.

Lifelong Vitality Pack® Necessary

Additional Support
- Slim & Sassy® Softgels
- Coriander
- Fennel
- Celery Seed

Wrinkles

Age effects or trauma to the overall integrity of the skin.

Description
Restores skin integrity and appearance of fine lines and wrinkles.

Suggested Duration
Ongoing

Immortelle
Apply over wrinkles 2x daily.

Yarrow|Pom
Massage 2-4 drops eveninly over skin after washing.

xEO Mega®
Take 2 softgels 2x daily.

DDR Prime® Softgels
Take 2 softgels 2x daily

Lifelong Vitality Pack® Necessary

Additional Support
- Sandalwood
- Arborvitae
- Myrrh
- Blue Tansy
- Veráge® or Anti-Aging skincare line

Yeast Infection

Fungal infection often caused by the overuse of antibiotics.

Description
Combats fungal infection and restores balance in the gut and affected areas.

Suggested Duration
1-3 months

PB Assist®
Take 2 capsules morning and evening on an empty stomach.

Lemon Eucalyptus, Clove, Tea Tree
Apply 1 drop of each diluted over vaginal area or lower abdomen 6x daily.

On Guard+ Softgels
Take 2 softgels 2x daily after food.

Lifelong Vitality Pack® Necessary

Additional Support
- Arborvitae
- Green Mandarin
- Oregano
- Thyme

Lifelong Vitality Pack® should be the base of every protocol. Use as directed.

Section 7
Lifestyle *Protocols*

Lifestyle Protocols

Take your wellness experience to the next level with Lifestyle Protocols.

You've used the Ailments section and the Protocols by Ailments to troubleshoot health challenges. Now use Lifestyle Protocols to uplevel the parts of your life you want to enhance.

Choose a Lifestyle Protocol that matches where you want to go next with your wellness. Do the protocol for the suggested time, then evaluate your progress.

If you're satisfied, move onto the next Lifestyle Protocol that stands out to you. If you feel you have more work to do, stick with the one you're on!

You can't go wrong with choosing a Lifestyle Protocol. Each one will take you in a positive direction.

After all, anything that points you toward a natural solutions lifestyle is the right direction!

BTW - if things are good right now, use the *Good Life* protocol!

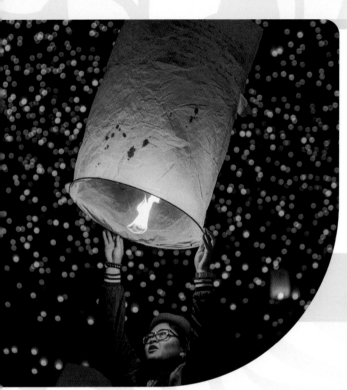

Abundance Generator

Sometimes life calls you to focus on more abundance. Whether it's abundance in money, health, or life-satisfaction, this protocol will help you draw good things to you.

Protocol Benefits
• Opens your first chakra (money & stability)
• Grounds your energy to the present moment
• Opens your mind to the story of new possibilities
• Creates an emotional set point for gratitude in your day

Time frame
*Do this protocol for **4 weeks**. Then reevaluate or switch to another Lifestyle Protocol.*

Abundant Atmosphere

Wild Orange
Diffuse 6-8 drops every day.

Elevation
Breathe a couple drops from your palms while focusing on your abundant future periodically each day.

First Chakra

Balance
Massage 2 drops into the heels of your feet each morning and night.

Vetiver & Rosemary
Add a drop of each to floor of your shower in the morning.

Dreamstorm

Get a special notebook to dreamstorm in once a day. It's best to do it first thing in the morning before the world takes over your attention.

Spend 10-15 minutes writing what you're grateful for and what you're excited to see unfold in your life.

Then review what you've written just before going to bed.

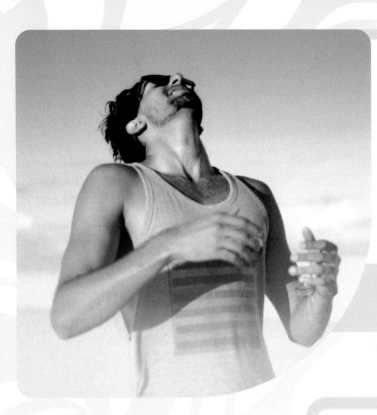

Addiction Recovery

Regain the satisfaction of being in control of your desires, cravings, and where you derive satisfaction in life with this protocol.

Protocol Benefits
- Helps curb cravings
- Uses activity as a healthy distraction
- Fortifies self-concept

Time frame
*Use this protocol for **8 weeks**. Then reevaluate to determine if you'll continue or move onto another Lifestyle Protocol.*

Confident Reflection

Align
Rub a drop over your heart during times of weakness.

Visualizing
Visualize yourself whole and complete while using the Align blend each day.

Craving Control

Black Pepper
Rub a drop on bottoms of feet (especially big toes), morning and night.

Grapefruit
Drink 4-8 drops in a glass or stainless steel water bottle throughout the day.

Purify
Diffuse 4-6 drops daily.

Active Distraction

Daily Physical Activity
Use walking, running, weight lifting, yoga, or other daily physical activity to keep endorphins and spirits high.

Mito2Max®
Take 2 capsules 30 minutes before physical activity.

Breathe
Rub 2 drops onto chest before and during physical activity.

Lifestyles

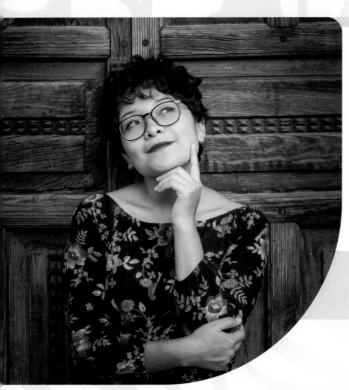

Age *Defier*

Aging is nothing more than the process of returning to childhood in many cultures. For those who choose youth over the temptation to slow down, this protocol keeps vitality from fading too quickly.

Protocol Benefits
- Decrease pain & inflammation
- Support cellular & organ health
- Improve digestion & elimination
- Reverse the appearance of aging

Time frame
*Use this protocol for **12 weeks,** then as desired for continued anti-aging benefits.*

Youthful Skin & Complexion

Immortelle
Roll on this blend daily to reduce age spots and wrinkles.

Essential Oil Skincare
Use Veráge® or Anti-Aging skincare products daily to provide anti-aging nutrients.

Pain Reducer

Deep Blue® Complex
Take 2 capsules whenever pain arises, or take 1 capsule 3x daily.

Deep Blue®
Massage a few drops into sore areas as often as needed.

Frankincense
Take a drop under the tongue. Also diffuse several drops.

Brain & Memory Booster

DDR Prime®
Take 2 softgels 2x daily.

Peppermint & Rosemary
Diffuse several drops of each daily. Also massage a couple drops onto back of neck.

Energy & Cellular Health

Lifelong Vitality Pack®
Take 2 of each bottle 2x daily.

Mito2Max®
Take 2 capsules 30 minutes before yoga or working out.

Citrus Bliss®
Inhale 2-4 drops from cupped hands as needed. Also diffuse several drops.

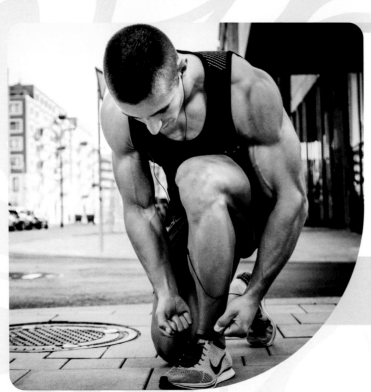

The *Athlete*

Life is about the hustle. For athletes of any kind, the hustle is sustainable when you care for your body and all the systems that make the machine work.

Protocol Benefits
- Eases stress on joints and connective tissue
- Soothes sore muscles & speeds recovery
- Provides full-body energy
- Boosts mood and motivation to increase likelihood of sticking with your routine

Time frame
*Use this protocol for **12 weeks** during training, then as desired to continually support your active lifestyle.*

Respiratory System Support

Breathe
Rub 2 drops onto chest before and during exercise.

Eucalyptus
Add 2 drops onto your shower floor during your post-workout shower.

Mood & Motivation Elevator

Motivate
Inhale 2 drops from your palms to prepare mentally for your routine.

Peppermint
Put a small dab on your tongue.

Full Body Energy Supply

Lifelong Vitality Pack®
Take 2 of each bottle 2x daily.

Mito2Max®
Take 2 capsules 30 minutes before yoga or working out.

Protein (Whey or Plant)
Drink a serving within 30 minutes of working out and as needed daily.

Muscle & Joint Support

Deep Blue® Complex
Take 2 capsules before working out.

Deep Blue®
Massage a few drops into muscles as a pre-workout. Also massage into sore areas post-workout.

Lemongrass
Rub 2 drops diluted into ligaments & joints that have been worked hard.

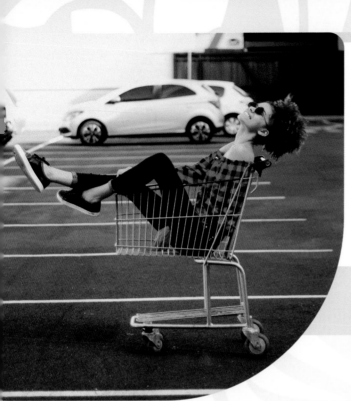

Auto-Immune-*Proof*

This protocol facilitates DNA repair, addresses unhealthy inflammatory issues, and gently supports regular immune function.

Protocol Benefits
- Focuses on long-term damaged DNA repair
- Helps balance and calm unhealthy inflammation
- Supports healthy immune function without stimulating hyper immune activity.

Time frame
*Do this protocol for **12 weeks**. Then reevaluate or switch to another Lifestyle Protocol.*

Immune System Fortification

PB Assist®
Take 1 capsule 3x daily with meals.

On Guard
Diffuse 4-6 drops daily, and rub 2 drops onto bottoms of feet in the morning.

Damaged DNA Repair

DDR Prime® Softgels
Take 2 softgels 2-3x daily.

DDR Prime®
Rub 2-4 drops into spine and or the bottoms of your feet every night before bed.

Inflammation Regulation

Lifelong Vitality Pack®
Take 2 of each bottle twice daily.

Deep Blue® Complex
Take 1 capsule 3x daily.

Frankincense, Turmeric & Copaiba
Use a drop of each under your tongue 2-3x daily. Also rub onto spine as needed.

Balance
Rub 2 drops on the bottoms of feet daily.

Lifestyles

217

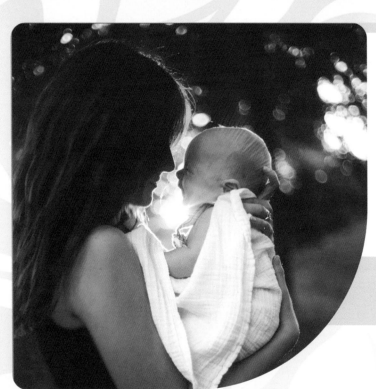

Babies: *Healthy and On-Track*

A healthy and happy baby brings happiness to the whole home. Use this protocol to address the basic elements of infant health.

Protocol Benefits
- Boosts baby's immune system
- Calms tummy troubles & solves digestive issues
- Keeps skin soothed and soft
- Helps baby feel calm and peaceful

Time frame
Use this protocol on an ongoing basis to maintain baby's health. Troubleshoot specific ailments in the other sections of this book as needed.

Happy Skin & Bums

Calmer
Rub gently with lotion onto baby's bum 2-3x daily to keep diaper rash away.

Also combine with baby lotion to soothe other areas of baby's skin.

Peaceful Mood

Lavender & Wild Orange
Let baby breathe a drop of each from your hands to soothe crying.

Peace
Diffuse 4-6 drops in baby's room to calm baby's temper.

Bolstered Immune System

On Guard
Diffuse 4-6 drops in the home daily to keep baby's immune system high. Rub a dab onto feet once a day for immune boost.

Lemon
Use as a gentle sanitizer on your hands and on commonly used objects.

Healthy Tummy

Tamer
Massage gently onto baby's tummy to calm digestive trouble (diarrhea, constipation, and tummy ache).

Bergamot
Rub a drop onto baby's feet 1-2x a day to stimulate healthy digestive function.

Babies: *Healthy Connection*

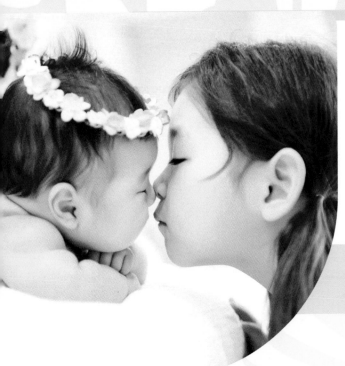

Sometimes baby can be inconsolable, detached, or overly attached. Healthy emotional connections set baby up for better overall health and a calmer home experience.

Protocol Benefits
- Promotes healthy maternal bond
- Promotes healthy paternal bond
- Calms anxiety and increases peaceful environment at home

Time frame
*Do this protocol for **2 weeks.** Then reevaluate or switch to another Lifestyle Protocol.*

Peaceful & Soothing Home

Peace or Console
Diffuse 4-6 drops of either blend to promote a peaceful atmosphere.

Combine with the power of music (classical music or new age piano) for powerful impact.

Soothing Maternal Bond

Myrrh & Geranium
Diffuse 2 drops of each during cuddle time with mom. Also rub a drop of each diluted over baby's back.

This is especially powerful during nursing or while singing to baby.

Soothing Paternal Bond

Patchouli & Frankincense
Diffuse 2 drops of each during cuddle time with dad. Also rub a drop of each diluted over baby's back.

This can be especially important if dad works out of the home.

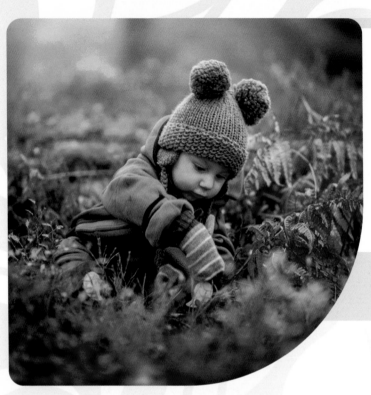

Babies: *Immunity Boosting*

This protocol is focused on babies who need extra support in developing a strong immune system.

Protocol Benefits
- Combats harmful pathogens in the air
- Sanitizes common surfaces naturally
- Improves immune system at the gut level
- Supercharges immune system through direct application

Time frame
*Do this protocol for **8 weeks**. Then reevaluate or switch to a different protocol.*

Immunity Supercharge

Stronger
Rub onto baby's spine and bottoms of feet 2-3x daily.

Frankincense
Rub a drop diluted into baby's spine nightly for full-body cellular support.

Healthy Gut for Healthy Immunity

Bergamot
Rub a drop neat onto baby's feet 1-2x daily.

PB Assist® Jr
Dissolve 1/2 sachet into baby's bottle once a day to improve immune system at the gut level (do not heat).

Clean & Safe Environment

Purify
Diffuse 4-6 drops to cleanse impurities from the air.

Lemon & On Guard
Combine several drops of each with water and a Tbs rubbing alcohol in a glass spray bottle to make a natural sanitizing surface cleaner.

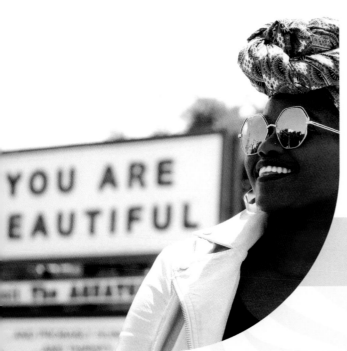

Beautifying

Beauty is a concept that starts from an internal perception. Use this protocol to nourish beauty on the outside and a healthy self-concept on the inside.

Protocol Benefits
- Uses oil-infused skincare to maintain healthy skin
- Repairs sun damage and signs of aging
- Provides extra nourishment to skin
- Encourages a healthy internal self-concept

Time frame
Do this protocol for **12 weeks.** *Then reevaluate, considering whether to continue your line of skincare products or to try another line of oil-infused skincare.*

Skin Enhancement

Immortelle
Massage into age spots, fine lines, and wrinkles daily as needed.

xEO Mega®
Double your daily dose of the omega complex to provide extra nourishment to your skin.

Beautiful Self-Concept

Beautiful
Apply to wrists and over heart during meditation, journaling, or while speaking positive affirmations in the mirror when you first wake up and right before bed.

Neroli & Rose
Wear as a perfume, remembering a few things you like about yourself each time you notice the fragrance.

Natural Skincare

Essential Oil Skincare
Use Veráge® or Anti-Aging skincare products daily to naturally protect skin from premature aging, to maintain suppleness, and to improve skin color.

Cleanser: *Use during morning shower and to remove makeup before bed.*
Toner: *Apply to restore skin nutrients after cleansing.*
Moisturizer: *Apply directly after toner.*
Serum: *Apply to improve fine lines and wrinkles as needed.*

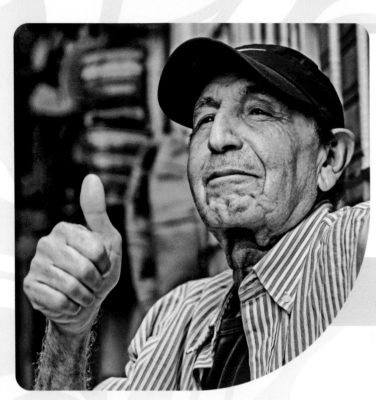

Brainiacs: *Mental Health*

This protocol supports healthy brains of all ages. It focuses on stimulating healthy neurological activity, brain chemistry, and a general sense of alertness.

Protocol Benefits
• Provides nutrients for brain and gut health
• Activates healthy neurological activity
• Stimulates mental activity aromatically
• Enhances memory

Time frame
Use this protocol for **12 weeks.** *Then reevaluate to continue use or switch to a different Lifestyle Protocol.*

Lifestyles

Aromatic Stimulant

Basil, Lavender, & Lime
Diffuse 2 drops of each to stimulate the mind and senses in the afternoons.

Neurological Activator

Vetiver
Rub a drop onto bottoms of feet and behind ears daily.

DDR Prime® & Copaiba
Massage 2 drops into spine or bottoms of feet daily.

Brain 1 & Brain 2 Fuel

Lifelong Vitality Pack®
Take 2 of each bottle 2x daily.

DDR Prime® Softgels
Take 2 softgels 2-3x daily.

PB Assist®
Take 1 capsule 3x daily to enhance the gut (the 2nd brain) and support neurotransmitter production.

Memory Enhancement

Rosemary & Peppermint
Diffuse several drops of each daily. Also massage a couple drops onto back of neck.

Peppermint
Use a drop of Peppermint on the tongue to awaken the mind as needed.

Frankincense
Hold a drop on your thumb to the roof of your mouth once daily.

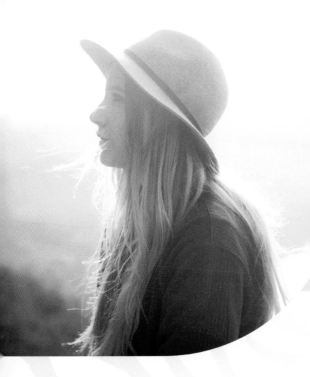

Cancer Combat

The body has the power to heal itself. While essential oils do not cure cancer, they facilitate a healthy alkaline environment, encourage proper cellular apoptosis, and support morale while combating cancer. These add up to a powerful cancer regimen.

Protocol Benefits
• Facilitates damaged DNA repair
• Promotes alkalinity & anti-carcinoma support
• Provides crucial and alkalizing nutrition
• Boosts morale & encouragement

Time frame
Do this protocol for **16 weeks**. *You may increase the frequency of any of the components. Reevaluate and continue as needed.*

Morale Booster

Elevation
Diffuse several drops or inhale from cupped hands as often as needed.

Damaged DNA Repair

DDR Prime® Softgels
Take 2 softgels 2-3x daily.

DDR Prime®
Massage 2 drops into spine and bottoms of feet twice daily.

Cellular Nutrition & Fuel

Lifelong Vitality Pack®
Take 2 capsules of each bottle twice daily.

Plant-Based Diet
Move to a completely plant-based diet. Avoid processed foods. Consume as much raw produce as possible.

Alkalinity & Anti-carcinoma Assist

Frankincense
Rub 2-4 drops Frankincense over or close to affected areas 4-8 times daily.

Sandalwood, Frankincense, & Siberian Fir:
Diffuse 2 drops of each throughout the day.

Cinnamon & Lemon
Drink 1 drop Cinnamon & 4 drops Lemon in water throughout the day.

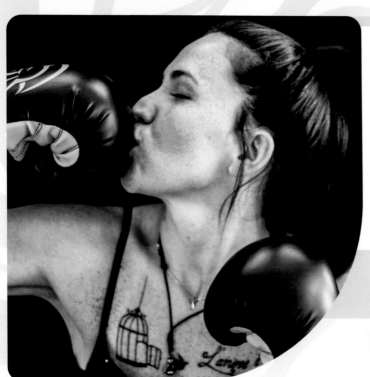

Confidence Overhaul

Self-confidence comes not from external validation, but from within. Use this protocol to process self-defeating emotions and patterns, to center your self-perception, and to reinforce a strong self-concept.

Protocol Benefits
- Grounds and centers your energy
- Opens your heart to vulnerability and possibility
- Redefines your perception of yourself and your future

Time frame
*Use this protocol for **21 days.** Then reevaluate and decide to continue or switch to a different Lifestyle Protocol.*

Grounding & Centering

Balance
Apply 2 drops to the bottoms of your feed each morning. Begin the day with prayer or gratitude, even if it's brief.

Align
Diffuse 4-6 drops in the home or office to keep your attention focused within.

Heart Opener

Beautiful
Apply over your heart 2-3x daily. Place your hand over your heart, and speak out loud a few things you appreciate about yourself.

Forgive or Console
Inhale a couple drops of either blend when you need to surrender old self-defeating patterns.

Self-Concept Reinforcement

Redefining Your Future Self
Spend 15 minutes each day visualizing or journaling about your ideal future self. Learn to define yourself not by what you see now, but by whom you know you're growing into.

Your Favorite Oil or Blend
Reinforce your concept of the new self by enjoying your favorite oil each time you do this exercise.

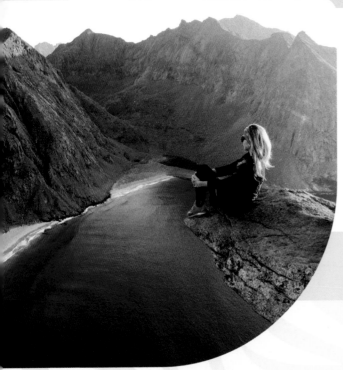

Emotional Detox

There are seasons to renew, and there are seasons to detox. Use this protocol to protect your energetic boundaries, purge pain and negativity from your body and energy, and to claim a more joyful state.

Protocol Benefits
- Cleanses the energy in your environment
- Trains your mind and soul to expect a new emotional set point
- Purges negativity from your physical body

Time frame
*Use this protocol for **21 days.** Then reevaluate and decide to continue or switch to a different Lifestyle Protocol.*

Negativity Purge

Deep Blue®
Use a few drops during daily exercise, focusing on allowing your body to release old pain and negative emotions.

Exercise that gets your heart rate up is ideal for this kind of release.

Purified Environment

Purify
Diffuse 4-6 drops daily, especially during meditation and journaling.

Tea Tree
Apply a drop to wrists after interactions with less-than-healthy relationships. This oil assists with "energetic vampirism."

Joy Infusion

Elevation
Add a couple drops to the floor of your shower each morning.

Motivate
Diffuse 4-6 drops or inhale a couple drops from your palms to elevate your mood.

Lemon, Lime, Grapefruit, Tangerine
Add 2 drops each to a glass or stainless steel water bottle. Contemplate a joyful emotional set point as you enjoy.

Lifestyles

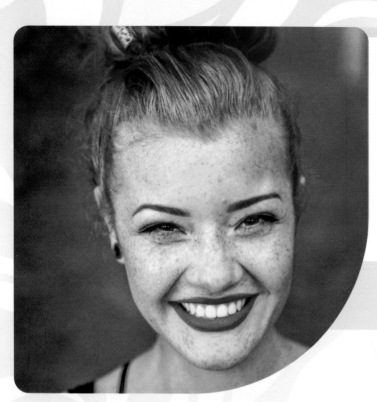

The *Good Life*

This is the master of all the Lifestyle Protocols. It addresses the fundamentals of continued health and wellness. Use it on its own or in addition to any other protocol.

Protocol Benefits
- Provides crucial nutrients to cells, organs, & body systems
- Promotes a sustainable healthy emotional state
- Allows the body to rejuvenate through meaningful sleep
- Increases energy naturally

Time frame
Treat this as an ongoing protocol. Use it in conjunction with any other protocol.

Energy Enhancement

Lemon
Drink a few drops in water throughout the day.

Greens
Add a serving to juice or a morning smoothie daily.

Meaningful Relaxation & Sleep

Serenity
Diffuse several drops, and rub a drop onto your temples before bed each night.

Serenity Complex
Take 2 softgels 30 minutes before bed.

Emotional Well-Being

Balance
Rub a drop onto the bottoms of feet each morning.

Citrus Bliss® or Elevation
Give yourself 60-second emotional resets throughout the day as you pause to breathe a couple drops from your palms.

Physical Wellness First

Lifelong Vitality Pack®
Take 2 of each bottle 2x daily.

TerraZyme®
Take 1-3 capsules with each meal.

PB Assist®
Take 1 capsule with each meal.

DDR Prime® Softgels
Take 1 softgel with each meal.

Lifestyles

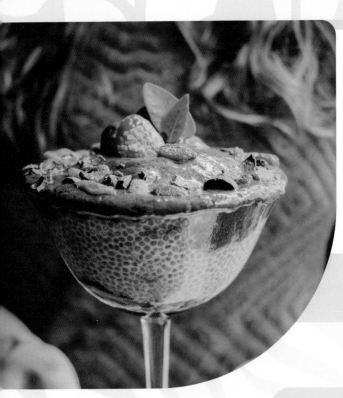

Gut Repair

Every body function is connected to the gut. A large part of the immune system is housed there, crucial neurotransmitters are produced, and nutrient assimilation happens. Repairing the gut repairs the mind and body.

Protocol Benefits
- Tames discomfort like gas, bloating, and indigestion
- Decreases inflammation
- Promotes internal tissue healing
- Encourages long-term mending and health

Time frame
Use the Tummy Tamer products on an ongoing basis. Use the Inflammation Challenger and the Long-term repair during separate 10-day sprees.

Tummy Tamer

DigestZen®
Drink a few drops in water or in a capsule, or rub two drops on the outside of the stomach for any stomach discomfort.

TerraZyme®
Take 1-3 capsules with each meal to experience easier digestive function.

Inflammation Challenger

Frankincense & Lemongrass
Take 2 drops each in a capsule 1-3 times a day. Only use Lemongrass internally for 10 days at a time (taking 2 week break before continuing).

Fiber
Mix one scoop with juice or water, or blend in a smoothie once daily or as needed.

Long-term Repair

GX Assist®
Purge the gut of Candida, fungus overgrowth, and unhealthy bacteria by taking 1 softgel with each meal for 10 days. Start with only 1 a day, and work your way to 3.

Bone Broth
Make homemade bone broth or buy from the health food store. Sip warm in a mug morning and night to nourish the gut. It's wise to cut inflammatory foods during this process as well (dairy, sugar, etc.)

Lifestyles

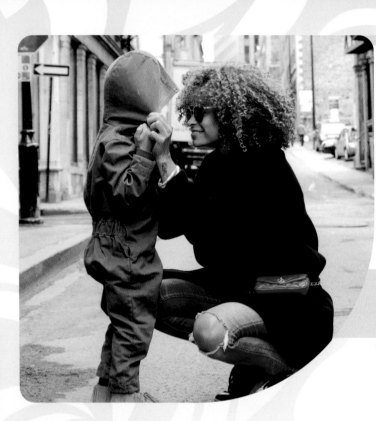

Home Holistic *Nurse*

Being the healer in your home means having the confidence to remedy the small things that can take away from enjoying life. Be prepared with this protocol to feel more empowered with your family's wellness.

Protocol Benefits
• Help the family feel peaceful and happy
• Remedy life's little emergencies
• Keep everyone's immune systems high

Time frame
This protocol is meant to be used on an ongoing basis. It can be used in conjunction with other protocols geared toward more specific wellness goals.

Preventative Wisdom

On Guard
Massage 2 drops diluted into sore joints and connective tissue.

Lemon
Add a few drops to a pitcher of water at dinner time to gently cleanse impurities.

Happy Moods All Around

Wild Orange
Diffuse several drops or let your child inhale from his/her own hands.

Peace
Apply a dab to the temples to calm quarrels and upset.

Life's Little Emergencies

Tea Tree
Use as an antiseptic and disinfectant for cuts and scrapes.

Lavender
Use to soothe rashes, bumps, bruises, and tears.

DigestZen®
Use to ease tummy aches and pain.

Helichrysum
Use to help cuts and scrapes heal.

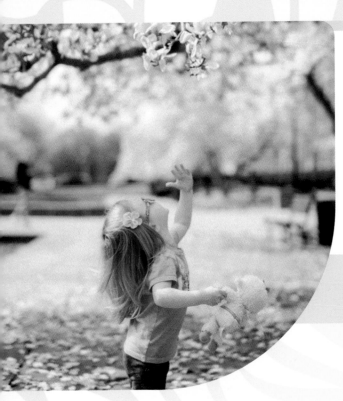

Kids : *Focused Energy*

Kids need energy to grow, play, and enjoy. Sometimes that energy simply needs to be focused in the right place at the right time. Use this protocol to help your child enjoy being a kid while also learning to focus in the right times.

Protocol Benefits
- Provides crucial nutrients to the brain and gut
- Grounds child's energy and improves focus & concentration
- Encourages energy that isn't hyperactive

Time frame
*Use this protocol for **4 weeks.** Then reevaluate and determine whether to continue or switch to another Lifestyle Protocol.*

Powerful Focus

Thinker
Roll onto the back of your child's neck when attention spans are short and focus is needed.

Steady
Rub a drop onto your child's feet each morning.

Kid's Brain Fuel

IQ Mega®
Use a double dose of Omegas to provide the brain with plenty of healthy fatty acids. Children's

PB Assist® Jr
Use 1-2 sachets daily to provide the gut (the 2nd brain) with plenty of healthy flora.

Balanced Energy

Wild Orange & Lavender
Diffuse 3 drops of each to stimulate a healthy level of energy that doesn't feel hyperactive.

Also combine 10 drops of each with FCO in a roller bottle for your child to use during playtime.

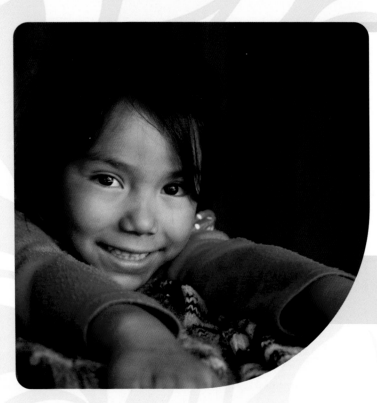

Kids: *Healthy and On – Track*

Healthy is an easier state to maintain when you've got the right components to support continued health! Use this protocol as a regular lifestyle standard to keep kids healthy and happy.

Protocol Benefits
- Provides crucial nutrients easy to miss in many modern diets
- Boost encouragement and focus
- Increase immunity

Time frame
Treat this as an ongoing protocol. It can be used in conjunction with other protocols targeted at more specific wellness goals.

Lifestyles

Healthy Immunity

Stronger
Rub a onto the bottoms of feet each morning to keep your child's immune system high.

Also diffuse several drops after school, and use On Guard or Abōde™ surface cleaner to keep common areas germ-free naturally.

Healthy Mind & Mood

Brave
Let your child breathe the oil from cupped hands to encourage a positive outlook and happy countenance.

Thinker
Roll onto the back of your child's neck to improve focus, especially during study and chore time.

Amazing Kid's Nutrition

a2z Chewable™
Take 1 daily for fundamental nutrients and a healthy body.

IQ Mega®
Take 1-2 Tbs daily by spoon, or mix into juice or a smoothie.

PB Assist® Jr
Consume 1 sachet daily to support healthy digestive & immune function.

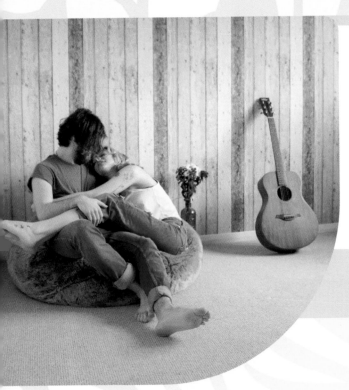

Love Life Boost

Whether seeking new love or fortifying an existing relationship, this protocol is designed to help you view yourself as beautiful and desirable, and to turn up the heat and attraction too.

Protocol Benefits
- Reinforces a positive self-concept
- Plumps lips to be more irresistible
- Leverages natural aphrodisiacs to boost attraction

Time frame
*Use this protocol for **2 weeks.** Then reevaluate or switch to a different Lifestyle Protocol.*

Positive Self - Reflection

Beautiful
Roll over heart daily. Enjoy the aroma as you speak out loud a few things you appreciate about yourself that you believe others will value too.

Rose
Roll over your wrists and heart while journaling about or visualizing your ideal relationship.

Tempting Aphrodisiacs

Fat Lips
Combine 2 drops each of Cinnamon, Geranium, and Cardamom with FCO in a small roller or empty 5ml bottle. This will plump your lips and make kissing a new adventure.

Passion
This blend is full of natural aphrodisiacs. Use it as a perfume, diffuse in the bedroom, or use with FCO in an intimate massage.

Ylang Ylang
This natural aphrodisiac serves as a beautiful perfume or cologne for men and women. Wear daily for increased sex appeal.

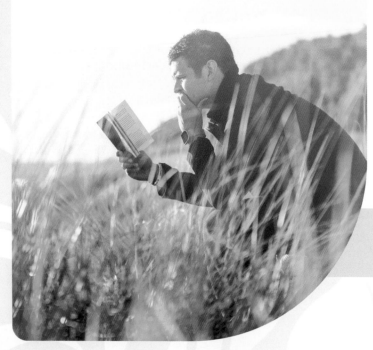

Mindfulness

To find your true self, go within. Turn anxiety & stress into peaceful introspection. This protocol takes your attention away from the outside world and to your inner world for self-discovery and more authentic personal expression.

Protocol Benefits
- Centers your mind and heart for meditation
- Turns your focus inward
- Clarifies the energy in your environment

Time frame
*Do this protocol for **4 weeks**. Then reevaluate or switch to another Lifestyle Protocol.*

Focused Introspection

Grapefruit & Siberian Fir
Rub a drop of each over your heart as you breathe deeply, taking your attention within. Use these moments to remind yourself what is real and what is perceived about yourself.

Sandalwood
Diffuse 4-6 drops during prayer, meditation, yoga, or chants.

Clarified Energy

Purify & Lemongrass
Diffuse 3-4 drops each daily to keep the energy in your space clean and open to new opportunity and discovery.

Centered Meditation

Vetiver & Ginger
Massage a drop of each onto the bottoms of feet, especially the big toes before meditation.

Anchor
Use a drop on wrists and temples during meditation, personal development reading, and journaling.

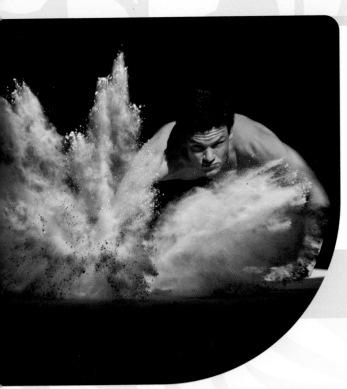

Musclemen: *Trimming, Toning, Bulking*

Building muscle happens from breaking down muscle tissue and refortifying it with the right macros, and this protocol supports components that make this process happen smoothly.

Protocol Benefits
- Manage inflammation while building muscle
- Cut body fat efficiently
- Support muscle development and recovery

Time frame
*Do this protocol for **4 weeks**. Then reevaluate or switch to another Lifestyle Protocol.*

Muscle Longevity

Siberian Fir & Marjoram
Massage a couple drops of each with FCO into fatigued muscles to restore and recover quickly.

Inflammation Manager

Deep Blue® Complex
Take 2 capsules before working out.

Deep Blue®
Massage a few drops into sore areas as often as needed.

Lemongrass
Take a drop under the tongue. Also diffuse several drops.

Trim & Bulk

Protein (Whey or Plant)
Drink a serving within 30 minutes of working out and as needed daily.

Grapefruit
Drink 4 drops in a glass or stainless steel water bottle daily to activate fat-burning enzymes produced by the liver.

Slim & Sassy®
Drink a few drops in water or chew Slim & Sassy® Gum to address cravings.

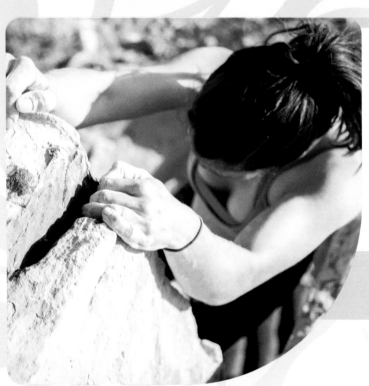

Pain & Inflammation – Away

Turn pain into peace by addressing inflammation at every level. This protocol is ideal for people with both temporary and chronic conditions.

Protocol Benefits
- Ease inflammation from the inside-out
- Soothe muscles, joints, & connective tissue
- Support healthy inflammatory response at a cellular and nervous system level

Time frame
*Do this protocol for **8 weeks.** Then reevaluate or switch to another Lifestyle Protocol.*

Body Restoration

Lifelong Vitality Pack®
Take 2 of each bottle twice daily to powerfully address inflammation on a cellular level.

Vetiver
Rub a drop into the bottoms of feet or spine for nervous system support.

Internal Inflammation Reduction

Deep Blue® Complex
Take 2 capsules whenever pain arises, or take 1 capsule 3x daily.

Frankincense & Copaiba
Use a drop of each under the tongue 2-3x daily.

DDR Prime® Softgels
Take 1 softgel with each meal.

Muscle, Joint, & Connective Tissue Help

Deep Blue®
Massage a few drops into painful areas as often as needed.

AromaTouch®
Massage a few drops with FCO to pull tension out of muscles.

Lemongrass
Rub a couple drops with FCO to soothe painful joints and ligaments.

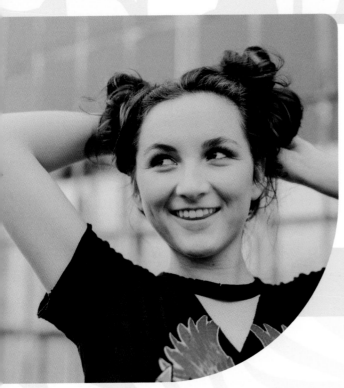

Teens: *Clear Skin*

Acne and blemishes arise from bacterial issues, hormone imbalance, or toxicity overload. This protocol addresses all three simultaneously.

Protocol Benefits
- Addresses bacterial issues on the surface
- Uses oil-infused skincare to safely address cosmetic issues
- Pulls toxicity overwhelm from endocrine system
- Helps balance hormone levels

Time frame
*Use this protocol for **8 weeks**. Then reevaluate and continue use as needed.*

HD Clear® Skincare Products

Use the HD Clear® face wash and moisturizer to help skin recover from acne and blemishes.

Toxicity Reduction

Zendocrine® Softgels
Take 1-2 softgels with each meal.

Zendocrine®
Rub a drop onto bottoms of feet 20 minutes before showering to pull toxins out of the body.

Hormone Balance

Ylang Ylang & Jasmine
Apply a dab of each to pulse points in the evening or in stressful moments.

Full Body Detox
Consider doing the 30-day Full Body Detox in this book to reset hormone balance in the body.

Topical Repair

HD Clear®
Apply a dab to affected areas.

Tea Tree
Alternate the HD Clear® with Tea Tree to see which oil your skin responds best to.

Helichrysum
Gently apply a dab to damaged skin.

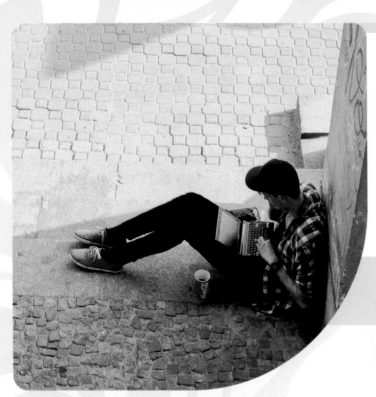

Teens: *Studiuos*

Students thrive when focus becomes easy. This protocol helps students laser in on what's important so they can keep priorities and also enjoy life outside of study.

Protocol Benefits
- Encourages focus & concentration
- Fuels the brain and body for optimal performance
- Fosters an environment conducive to productive studying

Time frame
*Do this protocol for **4 weeks.** Then reevaluate or continue on an ongoing basis.*

Studious Environment

Rosemary, Peppermint, & Lime
Diffuse 3 drops of each to promote memory retention and focus during study.

Focus Promoter

InTune®
Roll onto the back of neck and temples to improve state of concentration.

Balance
Rub a couple drops onto the bottoms of feet after showering each morning.

Brain & Body Fuel

Lifelong Vitality Pack®
Take 2 of each bottle 2x daily.

Mito2Max®
Take 1-2 capsules 30 minutes before study time.

PB Assist®
Take 1 capsule with each meal.

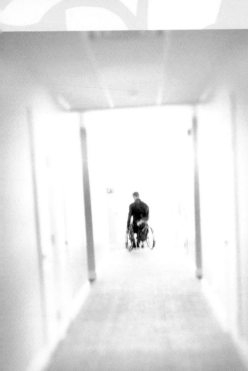

Trauma Recovery

Trauma of any kind - abuse, injury, or abrupt life transitions - can leave a sense of being broken or incomplete. Use this protocol to begin the process of realizing your wholeness, your perfection, and your possibility.

Protocol Benefits
• Provides body and mind with essential nutrients for physical and emotional recovery
• Boosts endorphins and positive mood neurotransmitters
• Facilitates the creation of a new story for the future

Time frame
*Do this protocol for **8 weeks.** Then reevaluate or switch to another Lifestyle Protocol.*

Return To True Self

Motivate
Diffuse several drops and inhale from cupped hands to return to a healthy sense of self.

Melissa
Use a drop under the tongue each day to improve serotonin production.

Whole Body Support

Lifelong Vitality Pack®
Take 2 of each bottle twice daily to provide crucial bio-available nutrients to cells, organs, and body systems.

Deep Blue® Complex
Take 1 capsule 3x daily to support a healthy inflammatory response.

DDR Prime®
Massage 2 drops into the spine each night.

Writing A New Story

Arise
Rub a couple drops over your heart and apply to pulse points.

Use this blend while journaling. Identify any self-defeating stories you might be telling yourself, and transform them into a story that empowers you to move into a future of new and improved possibility.

Consider working with a coach or counselor to guide your thoughts and processes.

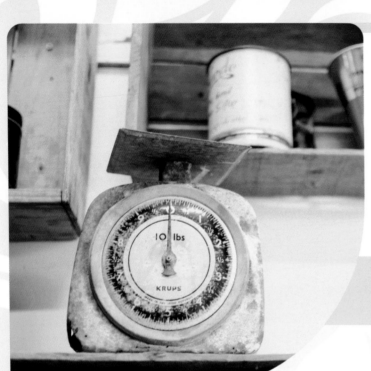

Weight Loss

Remember that healthy weight is subjective, not universal. Determine a weight goal you'll feel highly encouraged by, and use this protocol to help you achieve it.

Protocol Benefits
- Curb cravings naturally
- Keep your spirits & motivation high
- Release toxicity overload to eliminate the need for toxin-protecting fat stores

Time frame
*Do this protocol for **8 weeks.** Then reevaluate or switch to a different Lifestyle Protocol.*

Craving Control

Slim & Sassy® Softgels
Take 2-3 softgels 2-3x daily. Also chew Slim & Sassy® gum.

Slim & Sassy®
Massage several drops with FCO over fatty areas 30 minutes before showering.

Grapefruit
Drink a few drops in water throughout the day.

Internal Motivation

Lime & Rosemary
Diffuse 3 drops of each, or inhale a drop from your palms as needed.

Mito2Max®
Take 2 capsules 30 minutes before exercise to boost energy and determination.

Lifelong Vitality Pack®
Take 2 of each bottle 2x daily.

Endocrine, Organ, & Tissue Detox

Zendocrine® Complex
Take 1 capsule with each meal.

Zendocrine® Softgels
Take 1 softgel with each meal.

Slim & Sassy®
Massage several drops with FCO over fatty areas 30 minutes before showering. Wrap with muslin fabric for improved results.

Lifestyles

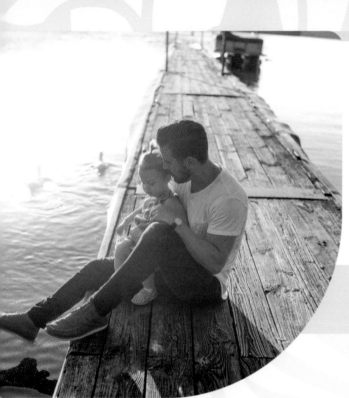

Whole Heart Healing

Whether life has presented a few bumps or it's simply time to return to wholeheartedness, hearts can always use healing.

Protocol Benefits
- Release crippling grief and sadness
- Transition anger and resentment into constructive emotions
- Return the heart to a state of hopefulness and renewal

Time frame
*Do this protocol for **8 weeks.** Then reevaluate or switch to another Lifestyle Protocol.*

Grief Release

Console
Rub a couple drops over the heart and also the pads of your feet. Breathe deeply, envisioning surrendering grief and pain to a higher power.

Heart & Soul Restoration

Forgive
Rub a couple drops over the heart, and inhale from cupped hands during prayer and meditation.

Hope
Wear as a perfume or cologne during the day, turning your thoughts to appreciation when you notice the aroma.

Anger & Resentment Transition

Wintergreen, Thyme, & Lemongrass
Place a dab of each on the corner of a paper where you can write out the negative emotions you'd like to transition.

Write silent letters that you can tear up or burn. Write to release, and then write to reposition your feelings into something constructive.

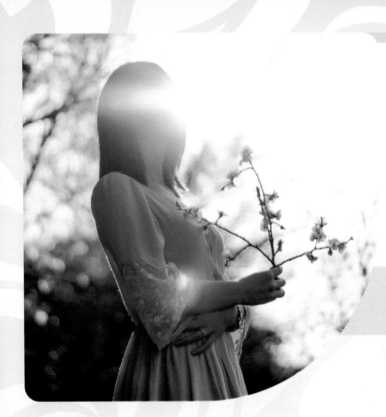

Whole *Life* Detox

You know it's time to purge what isn't serving when life gives you feedback in the form of conflict, health challenges, or difficulty seeing things differently. Use this protocol to jump start detoxing your life from many angles.

Protocol Benefits
- Remove toxicity from relationships
- Pull toxicity from your physical body
- Turn heart toxicity into connection with your heart
- Find a cooperative attitude through attitude detox

Time frame
Use this protocol for **2 weeks.** *Then reevaluate or switch to another Lifestyle Protocol.*

Attitude Detox

Bergamot & Cypress
Diffuse 3 drops each and apply to the bottoms of feet to encourage flexibility in perception while staying true to ethics and values.

Heart & Spirit Detox

Jasmine
Apply to pulse points and over heart to encourage a true sense of self.

Geranium & Arborvitae
Diffuse 2 drops each to reconnect to your heart center.

General Physical Detox

Lifelong Vitality Pack®
Take 2 of each bottle twice daily.

Zendocrine® Complex
Take 1 capsule with each meal.

Zendocrine® Softgels
Take 1 softgel with each meal.

Relationship Detox

Frankincense & Roman Chamomile
Breathe a drop of each from cupped hands as you contemplate relationships to determine their truth and purpose.

Douglas Fir
Diffuse several drops to facilitate surrendering unhealthy patterns.

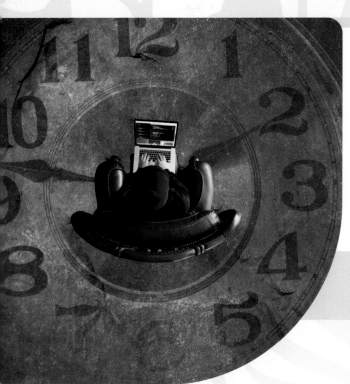

Working *Bee*

There is a season for diligent work, and this protocol supports being eagerly engaged in a worthy cause. Use it to be your best self so you can make your greatest contributions.

Protocol Benefits
- Keeps energy and focus grounded
- Supports the body with crucial nutrients for optimal performance and sustained energy
- Assists with mental clarity and creativity

Time frame
*Do this protocol for **4 weeks** or during intense periods of work and tight deadlines.*

Clarity & Creativity Spree

Peppermint & Frankincense
Hold a dab of each to the roof of your mouth for 30 seconds.

Citrus Bliss®
Diffuse several drops or inhale from cupped hands every few hours.

Energy Grounding

Balance
Rub 2 drops on bottoms of feet each morning to promote focus.

Patchouli, Bergamot, & Clary Sage
Diffuse 2 drops each during long work hauls to balance the soul.

Body Care & Maintenance

Lifelong Vitality Pack®
Take 2 of each bottle twice daily.

Mito2Max®
Take 2 capsules 30 minutes before yoga or working out.

Deep Blue® Complex
Take 2 capsules before working out, or 1 capsule 3x daily on non-workout days.

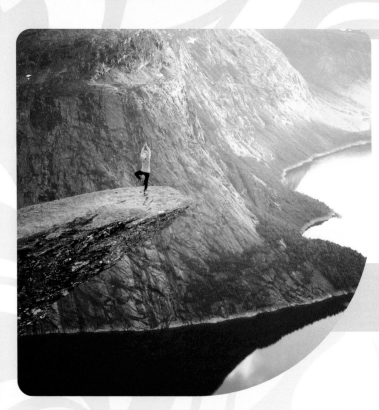

The *Yogi*

The Yogi yields a silent-but-powerful energy. He is dedicated to his practice and to his peace of mind. Above all else, he is committed to presence in every moment.

Protocol Benefits
- Increase presence of mind
- Maintain balanced energy
- Support muscles, joints, & connective tissue
- Boost physical and mental energy

Time frame
*Use this protocol on an **ongoing basis** as long as it serves your practice. Experiment using different oils during practice after a few weeks.*

Lifestyles

Intention, Prep, & Centerdness

Anchor
Apply a drop to bottoms of feet while setting intentions for your practice and in salutation poses.

Align
Rub a drop over the heart to bring your focus back to your center and the present moment.

Arise
Diffuse several drops and apply to pulse points to bring enlightenment to your most challenging poses and your most peaceful moments.

Zen for Joints & Ligaments

Lemongrass
Massage 2 drops diluted into sore joints and connective tissue.

Deep Blue®
Massage oil or rub to soothe muscles after a workout or yoga practice.

Physical Stamina

Lifelong Vitality Pack®
Take 2 of each bottle twice daily.

Mito2Max®
Take 2 capsules 30 minutes before yoga or working out.

Deep Blue® Complex
Take 2 capsules before working out, or 1 capsule 3x daily on non-workout days.

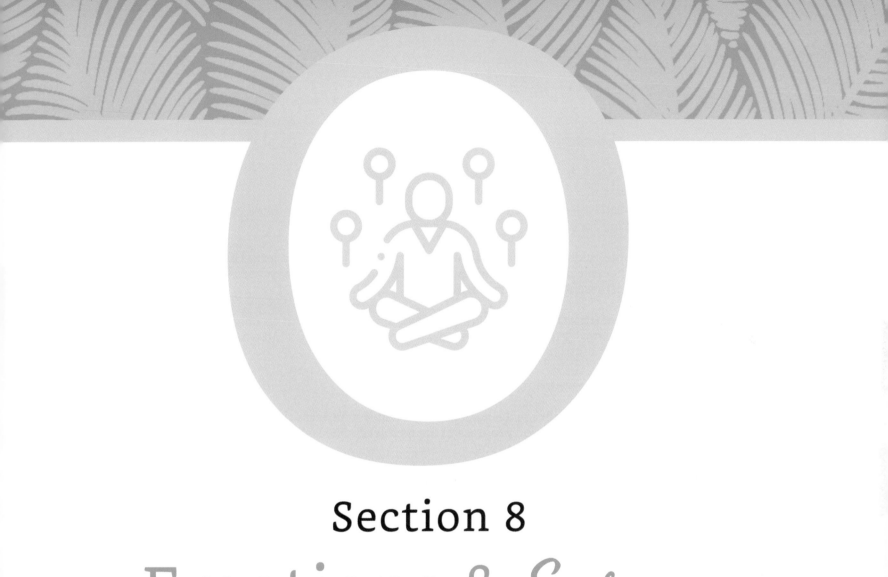

Section 8

Emotions & Energy

How to Use *Emotions & Energy*

This section addresses emotional and energetic health with an *emotional guidance scale* as a measuring stick.

The emotional guidance scale was developed by authors Esther and Jerry Hicks. The bottom of the scale indicates the lowest forms of emotion and energy, whereas the top of the scale represents the highest forms.

The premise of the scale is that making large leaps from a low point to a high point is usually impractical. Instead, take an honest emotional inventory. Find where you are, and see what it will take to progress upward just a little bit.

This is the fastest way to improve your emotions.

Each stage of the guidance scale includes oils to help you **process** the level where you are, as well as oils to help you **progress** to the next level. The last oil listed in each step is also the first oil of the following step.

You don't need to use all the oils listed. Use what feels best, or what you have on hand.

You'll also find powerful intentions you can speak or write as you use the suggested oils. These are designed to help meet you where you are in the moment, and to gently guide you to the next level.

Remember that you can't do it wrong. Discover what works for you, and enjoy climbing one step at a time.

Emotional Guidance Scale

Identify where you are on the scale. Use the suggested oils to process where you are and gently progress up the scale.

Blame, Justification
Discouragement
Disappointment
Overwhelmment
Frustration, Defensiveness
Pessimism
Boredom
Worry
Doubt
Contentment
Hopefulness
Anger
Optimism
Revenge
Positive Expectation, Belief
Hatred, Rage
Enthusiasm, Happiness
Jealousy
Passion
Insecurity, Guilt, Unworthiness
Fear, Grief, Depression,
Shame, Powerlessness, Despair
Knowledge, Empowerment,
Joy, Freedom, Gratitude, Love

Fear, Grief, Depression, Despair, Powerlessness, Shame

> *I can be okay right here, right now, for at least the next few moments. Then I can take the next few moments after that. I am safe. I can hold on.*

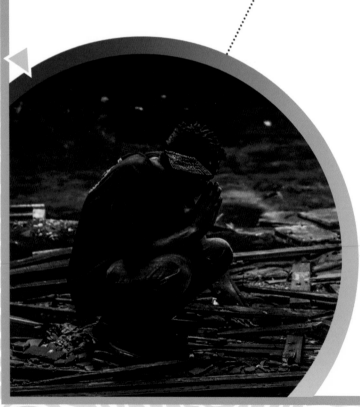

Oils to *Process Where You Are*

Balance
Rub 2 drops onto the bottoms of feet morning and evening to bring a sense of safety. However things may be, you are at least safe in the present moment.

Helichrysum
Apply to your wrists and solar plexus (above your naval) to initiate healing from shame and despair.

Slim & Sassy®
Add 4 drops to your glass or stainless steel water bottle throughout the day to help ease any desire to self-sabotage.

Oils to *Progress Up the Scale*

Melissa
Hold a drop to the roof of your mouth for 30 seconds to stimulate serotonin and dopamine production and receptivity, resulting in a lightened countenance.

Bergamot
Diffuse several drops throughout the day to begin returning to a sense of who you truly are.

Frankincense
Use a drop under your tongue 2-3 times daily to combat depression by facilitating proper neurotransmitter activity.

Insecurity, Guilt, Unworthiness

> *I have come this far, and I can go a little further. I don't need to know the exact journey. I'll do my best to make progress along the way.*

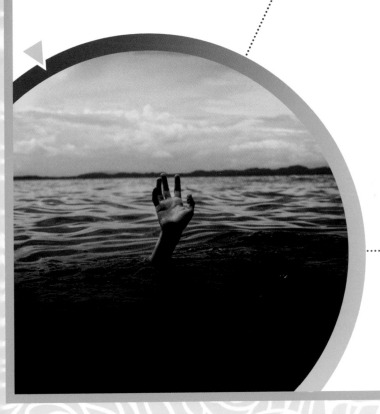

Oils to *Process Where You Are*

Frankincense & Myrrh
Insecurity and guilt can frequently be adopted from mother or father. Use Frankincense (father) or Myrrh (mother) on your wrists as you write out your feelings in a letter you can burn.

Jasmine
Apply over your heart, gently breathing in permission to be who you are.

Spearmint
Diffuse a few drops to lift the feeling of being unseen.

Oils to *Progress Up the Scale*

Peace
Apply a couple drops to pulse points during prayer, song, or meditation. Focus on turning thoughts about what's wrong into simply noticing the peace in the present moment.

Peppermint
Rub a drop over your heart to breathe life back into your heart.

Lemon
Inhale a few drops from your palms, offering your higher self permission to guide you to a truer self-concept.

Emotions

Jealousy

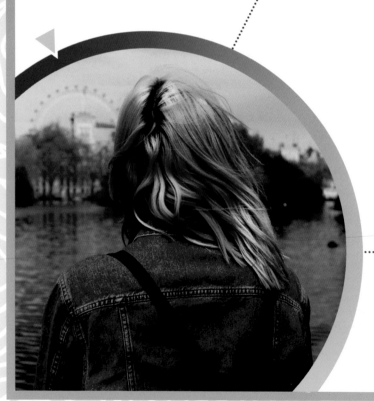

> *I am learning to find confidence within myself.*
> *I am learning to go within for the truth about me.*
> *I allow myself to grow and exist imperfectly.*

Oils to *Process Where You Are*

Lemon
Inhale a few drops from cupped hands to diffuse sharp feelings of jealousy or envy, including envy of the emotional state of others.

Birch
Add a few drops to a bath or shower. Allow yourself to release feelings of being unsupported.

Black Pepper
Diffuse a few drops to help clear emotional dishonesty and the temptation to mask insecurities with materialism.

Oils to *Progress Up the Scale*

Cinnamon
Put a dab on your tongue. Focus on exhaling jealousy and rejection of self.

Cedarwood
Massage a couple drops into the back of your neck and temples. Ask that you be met with a sense of community and support of those who really matter to you.

Cassia
Diffuse a few drops to transform feelings of embarrassment, humiliation, or being judged into a sense of self-assurance.

Hatred/Rage

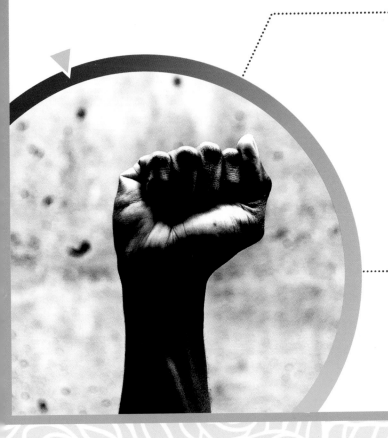

"
It is not my responsibility to hold others to what's right. I am in charge of showing up as my best self, and that is enough for right now.

Oils to *Process Where You Are*

Cassia
Diffuse a few drops, allowing the warmth to calm hatred and rage. Begin to see that your true desire is to feel safe and heard from within.

Thyme
Add a couple drops to your shower. Focus on washing away bitterness, resentment, and emotional bondage.

Tea Tree
Inhale a drop from your palms with the intention of releasing relationships that breach healthy boundaries.

Oils to *Progress Up the Scale*

Juniper Berry
Diffuse several drops to dilute irrational fears that become expressed as hate toward others.

Deep Blue®
Massage a few drops with FCO or lotion into sore and tense muscles where you may be storing unresolved pain.

Wintergreen
Inhale a drop from cupped hands with the intention of learning to surrender the need to control.

Revenge

> *This moment will pass, and future moments will yield solutions that I do not see perfectly now. I can be patient right now. I open myself to solutions that will serve in the long-term.*

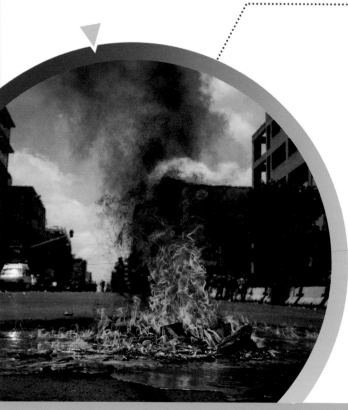

Oils to *Process Where You Are*

Wintergreen
Inhale a drop from your palms, visualizing negative emotions leaving your body and being absorbed by the earth or the sun.

Clary Sage
Put a dab over your third eye (between and right above your eyebrows), and ask the question, "Is there potentially another way to look at this scenario?"

Oregano
Add a toothpick swirl to a cup of hot tea. Acknowledge the desire for revenge, and then give it permission to fade.

Oils to *Progress Up the Scale*

Balance
Apply a drop behind and over your ears. Allow out-of-control feelings to begin to settle.

Console
Apply a drop to your pulse points and heart. Notice the slight improvement that comes from turning your attention from the outside world inward. Notice the inner pain that is asking to be acknowledged.

Cardamom
Drink a drop in water. Allow the sensation to remind you of what it feels like to be objective, to feel more responsible in your self-control.

Anger

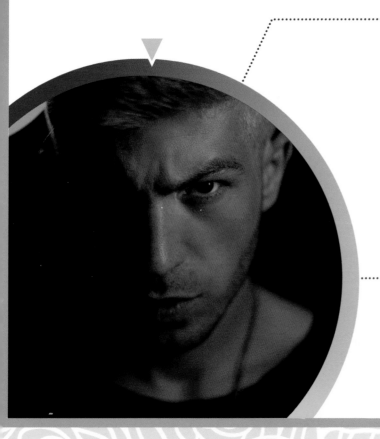

> I acknowledge and honor my feelings. I yield ones that do not serve to a higher power, and I claim my ability to be lighter and freer.

Oils to *Process Where You Are*

Cardamom
Diffuse a couple of drops. Let the aroma become the sensation of releasing angry feelings in a non-harmful way.

Peace
Apply a drop to your pulse points and heart. Turn your thoughts from whatever makes you angry, and focus just for a few moments only on your breath.

Balance
Apply a drop to your temples and the bottoms of your feet. Remember that feelings are temporal, and that even your anger is okay to acknowledge.

Oils to *Progress Up the Scale*

Douglas Fir
Inhale a few drops from your palms. Offer an intention to forgive any patterns of anger that have been passed from generations before you, and to be the end of that pattern.

Zendocrine®
Apply a couple drops to the bottoms of your feet 20 minutes before showering. Let your shower help wash away both physical and emotional toxicity.

Purify
Diffuse several drops to cleanse the energy of your space, and to begin cleansing emotion that has been harming more than it has been helping.

Discouragement

" *I live in a world with many possibilities. I don't need to see them all to know they are there because my life has had experiences where good things happened unexpectedly. I welcome more.*

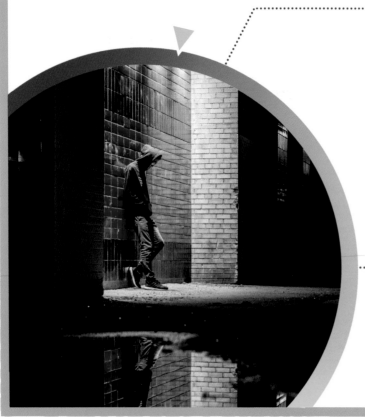

Oils to *Process Where You Are*

Purify
Inhale a few drops from cupped hands, remembering that patterns of the past do not determine the future.

Wild Orange
Diffuse several drops. Sense that there may be more opportunities and possibilities - even ones you aren't yet aware of.

Helichrysum
Apply a drop over your heart. Honor your hurt. Allow your feelings to be for the moment.

Oils to *Progress Up the Scale*

Cheer
Diffuse several drops, simply letting the beautiful aroma be enough in the now-moment.

Beautiful
Apply to your wrists and over your heart. Let yourself flow a little more effortlessly between breaths.

Eucalyptus
Inhale a drop from your palms. Allow feelings of being defeated or wanting to disappear from life to turn into trust that you can find a way to heal your life.

Blame, Justification

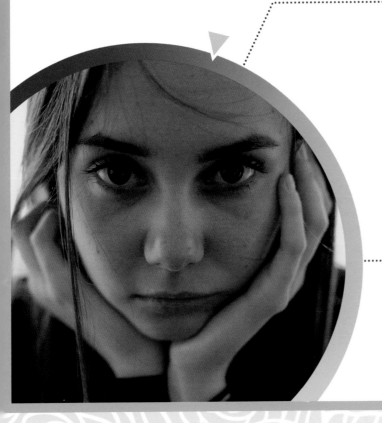

> *I care about myself enough to release others of the responsibility to make me feel good. I am feeling freer as I take my personal well-being back into my own hands.*

Oils to *Process Where You Are*

Eucalyptus
Inhale a couple drops from your palms, and rub a bit over your chest. Open your airways as you open your heart and surrender just a little bit of blame.

Ginger
Use a drop on the floor of your shower or in a bath. Gently release the desire to make others responsible for your experiences.

InTune®
Apply to the back of your neck. Write a page of ideas of things you (not others) can do for your situation.

Oils to *Progress Up the Scale*

Clove
Diffuse a couple drops, focusing on releasing feelings of being controlled and being co-dependent. Ask what it feels like to be in charge of your own feelings.

Cilantro
Use a toothpick swirl in cooking or add a bit to your diffuser blend. Let the taste symbolize feeling easier in your relationships.

Cypress
Inhale a couple drops from your palms, asking what it looks like to be more in flow.

Worry

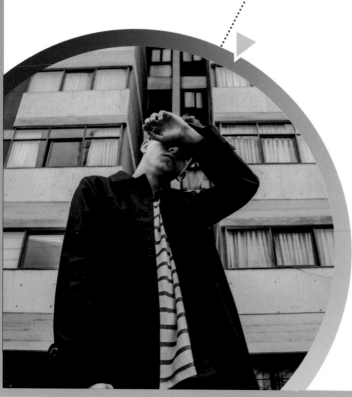

" *I care because I love, and I love enough to let go. I think about things I can do something about, and I focus on what I do want. I surrender everything else to my higher power.*

Oils to *Process Where You Are*

Cypress
Diffuse several drops, noticing the motion and flow of your breath. Remember that things work themselves out, and that life continues on.

Tea Tree
Inhale a drop from your palms. Release any unhealthy expectations you have of others.

Sandalwood
Use a drop on your temples during prayer and meditation. Surrender to higher guidance, and focus on the direction you want to go.

Oils to *Progress Up the Scale*

Rosemary
Diffuse a few drops as you learn to trust in a higher consciousness that has more answers and greater wisdom than your mind has alone.

Cilantro
Rub a drop to the bottoms of your feet before showering to detox the need to be in control.

DDR Prime®
Massage a few drops into your spine or bottoms of your feet to transform your body and emotions into operating with health and vitality.

Doubt

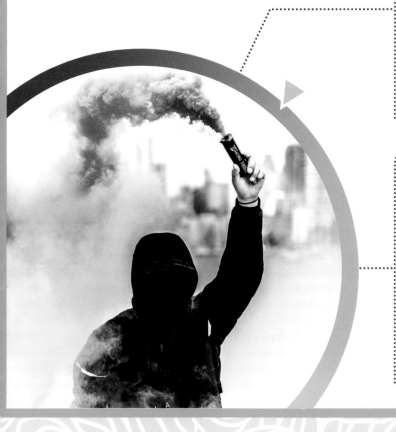

> *I embrace the wisdom of the unknown. I commit to showing up, keeping my word, and allowing things to work in my best interest today.*

Oils to *Process Where You Are*

DDR Prime®
Massage a few drops into your spine and your feet to support whole-body cellular health and emotional transformation.

Lemongrass
Diffuse a few drops to cleanse doubt from your energy, and commit to cleaning it up from your vocabulary.

Immortelle
Apply around your eyes and forehead to invite spiritual insight about how the greater good is unfolding.

Oils to *Progress Up the Scale*

Rose
Apply to your pulse points and over your heart to begin replacing self-doubt with divine love. Forces bigger than you have your best interest at heart.

Rosemary
Diffuse several drops to open your mind to ways you can transition from doubt into greater possibility.

Fennel
Dab a bit onto your tongue, and appreciate how this oil represents personal responsibility. All you can do is keep your agreements and do your best in any given day.

Emotions

Disappointment

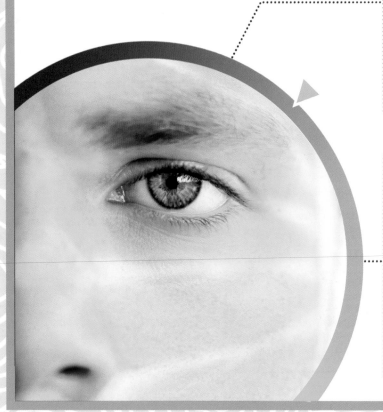

There is always a path forward for me. I am worthy of good things, and I open my mind to see the possibility of the next good thing. I take life one good thing at a time.

Oils to *Process Where You Are*

Fennel
Put a dab on your tongue, and consider the gift of being responsible for your life.

Cedarwood
Massage a few drops into your neck and shoulders, as well as anywhere you may have skin conditions. Remember that this aroma symbolizes community and the people who have your back.

Lemongrass
Diffuse several drops to cleanse disappointment from the air.

Oils to *Progress Up the Scale*

Arborvitae
Rub a drop onto your wrists and temples, looking for the connection between what you thought was disappointing and where you hope the road will take you.

HD Clear®
Apply to skin conditions where chronic disappointment may be manifesting physically.

Ylang Ylang
Wear as a perfume or cologne to remind yourself of your ability to be both intellectual and intuitive as you discover the way forward.

Emotions

Overwhelmment

"I am committed to saying yes to that which inspires me. I honor myself enough to say no to things that don't serve. I am committed to being well so I can make my greatest contributions.

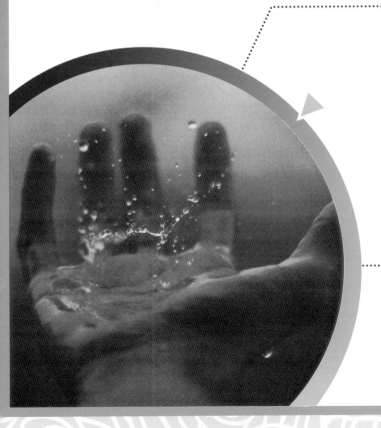

Oils to *Process Where You Are*

Ylang Ylang
Diffuse a few drops to soften your mood and emotional state.

DigestZen®
Drink a couple drops in water to help your physical digestion as well as your ability to digest emotions.

On Guard
Rub a couple drops on the bottoms of your feet to provide a protective energetic boundary as you prioritize and determine those things you will do best.

Oils to *Progress Up the Scale*

PastTense®
Massage onto muscles and areas where overwhelm has turned into pain and tension.

Basil
Diffuse a few drops with your favorite citrus oils to bring about a sense of renewal and refreshment.

ClaryCalm®
Apply to your wrists to help balance hormones and to experience the safety that lies in being vulnerable and say no to things that no longer serve (For men too. Be careful of photosensitivity for 48 hours.)

Emotions

Frustration, Irritation, Impatience, Defensiveness

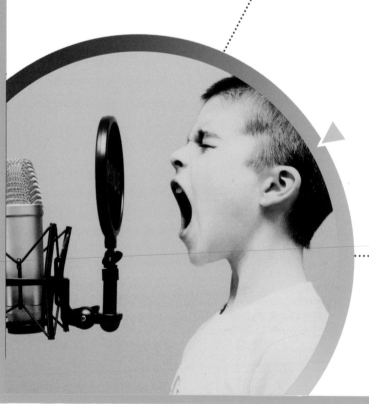

" *It's safe to be calm, and it's safe to be heard. I allow myself to see the humanity in others and in myself. I allow myself to be soft in my interactions with others.*

Oils to *Process Where You Are*

ClaryCalm®
Apply to pulse points (be careful of photosensitivity) to remember that force is the slowest way to bring about lasting change.

Vetiver
Apply a drop to the bottoms of your heels and behind your ears to calm the temptation to use irritation as a replacement for constructive communication.

Oregano
Add a toothpick swirl to a hot herbal tea to soothe desires to control others.

Oils to *Progress Up the Scale*

Breathe
Breathe a few drops from your palms, and rub some onto your chest. Inhale and exhale deeply as you release frustration through your breath.

Serenity
Rub a couple drops onto your temples and over your pillow to help you sleep peacefully and wake in a state of forgiveness.

Roman Chamomile
Diffuse a few drops to see the higher purpose in the things you're experiencing now.

Pessimism

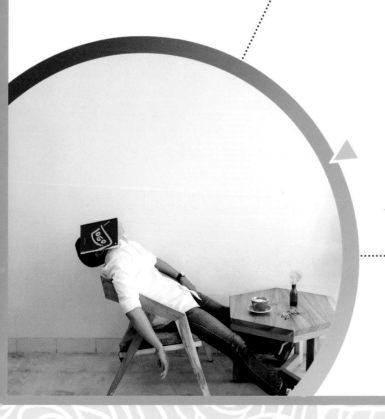

> *I release the past and surrender to what's unseen. I allow my mind to be calm, and to know that everything always works out.*

Oils to *Process Where You Are*

Roman Chamomile
Rub a drop over your forehead to encourage constructive insights that are authentic to the greater good.

Black Pepper
Use a drop in cooking or on the bottoms of your feet to release any sense of being controlled.

Vetiver
Apply a drop to your heels and behind your ears to root your attention to the present, rather than allowing it to run wild with unpleasant possibilities.

Oils to *Progress Up the Scale*

Wild Orange
Diffuse several drops throughout the day to regain the sense that there is enough abundance and prosperity.

Cheer
Breathe a couple drops from your palms as you shift pessimistic thoughts to thoughts that feel just a little lighter.

Peppermint
Hold a drop to the roof of your mouth to awaken your mind to other possibilities and outcomes.

Emotions

Boredom

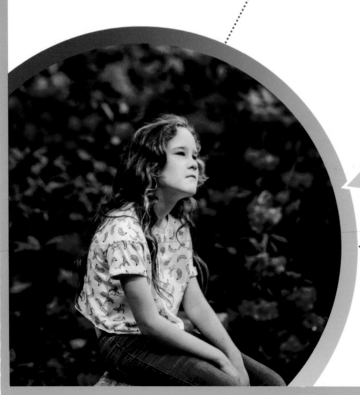

> I allow my thoughts to be peaceful and centered. I am easily seeing encouraging things on the horizon, and I lean into it.

Oils to *Process Where You Are*

Peppermint
Inhale a drop from cupped hands to find a bit of heartiness in this moment.

Cedarwood
Rub a couple drops onto pulse points, especially during journaling. This helps increase a sense of community and desire to connect with others.

Jasmine
Apply to pulse points to increase a sense of safety and desire to open up in close & intimate relationships.

Oils to *Progress Up the Scale*

Zendocrine®
Rub a couple drops on the bottoms of your feet 20 minutes before showering to pull out toxins that cause you to feel sluggish.

Citrus Bliss®
Inhale a few drops from your hands throughout the day to bring your energy a little bit higher.

Passion
Add a few drops to your body lotion to add inspiration to your day.

Contentment

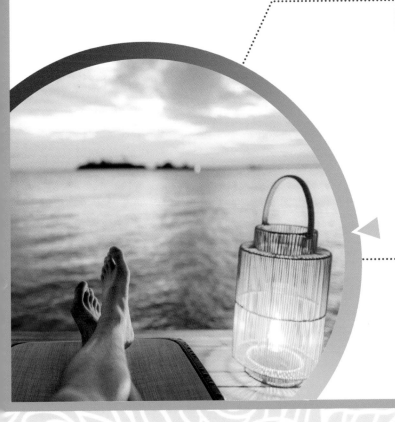

> *I am deeply present. I surrender to what is here and now, and I allow myself to be nurtured at every level.*

Oils to *Process Where You Are*

Passion
Diffuse a few drops to transition any agitation or lack of control into knowing that the present moment is all that matters.

Geranium
Rub a drop over your heart to indulge in a few things you appreciate about yourself in the here and now.

Roman Chamomile
Diffuse a couple drops or use in the bath to soak up what you love in the present moment.

Oils to *Progress Up the Scale*

Lemon
Use 4 drops in your drinking water throughout the day to add a little more light to your day-to-day experiences.

Sandalwood
Use a drop on the temples and wrists during gratitude prayers and meditation to see the divine unfolding through every hopeful feeling.

Immortelle
Apply around eyes and forehead to better sense the hope embedded in every variant of the future.

Hopefulness

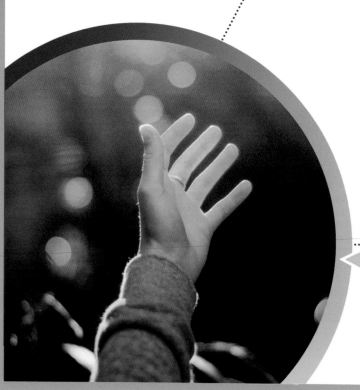

I take each day one moment at a time, allowing the best and highest good to blossom and guide me forward. I appreciate slight improvements often because I know they add up to a better life.

Oils to *Process Where You Are*

Immortelle
Apply this around your eyes and forehead to transition any remaining disparity into hopefulness.

Clary Sage
Use this oil in a bath to relax into seeing more of where you can allow hope to guide your life.

Serenity
Rub a couple drops onto your temples and over your pillow before bed to ease any troubled thoughts, drifting off with the intention to wake more hopeful.

Oils to *Progress Up the Scale*

Grapefruit
Drink a few drops in your glass or stainless steel water bottle throughout the day to facilitate a healthy relationship with your body and your mind.

Helichrysum
Apply a dab over the third eye (between and slightly above your eyebrows) to better see how hope can turn into continuous optimism.

Hope
Apply to pulse points and over the heart to feel the warmth of a more hopeful countenance.

Optimism

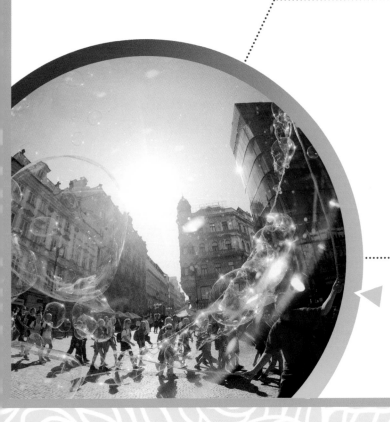

"

Possibility comes from within. I trust my intuition and inner guidance to find the best solutions. I relax into the ease of a satisfying future.

Oils to *Process Where You Are*

Hope
Apply to pulse points to gently invigorate the senses to recall feelings of seeing improvement and progress.

Cardamom
Inhale a drop from your palms to soothe remaining parts of the ego that want to stay focused on limitation rather than possibility.

Siberian Fir
Apply a few drops over your heart to lift any recurring family patterns of pessimism.

Oils to *Progress Up the Scale*

Melissa
Rub a drop onto the bottoms of your feet, focusing on the big toe, to shed light on the silver lining in every scenario.

Bergamot
Diffuse several drops to encourage a strong sense of self, knowing optimistic possibilities arise from within.

Tangerine
Put a few drops in your drinking water throughout the day to bring an air of fun to problem solving.

Emotions

Positive Expectation, Belief

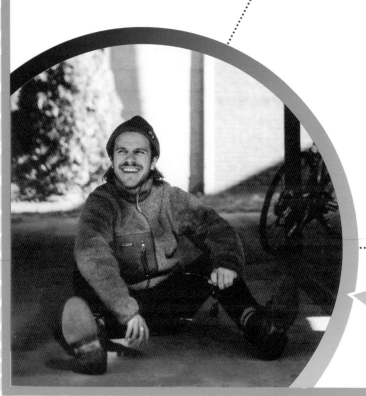

"I choose to see the future in a bright, encouraging light. I allow good things to come to me in unexpected and miraculous ways.

Oils to *Process Where You Are*

Tangerine
Diffuse several drops to keep a sense of playfulness. Remember that it can be fun and easy to expect positive things to unfold.

Peppermint
Rub a drop over the heart to improve buoyancy and a sense of optimism.

Cheer
Inhale a couple drops from cupped hands to find and lift those parts of you that doubt the future.

Oils to *Progress Up the Scale*

Citrus Bliss®
Diffuse several drops to invigorate the senses and see good things coming in your physical and spiritual surroundings.

Bergamot
Rub a drop over your solar plexus (just over your naval) to ignite belief in yourself. Belief in self opens belief to unlimited possibilities outside the self. (Avoid direct sunlight for 48 hours.)

Wild Orange
Inhale a couple drops from your hands to remember that abundance and well-being exist in unlimited supply.

Enthusiasm, Eagerness, Happiness

> *There is a space for happiness in every moment. I am worthy of happy feelings, and I show up in beautiful, eager pursuit of genuine happiness daily.*

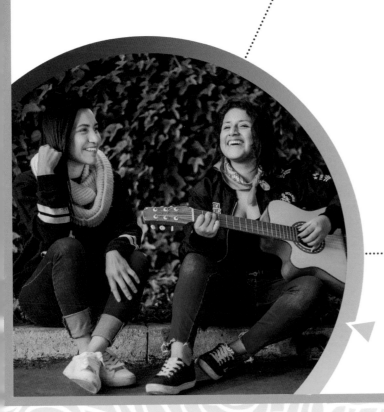

Oils to *Process Where You Are*

Wild Orange
Diffuse several drops to tap into the unlimited happiness that exists in the spaces you create your life in.

Lavender
Rub a couple drops over your throat to open your communication center and your willingness to speak enthusiasm.

Basil
Inhale a drop from your palms to ease self-limiting patterns of staying the same instead of being renewed.

Oils to *Progress Up the Scale*

Melissa
Hold a drop on the roof of your mouth to stimulate serotonin and dopamine production, boosting your feelings of elation.

Breathe
Rub a few drops over your heart to breathe new life into your daily experiences.

Motivate
Diffuse several drops to raise the vibration of your space, and to fuel the high energy of enthusiasm.

Emotions

265

Passion

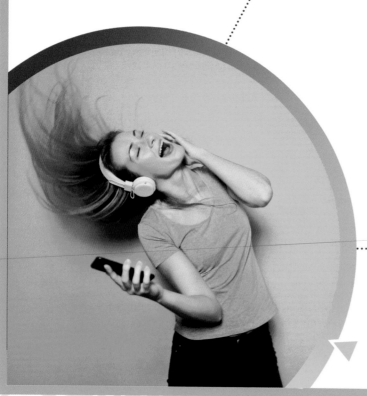

> *It is safe to be me, to be completely in love with who I am. What I love matters. I am free to pursue my true desires.*

Oils to *Process Where You Are*

Motivate
Diffuse several drops to acknowledge places where limited thinking gets in the way of passionately pursuing life.

Rosemary
Use a few drops in the shower or in a diffuser to inspire receptivity of new passionate possibilities.

Whisper
Apply to pulse points to tap into instinctive guidance. Sometimes you don't know all the answers; you only know what feels right.

Oils to *Progress Up the Scale*

Passion
Wear on pulse points as a perfume or cologne.

Jasmine
Apply over heart, taking several moments to breathe deeply and enjoy the building excitement that comes with living your passions.

Cheer
Use a few drops in water, or rub onto the bottoms of your feet 20 minutes before showering. A clean vessel (body) is conducive to a more passionate lifestyle.

Love, Joy, Knowledge, Empowerment, Freedom, Gratitude

> *I am connected to my true, inherent state of being. I am empowered in gratitude and a sense of freedom. I am loving and I am loved.*

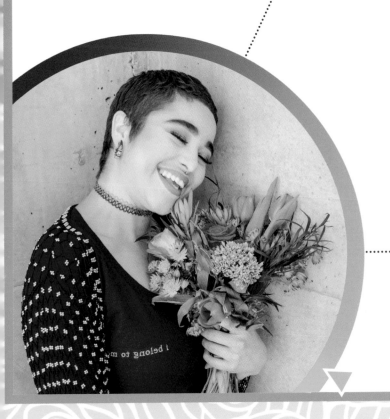

Oils to *Process Where You Are*

Cheer
Diffuse several drops to expand your knowing that all is well, joyful, purposeful, and divinely guided.

Arborvitae
Use a dab on the temples during gratitude prayers and gratitude journaling.

Ylang Ylang
Apply a drop to wrists and pulse points on the neck while doing something you love like singing in the car or shower.

Oils to *Progress Up the Scale*

Elevation
Inhale a drop from cupped hands during moments of reflection and appreciation.

Lime
Drink a few drops in a glass of ice water to sink further into your zest for life.

Rose
Apply over the heart to connect more deeply to unconditional self-love and love of others.

Emotions

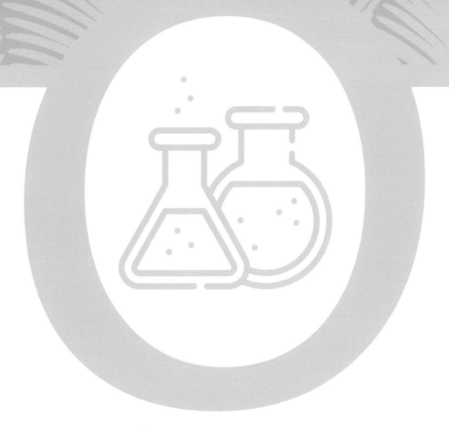

Section 9

Science & Research

How to Use *Science & Research*

While anecdotal evidence of essential oil benefits can be a powerful demonstration of what oils can do, science provides answers as to *why* they do what they do.

As of the publishing of this book, over 3,000 peer-reviewed studies have been documented by universities, hospitals, and research groups to discover and demonstrate the efficacy of essential oils and their constituents. These studies can be found in rapidly growing numbers through resources like www.pubmed.com and www.aromaticscience.com.

The treasure of essential oils is their chemistry. Each oil contains a unique and robust chemistry set and each chemical constituent provides various therapeutic benefits.

This section provides a breakdown of essential oils by common property and which naturally occurring chemical constituents provide the associated therapeutic benefits of each property. The science shared in this section has been drawn from the research and resources cited in the references section in this book.

Begin exploring this section by first becoming familiar with the common therapeutic properties essential oils have.

For an additional deep dive into the science and chemistry of essential oils, purchase "Essential Oils Unlocked" by PJ Hanks.

Therapeutic Properties *Glossary*

The following are the most common therapeutic properties of essential oils. The pages that follow expand on common chemical constituents that provide each of these therapeutic properties, and in which essential oils they can be found.

Analgesic	Reduces pain sensation	**Aphrodisiac**	Increases sexual desires
Anti-allergenic	Reduces allergic response	**Astringent**	Firms tissues, reduces secretions
Antiarthritic	Useful in treating arthritis	**Cardiotonic**	Vitalizes cardiovascular system
Antibacterial	Kills or prevents bacterial growth	**Carminative**	Reduces gas or bloating
Anticarcinogenic	Inhibits development of cancer cells	**Decongestant**	Reduces congestion and opens airways
Anticonvulsant	Reduces convulsions	**Digestive Stimulant**	Aids in proper digestive processes
Antidepressant	Alleviates depression symptoms	**Disinfectant**	Fights the spread of germs
Antiemetic	Eases nausea and vomiting	**Expectorant**	Removes excess mucus
Antifungal	Prevents fungal growth	**Immunostimulant**	Stimulates immune system activity
Anti-infectious	Prevents uptake of infection	**Nervine**	Beneficial effect on nerves
Anti-inflammatory	Alleviates inflammation	**Regenerative**	Promotes body tissue regeneration
Antioxidant	Reduces damage from free radicals	**Restorative**	Promotes restoration of body systems
Anti-parasitic	Destroys or inhibits growth of parasites	**Rubefacient**	Increases circulation & skin redness
Anti-rheumatic	Alleviates pain and stiffness	**Sedative**	Relaxes psychological and physical activity
Antispasmodic	Prevents or relieves spasms & convulsions	**Soporific**	Induces sleep
Antitumoral	Inhibits growth of tumors	**Stomachic**	Stimulates digestion & appetite
Antitussive	Relieves coughs	**Tonic**	Encourages feelings of vitality
Antiviral	Inhibits replication of viral RNA	**Vasodilator**	Relaxes blood vessels, lowers blood pressure

Other therapeutic properties *that have not been reviewed in this section due to redundancy or because less research has been done include anaphrodisiac, anti-carcinoma, anticatarrhal, anticoagulant, antimicrobial, antimutagenic, antiputrescent, antiseptic, antitoxic, calmative, cleanser, cytophylactic, deodorant, detoxifier, diuretic, emmenagogue, energizing, galactagogue, grounding, insecticidal, invigorating, laxative, mucolytic, neuroprotective, purifier, refreshing, relaxing, revitalizer, steroidal, stimulant, uplifting, vasoconstrictor, vermicide, vermifuge, and warming.*

Chemistry of *Essential Oils*

Essential oils are comprised of chemical compound groups. Each compound group is comprised of individual chemical constituents. Compound groups are defined by both the number of carbon atoms they have and the type of functional group assigned to them.

Constituents tend to have similar and complimentary therapeutic properties with other constituents found in their same group.

Monoterpene Hydrocarbons	Therapeutic properties include detoxifying, anti-inflammatory, antiseptic, sedative, insecticidal, anti-tumoral, restorative, and mood-enhancing.
Sesquiterpene Hydrocarbons	Therapeutic properties include anti-inflammatory, anti-microbial, analgesic, digestive stimulant, vasodilator, endocrine support, and calmative.
Chamazulene	Chamazulene is not a naturally occurring constituent in plants, but rather occurs during distillation as the constituent Matricene decomposes. Therapeutic properties include antioxidant and regenerative.
Monoterpene Alcohols	Therapeutic properties include antiseptic, anti-fungal, anti-microbial, analgesic, antioxidant, antispasmodic, and integumentary restorative.
Sesquiterpene Alcohols	Therapeutic properties include anti-microbial, anti-inflammatory, endocrine support, nervine, astringent, vasodilator, antispasmodic, sedative, and soporific.
Aldehydes	Therapeutic properties include calmative, anti-microbial, anti-inflammatory, analgesic, nervine, and hypotensive.
Esters	Therapeutic properties include calmative, analgesic, antispasmodic, anti-fungal, and nervine.
Ketones	Therapeutic properties include mucolytic, regenerative, analgesic, sedative, and anti-inflammatory.
Oxides	Therapeutic properties include anti-microbial, expectorant, mucolytic, and analgesic.

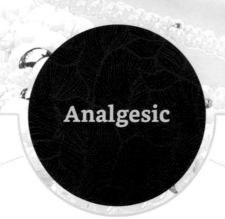

Analgesic

Reduces pain sensation

β-Caryophyllene

Constituent Details
- Sesquiterpene Alkene
- This constituent is a member of the cannabinoid family

Common Oils
- Copaiba (45-65%)
- Black Pepper (8-46%)
- Ylang Ylang (5-25%)
- Melissa (1-22%)
- Clove (0.6-20%)
- Magnolia (4.2%)
- Thyme (0.1-15%)
- Frankincense (0.1-10%)

δ-3-Carene

Constituent Details
- Monoterpene Alkene

Common Oils
- Cypress 7-30%
- Siberian Fir 5-20%
- Black Pepper 0.01-21%

Methyl Salicylate

Constituent Details
- Ester

Common Oils
- Birch (98%)
- Wintergreen (98%)
- Ylang Ylang (0-10.4%)

α-Pinene

Constituent Details
- Monoterpene Alkene

Common Oils
- Frankincense (25-65%)
- Cypress (20-65%)
- Juniper Berry (24-55%)
- Black Spruce (13.7%)
- Coriander (5-20%)
- Helichrysum 5-20%
- Rosemary (5-20%)
- Siberian Fir (5-20%)
- Black Pepper (1-20%)
- Fennel (1-15%)

Science

de Cássia da Silveira E, *Int J Mol Sci*, 2017 | Zalachoras, *Planta Medica*, 2010 | Jimenez, *Die Pharmazie*, 1989

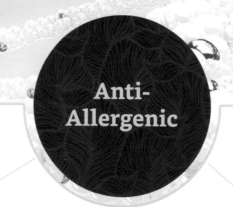

Anti-Allergenic

Reduces allergic response

Neral

Constituent Details
- Monoterpene Alkene Aldehyde

Common Oils
- Lemongrass (25-36%)
- Melissa (9-26%)
- Lemon (0.4-2%)
- Wild Orange (<1.3%)
- Geranium (0-1.1%)

Geranial

Constituent Details
- Monoterpene Alkene Aldehyde

Common Oils
- Lemon Myrtle (46-60%)
- Lemongrass (36-55%)
- Melissa (12-38%)
- Lemon (0.5-4.3%)
- Lime (2.2-3.9%)
- Wild Orange (<1.8%)

Citral

Constituent Details
- Monoterpene Aldehyde

Common Oils
- Lemon Myrtle (90%)
- Litsea (70-85%)
- Lemongrass (65-85%)
- Melissa (64%)
- Petitgrain (36%)
- Lime (6-9%)
- Lemon (2-5%)
- Bergamot (3%)

Mckay, *Phytotherapy Research*, 2006
Emílio-Silva, *Inflammation*, 2017

Science

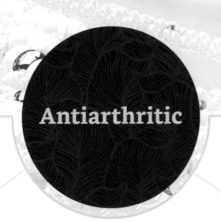

Antiarthritic

Useful in treating arthritis

Bornyl Acetate

Constituent Details
· Monoterpene Ester

Common Oils
· Black Spruce (36%)
· Siberian Fir (20-40%)
· Rosemary (11-15%)
· Douglas Fir (10%)
· Hinoki (7.2%)

Carvone

Constituent Details
· Monoterpene Ketone

Common Oils
· Spearmint (20-80%)
· Dill (40-65%)

α-Pinene

Constituent Details
· Monoterpene Alkene

Common Oils
· Frankincense (25-65%)
· Cypress (20-65%)
· Juniper Berry (24-55%)
· Black Spruce (13.7%)
· Coriander (5-20%)
· Helichrysum 5-20%
· Rosemary (5-20%)
· Siberian Fir (5-20%)
· Black Pepper (1-20%)
· Fennel (1-15%)

Naseri, *Iran Journal of Pharmaceutical Research*, 2012
Kim, *The American Journal of Chinese Medicine*, 2015

Science

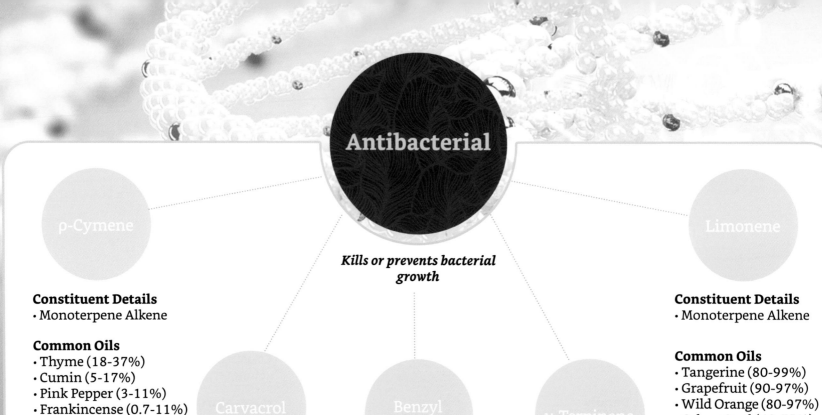

Antibacterial

Kills or prevents bacterial growth

ρ-Cymene

Constituent Details
· Monoterpene Alkene

Common Oils
· Thyme (18-37%)
· Cumin (5-17%)
· Pink Pepper (3-11%)
· Frankincense (0.7-11%)
· Oregano (3-10%)
· Coriander (0-8.4%)
· Rosemary (2.4-6%)
· Marjoram (2.2-5.3%)

Carvacrol

Constituent Details
· Monoterpene Phenol

Common Oils
· Oregano (60-80%)
· Thyme (0.2-16%)

Benzyl Acetate

Constituent Details
· Ester

Common Oils
· Jasmine (5-25%)
· Ylang Ylang (0.4-12%)

γ-Terpinene

Constituent Details
· Monoterpene Alkene

Common Oils
· Tea Tree (10-55%)
· Cumin (3-35%)
· Lime (5-20%)
· Marjoram (0.5-20%)
· Lemon (3-16%)
· Bergamot (3-12%)
· Coriander (0.1-10%)

Limonene

Constituent Details
· Monoterpene Alkene

Common Oils
· Tangerine (80-99%)
· Grapefruit (90-97%)
· Wild Orange (80-97%)
· Celery Seed (68-75%)
· Lemon (55-75%)
· Lime (40-70%)
· Dill (30-55%)
· Bergamot (20-55%)
· Spearmint (5-30%)
· Black Pepper (9-25%)
· Frankincense (5-20%)

Magi, *Frontiers in Microbiology,* 2015 | Cristani, *Journal of Agricultural and Food Chemistry,* 2007 | Rath, *Indian Journal of Pharmaceutical Sciences,* 2008

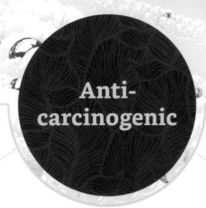

Anti-carcinogenic

Inhibits development of cancer cells

Limonene

Constituent Details
• Monoterpene Alkene

Common Oils
• Grapefruit (84-95%)
• Tangerine (87-91%)
• Wild Orange (93-96%)
• Lemon (56-76%)
• Lime (40-70%)
• Dill (35-68%)
• Bergamot (20-55%)
• Spearmint (5-30%)
• Black Pepper (9-25%)
• Frankincense (5-20%)

Lanceol

Constituent Details
• Sesquiterpene Alcohol

Common Oils
• Hawaiian Sandalwood (2-16%)
• Indian Sandalwood (1.5-1.7%)
• Helichrysum (.2%)
• Clary Sage (.1%)

p-Cymene

Constituent Details
• Monoterpene Alkene

Common Oils
• Thyme (18-37%)
• Cumin (5-17%)
• Pink Pepper (3-11%)
• Frankincense (0.7-11%)
• Oregano (3-10%)
• Coriander (0-8.4%)
• Rosemary (2.4-6%)
• Marjoram (2.2-5.3%)

Chen, *Oncology Letters*, 2013 | Elson, *Carcinogenesis*, 1988 | Marchese, *Materials*, 2017

Science

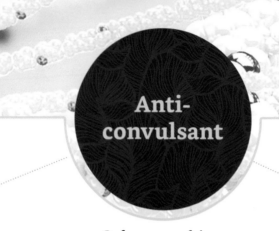

Anti-convulsant

Reduces convulsions

α-Thujene

Constituent Details
• Monoterpene Ketone

Common Oils
• Frankincense (1-19.3%)
• Juniper Berry (1.8%)

Thymol

Constituent Details
• Phenol

Common Oils
• Thyme (48-62%)
• Oregano (0.3-4%)
• Blue Tansy (0.8-1.8%)

E-Anethole

Constituent Details
• Ester

Common Oils
• Star Anise (71-91%)
• Fennel (58-92%)

Limonene

Constituent Details
• Monoterpene Alkene

Common Oils
• Tangerine (80-99%)
• Grapefruit (90-97%)
• Wild Orange (80-97%)
• Celery Seed (68-75%)
• Lemon (55-75%)
• Lime (40-70%)
• Dill (30-55%)
• Bergamot (20-55%)
• Spearmint (5-30%)
• Black Pepper (9-25%)
• Frankincense (5-20%)

Karimzadeh, *BMC Complementary and Alternative Medicine*, 2012
Aliabadi, *International Journal of Medical Laboratory*, 2016
Viana, *Biological & Pharmaceutical Bulletin*, 2000

Science

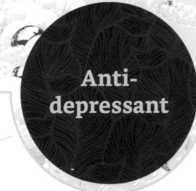

Anti-depressant

Alleviates depression symptoms

Neral

Constituent Details
· Monoterpene Alcohol

Common Oils
· Lemongrass (25-50%)
· Melissa (1-32%)

Benzyl Acetate

Constituent Details
· Ester

Common Oils
· Jasmine (5-25%)
· Ylang Ylang (0.4-12%)

αPhelland-rene

Constituent Details
· Monoterpene Alkede

Common Oils
· Dill (6.5%)
· Pink Pepper (5-17%)
· Frankincense (0-5.9%)

1,8-Cineole

Constituent Details
· Monoterpene Ether

Common Oils
· Eucalyptus (55-85%)
· Rosemary (30-60%)
· Cardamom (26-44%)
· Tulsi (12-16%)
· Tea Tree (3-15%)
· Basil (6-6.7%)
· Peppermint (1-10%)
· Spearmint (0.1-10%)
· Frankincense (0-2.9%)

Piccinelli, *Nutritional Neuroscience*, 2014
Kim, *Evidence-Based Complementary and Alternative Medicine*, 2014

Science

Constituent Details
- Monoterpene Alcohol

Common Oils
- Rose (10-30%)
- Citronella (16-29%)
- Geranium (5-25%)
- Lemongrass (1-15%)
- Melissa (1-8.1%)
- Neroli (0.8-3%)

Constituent Details
- Monoterpene Alkene

Common Oils
- Blue Tansy (10-30%)
- Douglas Fir (5-25%)
- Marjoram (0.4-33%)
- Juniper Berry(0.0-30%)
- Black Pepper (0.1-23%)

Geraniol

Sabinene

Gurjunene

Constituent Details
- Sesquiterpene Alkene

Common Oils
- Spikenard (3-13%)

Menthol

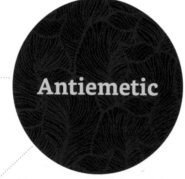

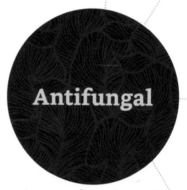

Neryl Acetate

Constituent Details
- Monoterpene Alcohol

Common Oils
- Peppermint (19-54%)

Antiemetic

Eases nausea and vomiting

Antifungal

Prevents fungal growth

Constituent Details
- Monoterpene Ester

Common Oils
- Helichrysum (25-50%)

Menthone

Constituent Details
- Monoterpene Ketone

Common Oils
- Peppermint (8-31%)
- Geranium (0.1-2.4%)
- Spearmint (0.1-1.7%)

Constituent Details
- Monoterpene Alkene

Common Oils
- Neroli (4.6-7%)
- Tulsi (3.4-6.2%)
- Lavender (0.3-10%)

β-Ocimene

Oz, *Frontiers in Pharmacology,* 2017
Sadraei, *Research in Pharmaceutical Sciences,* 2013

Djihane, *Saudi Pharmaceutical Journal,* 2017
Valente, *Food and Chemical Toxicology,* 2013
Flach, *Planta Medica,* 2002

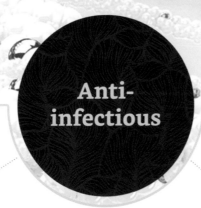

Anti-infectious

Prevents uptake of infection

Geranial

Constituent Details
- Monoterpene Aldehyde

Common Oils
- Lemon Myrtle (46-60%)
- Lemongrass (36-55%)
- Melissa (12-38%)
- Lemon (0.5-4.3%)
- Lime (2.2-3.9%)
- Wild Orange (<1.8%)

δ-3-Carene

Constituent Details
- Monoterpene Alkene

Common Oils
- Cypress (7-30%)
- Siberian Fir (5-20%)
- Black Pepper (0.01-21%)

Limonene

Constituent Details
- Monoterpene Alkene

Common Oils
- Tangerine (80-99%)
- Grapefruit (90-97%)
- Wild Orange (80-97%)
- Celery Seed (68-75%)
- Lemon (55-75%)
- Lime (40-70%)
- Dill (30-55%)
- Bergamot (20-55%)
- Spearmint (5-30%)
- Black Pepper (9-25%)
- Frankincense (5-20%)

Kon KV, *Expert Rev Anti Infect Ther*, 2012
Astani, *Iranian Journal of Microbiology*, 2014

Science

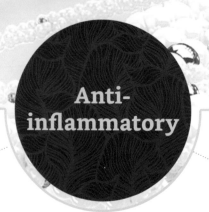

Anti-inflammatory

Alleviates Inflammation

Camphene

Constituent Details
· Monoterpene Alkene

Common Oils
· Siberian Fir (10-30%)
· Black Spruce (8.1%)
· Ginger (1-10%)

Camphor

Constituent Details
· Monoterpene Ketone

Common Oils
· Blue Tansy (5-20%)
· Rosemary (5-15%)
· Coriander (2-8%)

Methyl Salicylate

Constituent Details
· Ester

Common Oils
· Birch (98%)
· Wintergreen (98%)
· Ylang Ylang (0-10.4%)

β-Caryophyllene

Constituent Details
· Sesquiterpene Alkene

Common Oils
· Copaiba (45-65%)
· Black Pepper (8-46%)
· Ylang Ylang (5-25%)
· Melissa (1-22%)
· Clove (0.6-20%)
· Magnolia (4.2%)
· Thyme (0.1-15%)
· Frankincense (0.1-10%)

Oliveira-Tintino, *Phytomedicine,* 2018
Bayala, *PLoS ONE,* 2014

Science

Antioxidant

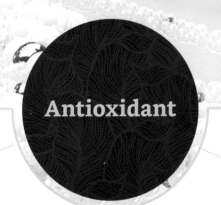

Reduces damage from free radicals

Bergamotene

Constituent Details
· Sesquiterpene Alkene

Common Oils
· Copaiba (2-12%)
· Basil (1-7%)

Camphene

Constituent Details
· Monoterpene Alkene

Common Oils
· Siberian Fir (10-30%)
· Black Spruce (8.1%)
· Ginger (1-10%)

Cinnamaldehyde

Constituent Details
· Aldehyde

Common Oils
· Cassia (75-97%)
· Cinnamon (45-80%)

β-Caryophyllene

Constituent Details
· Sesquiterpene Alkene

Common Oils
· Copaiba (45-65%)
· Black Pepper (8-46%)
· Ylang Ylang (5-25%)
· Melissa (1-22%)
· Clove (0.6-20%)
· Magnolia (4.2%)
· Thyme (0.1-15%)
· Frankincense (0.1-10%)

Pandey, *Medicines*, 2017
Li, *Journal of Food Science and Technology*, 2017

Science

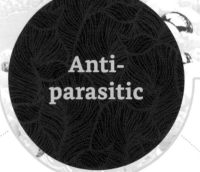

Anti-parasitic

Destroys or inhibits growth of parasites

ρ-Cymene

Methyleuge-nol

Limonene

Constituent Details
· Monoterpene Hydrocarbon

Common Oils
· Thyme (18-37%)
· Cumin (5-17%)
· Pink Pepper (3-11%)
· Frankincense (0.7-11%)
· Oregano (3-10%)
· Coriander (0-8.4%)
· Rosemary (2.4-6%)
· Marjoram (2.2-5.3%)

Constituent Details
· Phenylpropenoid Ether

Common Oils
· Clove (0.2%)
· Basil (0.1%)
· Tea Tree (.06%)

Constituent Details
· Monoterpene Alkene

Common Oils
· Tangerine (80-99%)
· Grapefruit (90-97%)
· Wild Orange (80-97%)
· Celery Seed (68-75%)
· Lemon (55-75%)
· Lime (40-70%)
· Dill (30-55%)
· Bergamot (20-55%)
· Spearmint (5-30%)
· Black Pepper (9-25%)
· Frankincense (5-20%)

Sena-Lopes, *Plos One*, 2018
Gomes, *American Journal of Plant Sciences*, 2014
Escobar, *Memórias Do Instituto Oswaldo Cruz*, 2010

Science

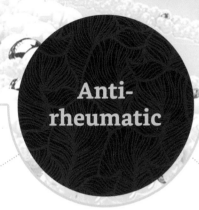

Anti-rheumatic

Alleviates pain & stiffness

Bornyl Acetate

Constituent Details
• Ester

Common Oils
• Black Spruce (36%)
• Siberian Fir (20-40%)
• Rosemary (11-15%)
• Douglas Fir (10%)
• Hinoki (7.2%)

Methyl Salicylate

Constituent Details
• Ester

Common Oils
• Birch (98%)
• Wintergreen (98%)
• Ylang Ylang (0-10.4%)

Geranial

Constituent Details
• Monoterpene Aldehyde

Common Oils
• Lemon Myrtle (46-60%)
• Lemongrass (36-55%)
• Melissa (12-38%)
• Lemon (0.5-4.3%)
• Lime (2.2-3.9%)
• Wild Orange (<1.8%)

Shakeel-u-Rehman, *EC Microbiology*, 2018
Mitoshi, *International Journal of Molecular Medicine*, 2014

Science

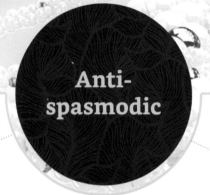

Anti-spasmodic

Prevents or relieves spasms, convulsions, & contractions

Linalyl Acetate

Constituent Details
· Monoterpene Ester

Common Oils
· Clary Sage (45-73%)
· Lavender (25-46%)
· Bergamot (17-40%)
· Marjoram (7-10%)
· Neroli (0.6-10%)
· Cardamom (6.5%)

Camphor

Constituent Details
· Monoterpene Ketone

Common Oils
· Blue Tansy (5-20%)
· Rosemary (5-15%)
· Coriander (2-8%)

Benzyl Benzoate

Constituent Details
· Ester

Common Oils
· Jasmine (8-20%)
· Ylang Ylang (4-14%)
· Cassia (1%)
· Cinnamon (1%)

β-Caryophyllene

Constituent Details
· Sesquiterpene Alkene

Common Oils
· Copaiba (45-65%)
· Black Pepper (8-46%)
· Ylang Ylang (5-25%)
· Melissa (1-22%)
· Clove (0.6-20%)
· Magnolia (4.2%)
· Thyme (0.1-15%)
· Frankincense (0.1-10%)

Leonhardt, *Fundam Clin Pharmacol*, 2010 | Andrade, *Journal of Medicinal Plants Research*, 2011 | Astudillo, *Phytotherapy Research*, 2004

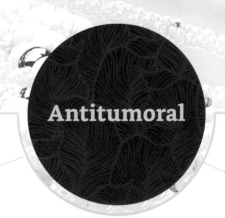

Antitumoral

Inhibits growth of tumors

α-Terpinene

α-Thujene

Carvacrol

α-Pinene

Constituent Details
· Monoterpene Alkene

Common Oils
· Tea Tree (5-13%)
· Marjoram (3-5.9%)
· Roman Chamomile (0-4.5%)
· Juniper Berry (0-2.6%)
· Douglas Fir (2%)

Constituent Details
· Monoterpene Ketone

Common Oils
· Frankincense (1-19.3%)
· Juniper Berry (1.8%)

Constituent Details
· Monoterpene Phenol

Common Oils
· Oregano (61-83%)
· Marjoram (76-81%)
· Thyme (41%)

Constituent Details
· Monoterpene Alkene

Common Oils
· Frankincense (25-65%)
· Cypress (20-65%)
· Juniper Berry (24-55%)
· Black Spruce (13.7%)
· Coriander (5-20%)
· Helichrysum 5-20%
· Rosemary (5-20%)
· Siberian Fir (5-20%)
· Black Pepper (1-20%)
· Fennel (1-15%)

Yin, *Cytotechnology*, 2011 | Biswas, *Evidence-Based Complementary and Alternative Medicine*, 2011 | Fernandes, *Bioactive Essential Oils and Cancer*, 2015

Science

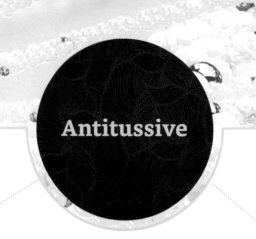

Antitussive

Relieves Coughs

1,8-Cineole

Constituent Details
• Monoterpene Ether

Common Oils
• Eucalyptus (55-85%)
• Rosemary (30-60%)
• Cardamom (26-44%)
• Tulsi (12-16%)
• Tea Tree (3-15%)
• Basil (6-6.7%)
• Peppermint (1-10%)
• Spearmint (0.1-10%)
• Frankincense (0-2.9%)

Menthol

Constituent Details
• Monoterpene Alcohol

Common Oils
• Peppermint (20-60%)

Khusimol

Constituent Details
• Sesquiterpene Alcohol

Common Oils
• Vetiver (5-15%)

Takaishi, *Molecular Pain*, 2012
Jirovetz, *Scientia Pharmaceutica*, 2003
Laude, *Pulmonary Pharmacology*, 1994

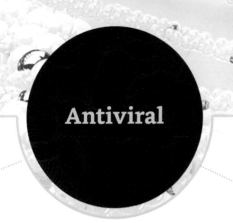

Antiviral

Prevents the replication of viral RNA

Citral

Constituent Details
· Monoterpene Alkene Aldehyde

Common Oils
· Lemon Myrtle (90%)
· Litsea (70-85%)
· Lemongrass (65-85%)
· Melissa (64%)
· Petitgrain (36%)
· Lime (6-9%)
· Lemon (2-5%)
· Bergamot (3%)

Lindestrene

Constituent Details
· Sesquiterpene Ether

Common Oils
· Myrrh (1-20%)

Geranial

Constituent Details
· Monoterpene Aldehyde

Common Oils
· Lemon Myrtle (46-60%)
· Lemongrass (36-55%)
· Melissa (12-38%)
· Lemon (0.5-4.3%)
· Lime (2.2-3.9%)
· Wild Orange (<1.8%)

Geraniol

Constituent Details
· Monoterpene Alcohol

Common Oils
· Rose (10-30%)
· Citronella (16-29%)
· Geranium (5-25%)
· Lemongrass (1-15%)
· Melissa (1-8.1%)
· Neroli (0.8-3%)
· Ylang Ylang (0-3%)
· Eucalyptus (0.2-2%)

Pourghanbari, *VirusDisease*, 2016
Farhath, *Avicenna Journal of Phytomedicine*, 2013
Astani, *Phytotherapy Research*, 2009

Science

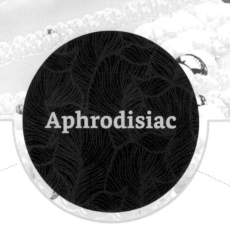

Aphrodisiac

Increases sexual desires

Carvacrol

Constituent Details
- Monoterpene Phenol
- Increases concentration of Follicle Stimulating Hormone and Testosterone

Common Oils
- Oregano (61-83%)
- Thyme (41%)

Benzyl Acetate

Constituent Details
- Ester

Common Oils
- Jasmine (5-25%)
- Ylang Ylang (0.4-12%)

Phytol Acetate

Constituent Details
- Diterpenoid Alkene Alcohol

Common Oils
- Jasmine (7-12%)

Nerol

Constituent Details
- Monoterpene Alkene Aldehyde

Common Oils
- Helichrysum (14.6%)
- Rose (0.8-8%)
- Melissa (0.6-1.3%)
- Neroli (0.3-1.3%)
- Geranium (0-1.2%)

Ali, *Asian Pacific Journal of Tropical Biomedicine*, 2015

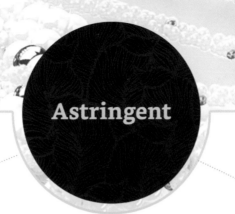

Astringent

Firms tissues & organs, reduces secretions

δ-3-Carene

Constituent Details
· Monoterpene Alkene

Common Oils
· Cypress (7-30%)
· Siberian (Fir 5-20%)
· Black Pepper (0.01-21%)

Fenchone

Constituent Details
· Monoterpene Ketone

Common Oils
· Fennel (1-20%)

Phytol

Constituent Details
· Alcohol

Common Oils
· Jasmine (3-50%)

α & β Santalol

Constituent Details
· Sesquiterpene Alcohol

Common Oils
· Hawaiian Sandalwood (10-60%)
· Indian Sandalwood (10-60%)

Sripathi, *National Product Research*, 2017
Raina AP, *Journal of Medicinal Plants Research*, 2013

Science

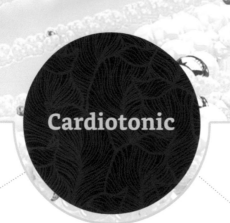

Cardiotonic

Vitalizes cardiovascular system, tones the heart

β-Caryophyllene

Constituent Details
- Sesquiterpene Alkene

Common Oils
- Copaiba (45-65%)
- Black Pepper (8-46%)
- Ylang Ylang (5-25%)
- Melissa (1-22%)
- Clove (0.6-20%)
- Magnolia (4.2%)
- Thyme (0.1-15%)
- Frankincense (0.1-10%)

Eugenol

Constituent Details
- Phenol/Phenylpropanoid

Common Oils
- Clove (63-95%)
- Basil (33.7%)
- Tulsi (31-50%)
- Cinnamon (1-10%)
- Laurel Leaf (1.2-3%)
- Jasmine (1.1-3%)
- Rose (1.3%)

Linalyl Acetate

Constituent Details
- Monoterpene Ester

Common Oils
- Clary Sage (40-75%)
- Petitgrain (40-65%)
- Lavender (25-45%)
- Bergamot (10-45%)
- Marjoram (7-10%)
- Neroli (0.6-10%)
- Cardamom (6.5%)

Lavdeep, *Pharmacologia*, 2013
Khair-Ul-Bariyah, *Pakistan Journal of Chemistry*, 2012
Unnikrishnan, *International Ayurvedic Medical Journal*, 2015

Carminative

Reduces gas or bloating

Bornyl Acetate

Constituent Details
• Monoterpene Ester

Common Oils
• Black Spruce (36%)
• Siberian Fir (20-40%)
• Rosemary (11-15%)
• Douglas Fir (10%)
• Hinoki (7.2%)

Menthol

Constituent Details
• Monoterpene Alcohol

Common Oils
• Peppermint (20-60%)

Zingiberene

Constituent Details
• Sesquiterpene Alkene

Common Oils
• Ginger (20-40%)

Curcumene

Constituent Details
• Sesquiterpene Alkene

Common Oils
• Helichrysum (2-20%)
• Ginger (0.1-10%)

Anethole

Constituent Details
• Phenylpropene

Common Oils
• Star Anise (71-91%)
• Fennel (50-90%)

Peana, *Phytomedicine*, 2002
Mustafa, *Journal of Essential Oil Research*, 2005

Science

Decongestant

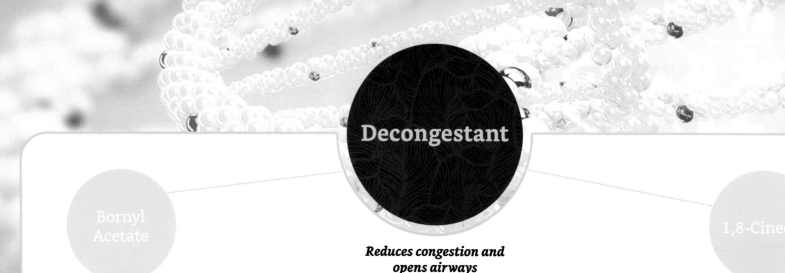

Reduces congestion and opens airways

Bornyl Acetate

Constituent Details
· Monoterpene Ester

Common Oils
· Black Spruce (36%)
· Siberian Fir (20-40%)
· Rosemary (11-15%)
· Douglas Fir (10%)
· Hinoki (7.2%)

1,8-Cineole

Constituent Details
· Monoterpene Ether

Common Oils
· Eucalyptus (55-85%)
· Rosemary (30-60%)
· Cardamom (26-44%)
· Tulsi (12-16%)
· Tea Tree (3-15%)
· Basil (6-6.7%)
· Peppermint (1-10%)
· Spearmint (0.1-10%)
· Frankincense (0-2.9%)

β-Pinene

Constituent Details
· Monoterpene Alkene

Common Oils
· Douglas Fir (20-40%)
· Black Spruce (14.2%)
· Cumin (4-35%)
· Lime (10-25%)
· Lemon (6-18%)
· Black Pepper (2-20%)
· Bergamot (3-12%)
· Blue Tansy (2-10%)

Camphor

Constituent Details
· Monoterpene Ketone

Common Oils
· Blue Tansy (5-20%)
· Rosemary (5-15%)
· Coriander (2-8%)

Camphene

Constituent Details
· Monoterpene Alkene

Common Oils
· Siberian Fir (10-30%)
· Black Spruce (8.1%)
· Ginger (1-10%)

Juergens, *Drug Research*, 2014
Santos, *Phytotherapy Research*, 2000
Peana, *Phytomedicine*, 2002

Science

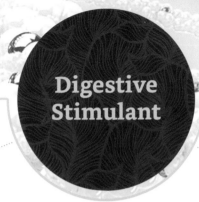

Digestive Stimulant

Aids in proper digestive processes

Linalyl Acetate

Constituent Details
· Monoterpene Ester

Common Oils
· Clary Sage (40-75%)
· Petitgrain (40-65%)
· Lavender (25-45%)
· Bergamot (10-45%)
· Marjoam (7-10%)
· Neroli (0.6-10%)
· Cardamom (6.5%)

Anethole

Constituent Details
· Phenylpropene

Common Oils
· Star Anise (71-91%)
· Fennel (50-90%)

Cinnamaldehyde

Constituent Details
· Aldehyde

Common Oils
· Cassia (75-97%)
· Cinnamon (45-80%)

β-Caryophyllene

Constituent Details
· Sesquiterpene Alkene

Common Oils
· Copaiba (45-65%)
· Black Pepper (8-46%)
· Ylang Ylang (5-25%)
· Melissa (1-22%)
· Clove (0.6-20%)
· Magnolia (4.2%)
· Thyme (0.1-15%)
· Frankincense (0.1-10%)

Asano, *Biochem Biophys Res Commun*, 2016
Dahham, *Molecules*, 2015

Science

Disinfectant

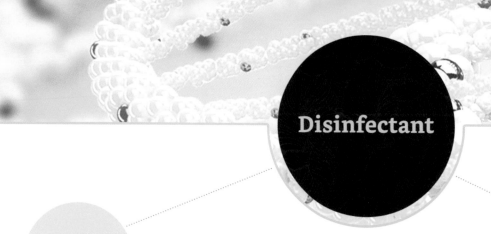

Fights the spread of germs

Aromadendrene

Constituent Details
· Sesquiterpene Alkene

Common Oils
· Patchouli (2-25%)
· Copaiba (1.8%)

Citronellyl Formate

Constituent Details
· Monoterpene Ester

Common Oils
· Geranium (1-15%)

α-Cedrene

Constituent Details
· Sesquiterpene Alkene

Common Oils
· Cedarwood (10-47%)

δ-3-Carene

Constituent Details
· Monoterpene Alkene

Common Oils
· Cypress (7-30%)
· Siberian Fir (5-20%)
· Black Pepper (0.01-21%)

Mulyaningsih, *Phytomedicine*, 2010
Mulyaningsih, *Pharm Biol*, 2011
Ouedrhiri, *Environ Sci Pollut Res Int*, 2017

Expectorant

Reduces pain sensation

Terpinyl Acetate

Constituent Details
Monoterpene Ester

Common Oils
- Cardamom (25-50%)
- Hinoki (9.1%)
- Laurel Leaf (4-7%)
- Cypress (4-6%)

Curzerene

Constituent Details
- Sesquiterpene Ether

Common Oils
Myrrh (15-35%)

Menthol

Constituent Details
- Monoterpene Alcohol

Common Oils
- Peppermint (20-60%)

α-Pinene

Constituent Details
- Monoterpene Alkene

Common Oils
- Frankincense (25-65%)
- Cypress (20-65%)
- Juniper Berry (24-55%)
- Black Spruce (13.7%)
- Coriander (5-20%)
- Helichrysum 5-20%
- Rosemary (5-20%)
- Siberian Fir (5-20%)
- Black Pepper (1-20%)
- Fennel (1-15%)

Rivas da Silva, *Molecules*, 2012
Yang, *Molecules*, 2011

Science

Immuno-stimulant

Stimulates immune system activity

Bornyl Acetate

Constituent Details
• Monoterpene Ester

Common Oils
• Black Spruce (36%)
• Siberian Fir (20-40%)
• Rosemary (11-15%)
• Douglas Fir (10%)
• Hinoki (7.2%)

Neral

Constituent Details
• Monoterpene Alcohol

Common Oils
• Lemongrass (25-50%)
• Melissa (1-32%)

Chamazulene

Constituent Details
• Sesquiterpene Polyalkene

Common Oils
• Blue Tansy (17-38%)
• Yarrow|Pom (19.7%)
• Roman Chamomile (0-4.4%)

Myrcene

Constituent Details
• Monoterpene Alkene

Common Oils
• Pink Pepper (5-20%)
• Juniper Berry (0-25%)
• Tangerine (0.5-8%)
• Wild Orange (0.5-5%)

Eugenol

Constituent Details
• Phenol/Phenylpro-panoid

Common Oils
• Clove (63-95%)
• Basil (33.7%)
• Tulsi (31-50%)
• Cinnamon (1-10%)
• Laurel Leaf (1.2-3%)
• Jasmine (1.1-3%)
• Rose (1.3%)

Dibazar, *Journal of Immunotoxicology*, 2015
Uyeda, *Asian Pacific Journal of Allergy and Immunology*, 2016

Constituent Details
• Monoterpene Alkene

Common Oils
• Tangerine (80-99%)
• Grapefruit (90-97%)
• Wild Orange (80-97%)
• Celery Seed (68-75%)
• Lemon (55-75%)
• Lime (40-70%)
• Dill (30-55%)
• Bergamot (20-55%)
• Spearmint (5-30%)
• Black Pepper (9-25%)

Limonene

Constituent Details
• Sesquiterpene Alkene

Common Oils
• Copaiba (45-65%)
• Black Pepper (8-46%)
• Ylang Ylang (5-25%)
• Melissa (1-22%)
• Clove (0.6-20%)
• Magnolia (4.2%)
• Thyme (0.1-15%)
• Frankincense (0.1-10%)

β-Caryophyl-lene

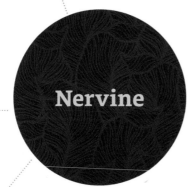

Nervine

Beneficial effect on nerves

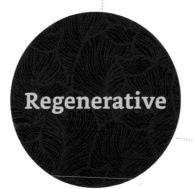

Regenerative

Promotes body tissue regeneration

Chamazulene

Constituent Details
• Sesquiterpene Poly-alkene

Common Oils
• Blue Tansy (2-15%)

Isovalencenol

Constituent Details
• Sesquiterpene Alcohol
• This Constituent is responsible for much of Vetiver's beautiful perfume-like aroma

Common Oils
• Vetiver (5-20%)

Constituent Details
• Monoterpene Alkene

Common Oils
• Siberian Fir (10-30%)
• Black Spruce (8.1%)
• Ginger (1-10%)

Camphene

Lenardão, *Journal of the Brazilian Chemical Society*, 2015

Viveros-Paredes, *Pharmaceuticals*, 2017
Tiwari, *Toxicology in Vitro*, 2009

Science

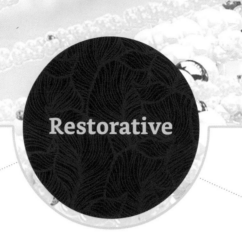

Restorative

Promotes restoration and recovery of body systems

Chamazulene

Constituent Details
- Sesquiterpene Polyalkene

Common Oils
- Blue Tansy (17-38%)
- Yarrow|Pom (19.7%)
- Roman Chamomile (0-4.4%)

Curzerene

Constituent Details
- Sesquiterpene Ether

Common Oils
- Myrrh (15-35%)

Citronellol

Constituent Details
- Monoterpene Alcohol

Common Oils
- Geranium (30-45%)
- Rose (20-40%)
- Citronella (3-22%)
- Lemon Eucalyptus (5.4%)

Linalool

Constituent Details
- Monoterpene Alcohol

Common Oils
- Magnolia (69.9%)
- Coriander (60-75%)
- Basil (40-80%)
- Lavender (20-47%)
- Petitgrain (15-30%)
- Clary Sage (8-40%)
- Cilantro (10-35%)
- Bergamot (3-20%)

Chien, *Evidence-Based Complementary and Alternative Medicine*, 2012
Al-Mobeeriek, *Clinical, Cosmetic and Investigational Dentistry*, 2011
Bowles, *International Journal of Aromatherapy*, 2002

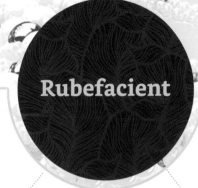

Rubefacient

Increases circulation & skin redness

Linalyl Acetate

Constituent Details
• Monoterpene Ester

Common Oils
• Clary Sage (40-75%)
• Petitgrain (40-65%)
• Lavender (25-45%)
• Bergamot (10-45%)
• Marjoram (7-10%)
• Neroli (0.6-10%)
• Cardamom (6.5%)

Myrcene

Constituent Details
• Monoterpene Alkene

Common Oils
• Pink Pepper (5-20%)
• Juniper Berry (0-25%)
• Tangerine (0.5-8%)
• Wild Orange (0.5-5%)

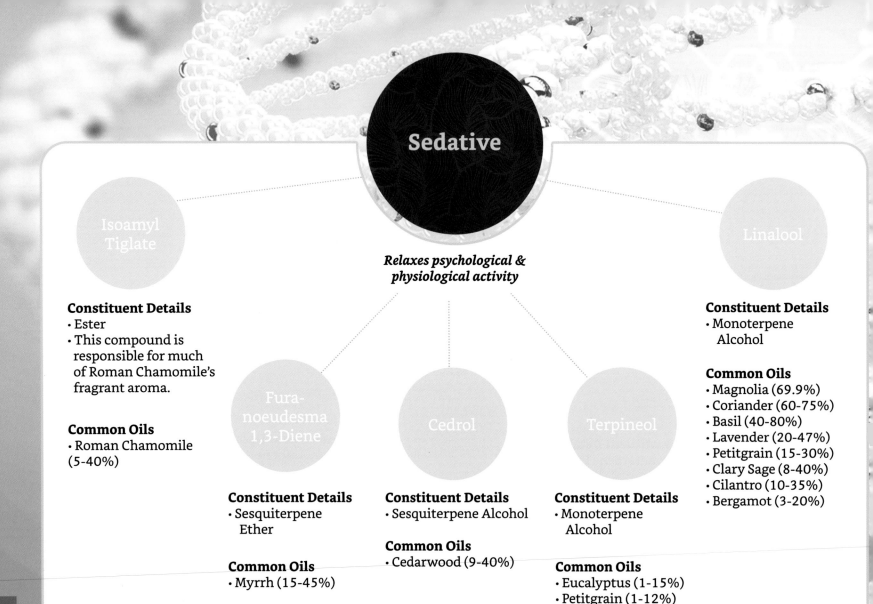

Sedative

Relaxes psychological & physiological activity

Isoamyl Tiglate

Constituent Details
· Ester
· This compound is responsible for much of Roman Chamomile's fragrant aroma.

Common Oils
· Roman Chamomile (5-40%)

Fura-noeudesma 1,3-Diene

Constituent Details
· Sesquiterpene Ether

Common Oils
· Myrrh (15-45%)

Cedrol

Constituent Details
· Sesquiterpene Alcohol

Common Oils
· Cedarwood (9-40%)

Terpineol

Constituent Details
· Monoterpene Alcohol

Common Oils
· Eucalyptus (1-15%)
· Petitgrain (1-12%)

Linalool

Constituent Details
· Monoterpene Alcohol

Common Oils
· Magnolia (69.9%)
· Coriander (60-75%)
· Basil (40-80%)
· Lavender (20-47%)
· Petitgrain (15-30%)
· Clary Sage (8-40%)
· Cilantro (10-35%)
· Bergamot (3-20%)

Han, *Biochimie Open*, 2017
Kagawa, *Planta Medica*, 2003
Sharafzadeh, *Journal of Applied Pharmaceutical Science*, 2011

Science

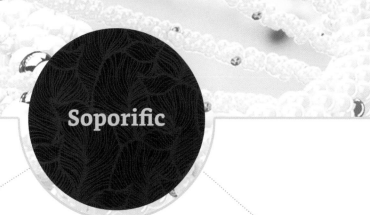

Soporific

Induces sleep

Benzyl Acetate

Constituent Details
• Ester

Common Oils
• Jasmine (5-25%)
• Ylang Ylang (0.4-12%)

Isobutyl Angelate

Constituent Details
• Ester

Common Oils
• Roman Chamomile (5-40%)

Cedrol

Constituent Details
• Sesquiterpene Alcohol

Common Oils
• Cedarwood (9-40%)

Takeda, *Evidence-Based Complementary and Alternative Medicine*, 2017
Cho, *Evidence-Based Complementary and Alternative Medicine*, 2013
Sayowan, *Journal of Health Research*, 2013

Science

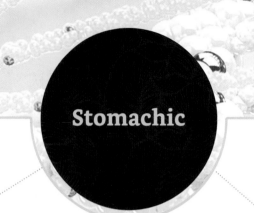

Stomachic

Stimulates digestion & appetite

Limonene

Constituent Details
• Monoterpene Alkene

Common Oils
• Tangerine (80-99%)
• Grapefruit (90-97%)
• Wild Orange (80-97%)
• Celery Seed (68-75%)
• Lemon (55-75%)
• Lime (40-70%)
• Dill (30-55%)
• Bergamot (20-55%)
• Spearmint (5-30%)
• Black Pepper (9-25%)
• Frankincense (5-20%)

Anethole

Constituent Details
• Phenylpropene

Common Oils
• Star Anise (71-91%)
• Fennel (50-90%)

Curcumene

Constituent Details
• Sesquiterpene Alkene

Common Oils
• Helichrysum (2-20%)
• Ginger (0.1-10%)

Yamahara, *Yakugaku Zasshi*, 1992
Asano, *Biochemical and Biophysical Research Communications*, 2016

Science

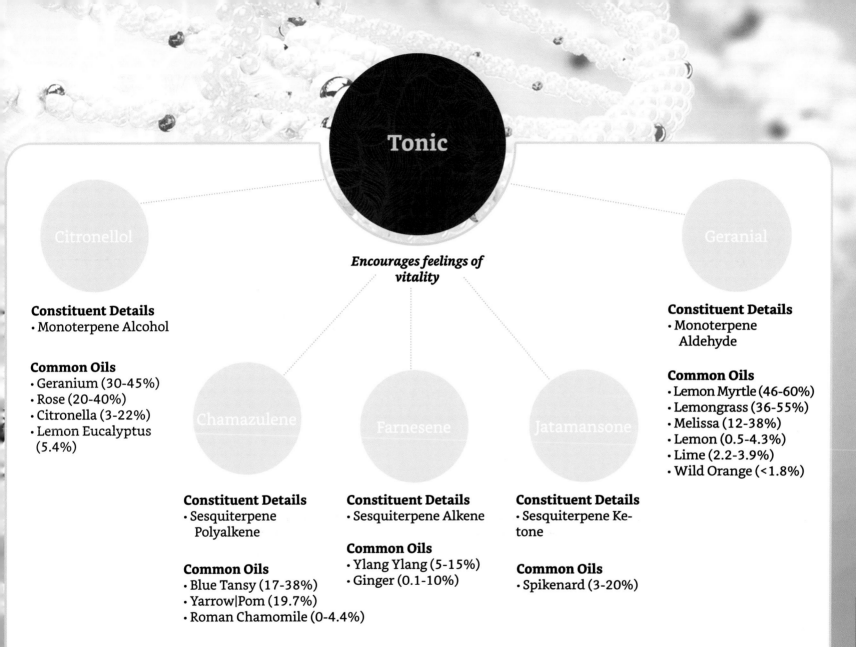

Tonic

Encourages feelings of vitality

Citronellol

Constituent Details
- Monoterpene Alcohol

Common Oils
- Geranium (30-45%)
- Rose (20-40%)
- Citronella (3-22%)
- Lemon Eucalyptus (5.4%)

Chamazulene

Constituent Details
- Sesquiterpene Polyalkene

Common Oils
- Blue Tansy (17-38%)
- Yarrow|Pom (19.7%)
- Roman Chamomile (0-4.4%)

Farnesene

Constituent Details
- Sesquiterpene Alkene

Common Oils
- Ylang Ylang (5-15%)
- Ginger (0.1-10%)

Jatamansone

Constituent Details
- Sesquiterpene Ketone

Common Oils
- Spikenard (3-20%)

Geranial

Constituent Details
- Monoterpene Aldehyde

Common Oils
- Lemon Myrtle (46-60%)
- Lemongrass (36-55%)
- Melissa (12-38%)
- Lemon (0.5-4.3%)
- Lime (2.2-3.9%)
- Wild Orange (<1.8%)

Bastos, *Basic & Clinical Pharmacology & Toxicology*, 2009
Mckay, *Phytotherapy Research*, 2006
Nishteswar, *AYU*, 2014

Science

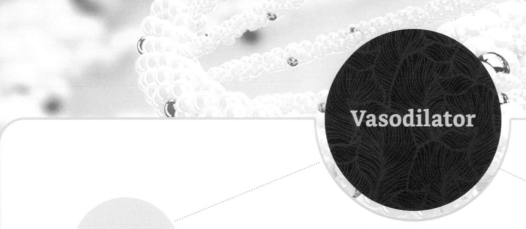

Vasodilator

Relaxes blood vessels, lowers blood pressure

Citronellol

Constituent Details
· Monoterpene Alcohol

Common Oils
· Geranium (30-45%)
· Rose (20-40%)
· Citronella (3-22%)
· Lemon Eucalyptus (5.4%)

Anethole

Constituent Details
· Phenylpropene

Common Oils
· Star Anise (71-91%)
· Fennel (50-90%)

Bulnesene

Constituent Details
· Sesquiterpene Alkene

Common Oils
· Patchouli (1-20%)

Cinnamaldehyde

Constituent Details
· Aldehyde

Common Oils
· Cassia (75-97%)
· Cinnamon (45-80%)

Tognolini, Pharmacological Research, 2007
Soares, *Life Sciences*, 2007
Ribeiro-Filho, *European Journal of Pharmacology*, 2016

Science

Section 10

References & Index

Bibliography

Aromatic Science. AromaticScience, LLC. Web. July, 2017. <www.aromaticscience.com>

AromaTools. Modern Essentials: a Contemporary Guide to the Therapeutic Use of Essential Oils. AromaTools, 2018.

Enlighten Alternative Healing. Emotions and Essential Oils: A Modern Resource for Healing: Emotional Reference Guide. 4th ed., Enlighten Alternative Healing, 2017.

Harding, Jennie: The Essential Oils Handbook. Duncan Baird Publishers Ltd, 2008.

Hill, David K: The dōTERRA Essential Oil Chemistry Handbook. 3rd ed., 2019

Lawless, Julia: The Encyclopedia of Essential Oils: The Complete Guide to the Use of Aromatic Oils In Aromatherapy, Herbalism, Health, and Well Being. Conari Press, 2013.

Schiller, Carol & Schiller, David: The Aromatherapy Encyclopedia: A Concise Guide to Over 395 Plant Oils. Basic Health Publications Inc, 2008.

Schnaubelt, Kurt. The Healing Intelligence of Essential Oils: the Science of Advanced Aromatherapy. Healing Arts Press, 2011.

Tisserand, Robert, et al. Essential Oil Safety: A Guide for Health Care Professionals. 2nd ed., Churchill Livingstone/Elsevier, 2014.

Total Wellness Publishing. The Essential Life: A Simple Guide to Living the Wellness Lifestyle. Total Wellness Publishing, 2017.

Worwood, Valerie Ann. The Complete Book of Essential Oils and Aromatherapy, Revised and Expanded: Over 800 Natural, Nontoxic, and Fragrant Recipes to Create Health, Beauty, And Safe Home and Work Environments. New World Library, 2016.

References

Al-Howiriny T, et al., "Gastric antiulcer, antisecretory and cytoprotective properties of celery (Apium graveolens) in rats", Pharmaceutical Biology (2010); 48(7)

Al-Mobeeriek, Azizah. "Effects of Myrrh on Intra-Oral Mucosal Wounds Compared with Tetracycline- and Chlorhexidine-Based Mouthwashes." *Clinical, Cosmetic and Investigational Dentistry*, 2011, p. 53., doi:10.2147/cciden.s24064.

Ali, B., Al-Wabel, N. A., Shams, S., Ahamad, A., Khan, S. A., & Anwar, F. (2015, August). Essential oils used in aromatherapy: A systemic review. *Asian Pacific Journal of Tropical Biomedicine*, 5(8), 601-611. doi:https://doi.org/10.1016/j.apjtb.2015.05.007

Aliabadi, Ali, et al. "Effects of Thymol on Serum Biochemical and Antioxidant Indices in Kindled Rats." *International Journal of Medical Laboratory*, vol. 3, no. 1, Feb. 2016, pp. 43-49.

Almeida, Reinaldo Nóbrega De, et al. "Essential Oils and Their Constituents: Anticonvulsant Activity." *Molecules*, vol. 16, no. 3, 2011, pp. 2726-2742., doi:10.3390/molecules16032726.

Andrade, Luciana N. "Spasmolytic Activity of p-Menthane Esters." *Journal of Medicinal Plants Research*, vol. 5, no. 32, 2011, doi:10.5897/jmpr11.1074.

Asano T., Aida S., Suemasu S., et al. "Anethole Restores Delayed Gastric Emptying and Impaired Gastric Accommodation in Rodents." *Biochem Biophys Res Commun.* 2016;472(1):125-30

Asano, Teita, et al. "Anethole Restores Delayed Gastric Emptying and Impaired Gastric Accommodation in Rodents." *Biochemical and Biophysical Research Communications*, vol. 472, no. 1, 2016, pp. 125-130., doi:10.1016/j.bbrc.2016.02.078.

Astani, Akram, and Paul Schnitzler. "Antiviral Activity of Monoterpenes Beta-Pinene and Limonene against Herpes Simplex Virus in Vitro." *Iranian Journal of Microbiology*, vol. 6, no. 3, June 2014, pp. 149-155.

Astani, Akram, et al. "Comparative Study on the Antiviral Activity of Selected Monoterpenes Derived from Essential Oils." *Phytotherapy Research*, 2009, doi:10.1002/ptr.2955.

Astudillo, Adela, et al. "Antispasmodic Activity of Extracts and Compounds Of Acalypha Phleoides Cav." *Phytotherapy Research*, vol. 18, no. 2, 2004, pp. 102-106., doi:10.1002/ptr.1414.

Baananou S, et al., "Antiulcerogenic and antibacterial activities of Apium graveolens essential oil and extract", Natural Product Research (2013); 27(12)

Bastos, Joana F. A., et al. "Hypotensive and Vasorelaxant Effects of Citronellol, a Monoterpene Alcohol, in Rats." *Basic & Clinical Pharmacology & Toxicology*, vol. 106, no. 4, July 2009, pp. 331-337., doi:10.1111/j.1742-7843.2009.00492.x.

Bayala, Bagora, et al. "Chemical Composition, Antioxidant, Anti-Inflammatory and Anti-Proliferative Activities of Essential Oils of Plants from Burkina Faso." *PLoS ONE*, vol. 9, no. 3, 2014, doi:10.1371/journal.pone.0092122.

Biswas, Raktim, et al. "Thujone-Rich Fraction Of Thuja Occidentalis Demonstrates Major Anti-Cancer Potentials: Evidences From In Vitro Studies on A375 Cells." *Evidence-Based Complementary and Alternative Medicine*, vol. 2011, 2011, pp. 1-16., doi:10.1093/ecam/neq042.

Bowles, E Joy, et al. "Effects of Essential Oils and Touch on Resistance to Nursing Care Procedures and Other Dementia-Related Behaviours in a Residential Care Facility." *International Journal of Aromatherapy*, vol. 12, no. 1, July 2002, pp. 22-29., doi:10.1054/ijar.2001.0128.

Chen, Yingli, et al. "Composition and Potential Anticancer Activities of Essential Oils Obtained from Myrrh and Frankincense." *Oncology Letters*, vol. 6, no. 4, Aug. 2013, pp. 1140-1146., doi:10.3892/ol.2013.1520.

Chien, Li-Wei, et al. "The Effect of Lavender Aromatherapy on Autonomic Nervous System in Midlife Women with Insomnia." *Evidence-Based Complementary and Alternative Medicine*, vol. 2012, 2012, pp. 1-8., doi:10.1155/2012/740813.

Cho, Mi-Yeon, et al. "Effects of Aromatherapy on the Anxiety, Vital Signs, and Sleep Quality of Percutaneous Coronary Intervention Patients in Intensive Care Units." *Evidence-Based Complementary and Alternative Medicine*, vol. 2013, 2013, pp. 1-6., doi:10.1155/2013/381381.

Cristani, Mariateresa, et al. "Interaction of Four Monoterpenes Contained in Essential Oils with Model Membranes: Implications for Their Antibacterial Activity." *Journal of Agricultural and Food Chemistry*, vol. 55, no. 15, 2007, pp. 6300-6308., doi:10.1021/jf070094x.

Dahham, S.S., Tabana, Y.M., Iqbal, M.A., et al. "The Anticancer, Antioxidant and Antimicrobial Properties of the Sesquiterpene β-Caryophyllene from the Essential Oil of Aquilaria crassna." *Molecules*. 2015;20(7):11808-11829.

de Cássia da Silveira E, Sá R, Lima TC et al. Analgesic-Like Activity of Essential Oil Constituents: An Update. *Int J Mol Sci*. 2017 Dec 9;18(12). pii: E2392. doi: 10.3390/ijms18122392.

Djihane, Bouzid, et al. "Chemical Constituents of Helichrysum Italicum (Roth) G. Don Essential Oil and Their Antimicrobial Activity against Gram-Positive and Gram-Negative Bacteria, Filamentous Fungi and Candida Albicans." *Saudi Pharmaceutical Journal*, vol. 25, no. 5, 2017, pp. 780-787., doi:10.1016/j.jsps.2016.11.001.

Elson, Charles E., et al. "Anti-Carcinogenic Activity of d-Limonene during the Initiation and Promotion/Progression Stages of DMBA-Induced Rat Mammary Carcinogenesis." *Carcinogenesis*, vol. 9, no. 2, 1988, pp. 331-332., doi:10.1093/carcin/9.2.331.

Emílio-Silva, Maycon T., et al. "Antipyretic Effects of Citral and Possible Mechanisms of Action." *Inflammation*, vol. 40, no. 5, 2017, pp. 1735-1741., doi:10.1007/s10753-017-0615-4.

Escobar, Patricia, et al. "Chemical Composition and Antiprotozoal Activities of Colombian Lippia Spp Essential Oils and Their Major Components." *Memórias Do Instituto Oswaldo Cruz*, vol. 105, no. 2, 2010, pp. 184-190., doi:10.1590/s0074-02762010000200013.

Farhath, Seema, et al. "Immunomodulatory Activity of Geranial, Geranial Acetate, Gingerol, and Eugenol Essential Oils: Evidence for Humoral and Cell-Mediated Responses." *Avicenna Journal of Phytomedicine*, vol. 3, no. 3, 2013, pp. 224-230.

Fernandes, Janaina. "Antitumor Monoterpenes." *Bioactive Essential Oils and Cancer*, 2015, pp. 175-200., doi:10.1007/978-3-319-19144-7_8.

Flach, Adriana, et al. "Chemical Analysis and Antifungal Activity of the Essential Oil Of Calea Clematidea." *Planta Medica*, vol. 68, no. 9, 2002, pp. 836-838., doi:10.1055/s-2002-34414.

Gomes, Marcos S., et al. "Use of Essential Oils of the Genus Citrus as Biocidal Agents." *American Journal of Plant Sciences*, vol. 05, no. 03, Feb. 2014, pp. 299-305., doi:10.4236/ajps.2014.53041.

Han, Xuesheng, et al. "Chemical Composition Analysis and in Vitro Biological Activities of Ten Essential Oils in Human Skin Cells." *Biochimie Open*, vol. 5, 2017, pp. 1-7., doi:10.1016/j.biopen.2017.04.001.

Jimenez, J, et al. "Comparative Study of Different Essential Oils of Bupleurum Gibraltaricum Lamarck." *Die Pharmazie*, vol. 44, no. 4, 1 Apr. 1989, pp. 284-287.

Jirovetz, L., et al. "Medicinal Used Plants from India: Analysis of the Essential Oils of Sphaeranthus Indicus Flowers, Roots and Stems with Leaves." *Scientia Pharmaceutica*, vol. 71, 2003, pp. 251-259.

Juergens, U. "Anti-Inflammatory Properties of the Monoterpene 1.8-Cineole: Current Evidence for Co-Medication in Inflammatory Airway Diseases." *Drug Research*, vol. 64, no. 12, 2014, pp. 638-646., doi:10.1055/s-0034-1372609.

Kagawa, D, et al. "The Sedative Effects and Mechanism of Action of Cedrol Inhalation with Behavioral Pharmacological Evaluation." *Planta Medica*, vol. 69, no. 7, July 2003, pp. 637-641., doi:10.1055/s-2003-41114.

Karimzadeh, Fariba, et al. "Anticonvulsant and Neuroprotective Effects of Pimpinella Anisum in Rat Brain." *BMC Complementary and Alternative Medicine*, vol. 12, no. 1, 2012, doi:10.1186/1472-6882-12-76.

Khair-Ul-Bariyah, S., et al. "Ocimum Basilicum: A Review on Phytochemical and Pharmacological Studies." *Pakistan Journal of Chemistry*, vol. 2, no. 2, 2012, pp. 78-85., doi:10.15228/2012.v02.i02.p05.

Kim, Dae-Seung, et al. "Alpha-Pinene Exhibits Anti-Inflammatory Activity Through the Suppression of MAPKs and the NF-KB Pathway in Mouse Peritoneal Macrophages." *The American Journal of Chinese Medicine*, vol. 43, no. 04, 2015, pp. 731-742., doi:10.1142/s0192415x15500457.

Kim, Ka Young, et al. "The Effect of 1,8-Cineole Inhalation on Preoperative Anxiety: A Randomized Clinical Trial." *Evidence-Based Complementary and Alternative Medicine*, vol. 2014, 2014, pp. 1-7., doi:10.1155/2014/820126.

Kon KV, Rai MK. Plant essential oils and their constituents in coping with multidrug-resistant bacteria. *Expert Rev Anti Infect Ther*. 2012;10(7):775-790.

Laude, E.a., et al. "The Antitussive Effects of Menthol, Camphor and Cineole in Conscious Guinea-Pigs." *Pulmonary Pharmacology*, vol. 7, no. 3, 1994, pp. 179-184., doi:10.1006/pulp.1994.1021.

Lavdeep Banewal, Deepa Khanna and Sidharth Mehan. "Spices, Fruits, Nuts and Vitamins: Preventive Interventions for Myocardial Infarction."

Pharmacologia, vol. 4, 2013, p. 553-570, doi: 10..5567/pharmacologia.2013.553.570

Lenardão, Eder J., et al. "Antinociceptive Effect of Essential Oils and Their Constituents: an Update Review." *Journal of the Brazilian Chemical Society*, 2015, doi:10.5935/0103-5053.20150332.

Leonhardt V, Leal-Cardoso JH, Lahlou S, Et Al. Antispasmodic effects of essential oil of Pterodon polygalaeflorus and its main constituent β-caryophyllene on rat isolated ileum. *Fundam Clin Pharmacol*. 2010;24(6):749-758.

Li, Hailong, et al. "Evaluation of the Chemical Composition, Antioxidant and Anti-Inflammatory Activities of Distillate and Residue Fractions of Sweet Basil Essential Oil." *Journal of Food Science and Technology*, vol. 54, no. 7, Aug. 2017, pp. 1882-1890., doi:10.1007/s13197-017-2620-x.

Magi, Gloria, et al. "Antimicrobial Activity of Essential Oils and Carvacrol, and Synergy of Carvacrol and Erythromycin, against Clinical, Erythromycin-Resistant Group A Streptococci." *Frontiers in Microbiology*, vol. 6, Mar. 2015, doi:10.3389/fmicb.2015.00165.

Marchese, Anna, et al. "Update on Monoterpenes as Antimicrobial Agents: A Particular Focus on p-Cymene." *Materials*, vol. 10, no. 8, 2017, p. 947., doi:10.3390/ma10080947.

Mckay, Diane L., and Jeffrey B. Blumberg. "A Review of the Bioactivity and Potential Health Benefits of Peppermint Tea (Mentha Piperita L.)." *Phytotherapy Research*, vol. 20, no. 8, 2006, pp. 619-633., doi:10.1002/ptr.1936.

Mckay, Diane L., and Jeffrey B. Blumberg. "A Review of the Bioactivity and Potential Health Benefits of Chamomile Tea (Matricaria Recutita L.)." *Phytotherapy Research*, vol. 20, no. 7, 2006, pp. 519-530., doi:10.1002/ptr.1900.

Mencherini T, et al., "An extract of Apium graveolens var. Dulce leaves: structure of the major constituent, apiin, and its anti-inflammatory properties" The Journal of Pharmacy and Pharmacology (2007); 59(6)

Mitoshi, Mai, et al. "Suppression of Allergic and Inflammatory Responses by Essential Oils Derived from Herbal Plants and Citrus Fruits." *International Journal of Molecular Medicine*, vol. 33, no. 6, 2014, pp. 1643-1651., doi:10.3892/ijmm.2014.1720.

Mulyaningsih, S., Sporer F, Zimmermann, S., et al. "Synergistic Properties of the Terpenoids Aromadendrene and 1,8-cineole from the Essential Oil of Eucalyptus Globulus Against Antibiotic-Susceptible and Antibiotic-Resistant Pathogens." *Phytomedicine*. 2010;17(13):1061-1066.

Mulyaningsih, S., Sporer, F., Reichling, J., et al. "Antibacterial Activity of Essential Oils from Eucalyptus and of Selected Components Against Multidrug-Resistant Bacterial Pathogens." *Pharm Biol*. 2011;49(9):893-899.

Mustafa, Akhlaq, et al. "Volatile Oil Constituents of the Fresh Rhizomes of Curcuma Amada Roxb." *Journal of Essential Oil Research*, vol. 17, no. 5, 2005, pp. 490-491., www.tandfonline.com/doi/abs/10.1080/10412905.2005.9698974.

Naseri, Mohsen, et al. "The Study of Anti-Inflammatory Activity of Oil-Based Dill (Anethum Graveolens L.) Extract Used Topically in Formalin-Induced Inflammation Male Rat Paw." *Iran Journal of Pharmaceutical Research*, vol. 11, no. 4, 2012, pp. 1169-1174.

Nishteswar, K. "Credential Evidences of Ayurvedic Cardio-Vascular Herbs." *AYU (An International Quarterly Journal of Research in Ayurveda)*, vol. 35, no. 2, 2014, p. 111., doi:10.4103/0974-8520.146194.

Oliveira-Tintino, Cícera Datiane De Morais, et al. "Anti-Inflammatory and Anti-Edematogenic Action of the Croton Campestris A. St.-Hil (Euphorbiaceae) Essential Oil and the Compound ß-Caryophyllene in in Vivo Models." *Phytomedicine*, vol. 41, 2018, pp. 82-95., doi:10.1016/j.phymed.2018.02.004.

Ouedrhiri, W., Balouiri, M., Bouhdid, S., et al. "Antioxidant and Antibacterial Activities of Pelargonium Asperum and Ormenis Mixta Essential Oils and Their Synergistic Antibacterial Effect." *Environ Sci Pollut Res Int*. 2017 Jul 22. doi: 10.1007/s11356-017-9739-1.

Oz, Murat, et al. "Cellular and Molecular Targets of Menthol Actions." *Frontiers in Pharmacology*, vol. 8, 2017, doi:10.3389/fphar.2017.00472.

Pandey, Abhay K., and Pooja Singh. "The Genus Artemisia: a 2012-2017 Literature Review on Chemical Composition, Antimicrobial, Insecticidal and Antioxidant Activities of Essential Oils." *Medicines*, vol. 4, no. 3, Dec. 2017, p. 68., doi:10.3390/medicines4030068.

Peana AT, D'Aquila PS, Panin F, et al. "Anti-Inflammatory Activity of Linalool and Linalyl Acetate Constituents of Essential Oils." *Phytomedicine*. 2002;9(8):721-726.

Peana AT, D'Aquila PS, Panin F, et al. "Anti-Inflammatory Activity of Linalool and Linalyl Acetate Constituents of Essential Oils." *Phytomedicine*. 2002;9(8):721-726.

Piccinelli, Ana Claudia, et al. "Antihyperalgesic and Antidepressive Actions of (R)-( )-Limonene, α-Phellandrene, and Essential Oil From Schinus Terebinthifolius fruits in a Neuropathic Pain Model." *Nutritional Neuroscience*, vol. 18, no. 5, 2014, pp. 217-224., doi:10.1179/1476830514y.0000000119.

Pourghanbari, Gholamhosein, et al. "Antiviral Activity of the Oseltamivir and Melissa Officinalis L. Essential Oil against Avian Influenza A Virus (H9N2)." *Virus Disease*, vol. 27, no. 2, 2016, pp. 170-178., doi:10.1007/s13337-016-0321-0.

Raina AP, Negi KS, Dutta M. "Variability in Essential Oil Composition of Sage (Salvia officinalis L.) Grown Under North Western Himalayan Region of India." *Journal of Medicinal Plants Research*. 2013;7(11):683-688.

Rath, Cc, et al. "Antibacterial Potential Assessment of Jasmine Essential Oil against E. Coli." *Indian Journal of Pharmaceutical Sciences*, vol. 70, no. 2, 2008, p. 238., doi:10.4103/0250-474x.41465.

Ribeiro-Filho, Helder Veras, et al. "Biphasic Cardiovascular and Respiratory Effects Induced by ß-Citronellol." *European Journal of Pharmacology*, vol. 775, 2016, pp. 96-105., doi:10.1016/j.ejphar.2016.02.025.

Rivas da Silva, A.C., Lopes, P.M., Barros de Azevedo, M.M., et al. "Biological Activities of A-pinene and ß-pinene Enantiomers." *Molecules*. 2012;17(6):6305-6316.

Sadraei, H., et al. "Inhibitory Effect of Rosa Damascena Mill Flower Essential Oil, Geraniol and Citronellol on Rat Ileum Contraction." *Research in Pharmaceutical Sciences*, vol. 8, no. 1, Jan. 2013, pp. 17-23.

Santos, F. A., and V. S. N. Rao. "Anti-inflammatory and Antinociceptive Effects of 1,8-Cineole a Terpenoid Oxide Present in Many Plant Essential Oils." *Phytotherapy Research*, vol. 14, no. 4, 2000, pp. 240-244., doi:10.1002/1099-1573(200006)14:4<240::aid-ptr573>3.0.co;2-x.

Sayowan, Winai, et al. "The Effects of Jasmine Oil Inhalation on Brain Wave Activities and Emotions." *Journal of Health Research*, vol. 27, no. 2, Apr. 2013, pp. 73-77.

Sena-Lopes, Ângela, et al. "Chemical Composition, Immunostimulatory, Cytotoxic and Antiparasitic Activities of the Essential Oil from Brazilian Red Propolis." *Plos One*, vol. 13, no. 2, Jan. 2018, doi:10.1371/journal.pone.0191797.

Shaghayegh Pishkhan Dibazar, Shirin Fateh & Saeed Daneshmandi (2015) Immunomodulatory effects of clove (Syzygium aromaticum) constituents on macrophages: In vitro evaluations of aqueous and ethanolic components, Journal of Immunotoxicology, 12:2, 124-131, DOI: 10.3109/1547691X.2014.912698

Shakeel-u-Rehman., et al. "Essential Oil Composition of Rosmarinus officinalis L. from Kashmir (India)". *EC Microbiology* 14.2, 2018: 29-32.

Sharafzadeh, Shahram, and Omid Alizadeh. "German and Roman Chamomile." *Journal of Applied Pharmaceutical Science*, vol. 01, no. 10, 2011, pp. 01-05.

Singh A, Handa SS, "Hepatoprotective activity of Apium graveolens and Hygrophila auriculata against paracetamol and thioacetamide intoxication in rats", Journal of Ethnopharmacology (1995); 49(3)

Soares, Pedro Marcos G., et al. "Effects of Anethole and Structural Analogues on the Contractility of Rat Isolated Aorta: Involvement of Voltage-Dependent Ca2 -Channels." *Life Sciences*, vol. 81, no. 13, 2007, pp. 1085-1093., doi:10.1016/j.lfs.2007.08.027.

Sripathi R, Jayagopal D, Ravi S. "A Study on the Seasonal Variation of the Essential Oil Composition from Plectranthus Hadiensis and its Antibacterial Activity." *National Product Research*. 2017 Aug 8:1-4. doi: 10.1080/14786419.2017.1363748.

Takaishi, Masayuki, et al. "1,8-Cineole, a TRPM8 Agonist, Is a Novel Natural Antagonist of Human TRPA1." *Molecular Pain*, vol. 8, 2012, doi:10.1186/1744-8069-8-86.

Takeda, Ai, et al. "Effects of Inhalation Aromatherapy on Symptoms of Sleep Disturbance in the Elderly with Dementia." *Evidence-Based Complementary and Alternative Medicine*, vol. 2017, 2017, pp. 1-7., doi:10.1155/2017/1902807.

Tisserand, Robert, et al. *Essential Oil Safety: a Guide for Health Care Professionals*. Churchill Livingstone/Elsevier, 2014.

Tognolini, Massimiliano, et al. "Protective Effect of Foeniculum Vulgare Essential Oil and Anethole in an Experimental Model of Thrombosis." *Pharmacological Research*, vol. 56, no. 3, 2007, pp. 254-260., doi:10.1016/j.phrs.2007.07.002.

Tuetun B, et al., "Mosquito repellency of the seeds of celery (Apium graveolens L.)" Annals of Tropical Medicine and Parasitology (2004); 98(4)

Uyeda, Saori, et al. "Enhancement and Regulation Effect of Myrcene on Antibody Response in Immunization with Ovalbumin and Ag85B in Mice." *Asian Pacific Journal of Allergy and Immunology*, 2016, doi:10.12932/ap0734.

Valente, J., et al. "Antifungal, Antioxidant and Anti-Inflammatory Activities of Oenanthe Crocata L. Essential Oil." *Food and Chemical Toxicology*, vol. 62, 2013, pp. 349-354., doi:10.1016/j.fct.2013.08.083.

Vergara-Galicia Jorge, et al., "Vasorelaxant activity of extracts obtained from Apium graveolens: Possible source for vasorelaxant molecules isolation with potential antihypertensive effect", Asian Pacific Journal of Tropical Biomedicine (2013); 3(10)

Viana, Glauce Socorro De Barros, et al. "Anticonvulsant Activity of Essential Oils and Active Principles from Chemotypes of Lippia Alba(Mill.) N.E. Brown." *Biological & Pharmaceutical Bulletin*, vol. 23, no. 11, 2000, pp. 1314-1317., doi:10.1248/bpb.23.1314.

Vidhya Unnikrishnan, and K Nishteswar. "Cardio Protective Activities of Herbal Formulation of Bhavamishra - A Review." *International Ayurvedic Medical Journal*, vol. 3, no. 2320, Mar. 2015, pp. 850-861.

Viveros-Paredes, Juan, et al. "Neuroprotective Effects of ß-Caryophyllene against Dopaminergic Neuron Injury in a Murine Model of Parkinson's Disease Induced by MPTP." *Pharmaceuticals*, vol. 10, no. 4, June 2017, p. 60., doi:10.3390/ph10030060.

Yamahara, Johji, et al. "Stomachic Principles in Ginger. II. Pungent and Anti-Ulcer Effects of Low Polar Constituents Isolated from Ginger, the Dried Rhizoma of Zingiber Officinale ROSCOE Cultivated in Taiwan. The Absolute Stereostructure of a New Diarylheptanoid." *Yakugaku Zasshi*, vol. 112, no. 9, 1992, pp. 645-655., doi:10.1248/yakushi1947.112.9_645.

Yang, Z., Wu, N., Zu, Y., Et Al. "Comparative Anti-Infectious Bronchitis Virus (IBV) Activity of (-)-pinene: Effect on Nucleocapsid (N) Protein." *Molecules*. 2011;16(2):1044-1054.

Yin, Qing-Hua, et al. "Anti-Proliferative and pro-Apoptotic Effect of Carvacrol on Human Hepatocellular Carcinoma Cell Line HepG-2." *Cytotechnology*, vol. 64, no. 1, 2011, pp. 43-51., doi:10.1007/s10616-011-9389-y.

Zalachoras, Ioannis, et al. "Assessing the Local Anesthetic Effect of Five Essential Oil Constituents." *Planta Medica*, vol. 76, no. 15, 2010, pp. 1647-1653., doi:10.1055/s-0030-1249956.

Index

A

a2z Chewable™ 173, 230
Abōde™ 48, 128, 192
Abscess 21, 105
Absentmindedness 21
Abuse Recovery 21, 145
Aches 21, 68, 78, 81, 107,
    114, 116, 134, 159,
    183, 201
Acid Reflux 21, 71, 144,
    156, 183, 184
Acne 21, 64, 90, 107, 114,
    117, 119, 148, 183,
    184, 235
Actinic Keratosis 21
Adaptiv™ 24, 34, 41, 51,
    55, 129, 173, 186,
    188, 189, 193, 200,
    201, 203, 206
Adaptiv™ Complex 173,
    186, 188, 189, 193,
    200, 201, 203, 206
ADD/ADHD 21, 70, 121,
    157, 176, 180, 183,
    185
Addiction: Alcohol 21
Addiction: Caffeine 21
Addiction: Drugs 21
Addiction: Food 21
Addiction: Internet/Video
    Games 21
Addiction: Pain Medication
    22
Addiction: Sex/ Pornogra-
    phy 22
Addiction: Smoking 22
Addiction: Sugar 22
Addiction: Work 22
Addison's Disease 22
Adenitis 22, 111
Adrenal Fatigue 22, 63, 66,
    111, 134, 147, 158,
    169, 183, 185
Age Spots 22, 149
Aging 22, 96, 97, 110, 141,
    149, 215
Agitation 22, 132
AIDS 22, 88, 183, 185
Airborne Bacteria 22, 73,
    74, 94, 164
Air Pollution 22
Air-X™ 22, 130
Alertness 23, 106, 162
Align 131, 214, 224
Alkalosis 23
Allergies (Seasonal, Pet
    Dander) 23
Alpha CRS® 173
Alzheimer's/ Dementia 23
Amnesia 23
Analgesic 23, 65, 66, 76,
    77, 80, 83, 90, 93, 94,
    98, 100, 106, 109,
    113, 115, 119, 120,
    123, 271, 273, 297
Anchor 132, 188, 202, 232
Anemia 23, 49, 54
Aneurysm 23, 75, 79, 83,
    85, 117
Anger 23, 98, 135, 141,
    146, 159, 165, 239,
    251
Angina 23
Anguish 23
Animals: Bleeding 23
Animals: Bone Pain 23
Animals: Cancer (skin) 23
Animals: Colds & Cough 24
Animals: Stress & Anxiety
    24
Ankle Swelling 24
Ankylosing Spondylitis 24
Anorexia 24, 86, 109
Antibacterial 24, 62, 63,
    69, 72, 74, 79, 87, 88,
    91, 93, 96, 100, 101,
    104, 119, 122, 271,
    276
Anticoagulant 24, 88
Antidepressant 24, 64, 73,
    83, 84, 89, 96, 97,
    101, 103, 107, 110,
    112, 125, 271
Antifungal 24, 66, 74, 93,
    271, 280
Antioxidant 24, 65, 72, 73,
    76, 80, 97, 118, 142,
    166, 169, 174, 177,
    180, 271, 283
Antisocial 24
Antiviral 24, 65, 69, 76, 81,
    86, 92, 95, 96, 101,
    104, 119, 271, 289
Anxiety 24, 29, 34, 41, 65,
    67, 70, 72, 77, 83, 89,
    90, 91, 92, 96, 98,
    101, 102, 103, 110,
    113, 119, 120, 121,
    122, 125, 129, 135,
    138, 139, 145, 150,
    151, 154, 163, 165,
    172, 173, 179, 180,
    183, 186
Apathy 24, 89, 161
Aphrodisiac 25, 68, 97,
    110, 112, 140, 161,
    168, 271, 290
Appetite Stimulant 25
Appetite Suppressant 25,
    86
Arborvitae 21, 26, 30, 32,
    33, 34, 35, 37, 38, 39,
    40, 43, 45, 46, 50, 51,
    52, 53, 54, 55, 56,
    57, 58, 62, 128, 146,
    167, 190, 191, 192,
    194, 203, 206, 208,
    209, 240, 256, 267
Arise 133, 193, 237
AromaTouch® 21, 25, 30,
    32, 34, 36, 37, 39, 40,
    41, 44, 46, 47, 55, 57,
    134, 198, 201, 204,
    234
Arrhythmia 25
Arteriosclerosis 25
Artery Issues 25
Arthritic Pain 25
Asthma 25, 68, 81, 83, 93,
    101, 106, 107, 113,
    118, 130, 136, 158,
    183, 187
Atherosclerosis 25
Athlete's Foot 25, 74, 77,
    96, 99, 104, 117, 155
Autism/Asperger's 25
Autoimmune Disorders 25,
    160
Autointoxication 25

B

Back Pain 25, 112, 135,
    143, 183, 188
Back Stiffness 26
Bacterial Infection 26, 67,
    73, 95, 118, 148
Bags Under Eyes 26
Balance 21, 23, 24, 26, 34,
    36, 40, 41, 46, 47, 49,
    51, 52, 53, 54, 55, 56,
    57, 69, 75, 83, 84, 96,
    121, 125, 129, 134,
    135, 140, 141, 145,
    147, 150, 161, 165,
    168, 169, 172, 173,
    183, 186, 188, 199,
    200, 202, 203, 205,
    206, 207, 208, 213,
    217, 224, 226, 235,
    236, 241, 242, 246,
    250, 251
Balance Problems 26
Balding 26
Basal Cell Carcinoma 26
Basil 22, 23, 24, 25, 26, 28,
    29, 32, 34, 35, 36, 38,
    39, 41, 44, 45, 46, 48,
    49, 50, 51, 53, 54, 55,
    56, 57, 58, 59, 63,
    119, 131, 134, 139,
    158, 185, 189, 192,
    194, 198, 207, 222,
    257, 265, 279, 283,
    284, 288, 292, 294,
    298, 300, 302
Bed Bugs 26
Bed Sores 26
Bed-wetting 26
Bee Sting 26, 152
Bell's Palsy 26
Bergamot 21, 22, 23, 24,
    25, 27, 28, 30, 31, 32,
    35, 36, 37, 45, 46, 48,
    50, 51, 52, 54, 58, 59,
    64, 70, 78, 90, 96,
    122, 125, 128, 131,
    138, 140, 146, 147,
    161, 163, 168, 191,
    193, 195, 218, 220,
    240, 241, 246, 263,
    264, 274, 276, 277,
    281, 284, 286, 289,
    292, 294, 295, 299,
    300, 301, 302, 304
Bipolar Disorder 26, 132,
    173, 183, 188
Bites 26, 42, 56, 81, 91, 93,
    118, 139, 164
Black Pepper 21, 22, 26, 29,
    30, 31, 36, 37, 42, 44,
    46, 47, 50, 52, 54, 55,
    58, 65, 96, 132, 156,
    160, 177, 189, 191,
    192, 195, 200, 201,
    202, 206, 214, 248,
    259, 273, 275, 276,
    277, 278, 280, 281,
    282, 283, 284, 286,
    287, 291, 292, 294,
    295, 296, 297, 299,
    304
Black Spruce 22, 42, 45, 66,
    72, 159, 185, 199,
    200, 201, 202, 203,
    206, 273, 275, 278,
    282, 283, 285, 287,

Index

Index

DIY's, Roller Blends & Diffuser Recipe

DIY RECIPES

DIFFUSER RECIPES

ROLLER BOTTLE BLENDS

Photography Credits

Thank you to the up-and-coming artists on Unsplash for putting their work into the world. The following artists' beautiful photography is found throughout Advanced Oil Magic.

INTRO

Joshua Fuller
Eddie Hooiveld
Yasin Hoşgör
Liana Mikah
Katherine Hanlon
Holger Link
Ian Wagg
Joshua Coleman

AILMENTS

Mehrshad Rajabi
Christin Hume
Rizky Subagja
Jeshoots.com
Evelyn Mostrom
Iler Stoe
Julie Johnson
Nik MacMillan
Stacey Rozells
Annie Spratt
Omar Lopez
Andrew Pons
A Fox
Oliver Sjöström
Tanja Heffner
Andrii Podilnyk
Fabio Spinelli
Xavier Mouton Photographie
Edward Virvel
Kelly Sikkema

Artem Bali
Matteo Vistocco
Rawpixel

SINGLE OILS

Tamara Garcevic
Francesca Hotchin
Milan Popovic
Grace Ho
Matteo Vistocco
Taya Iv
Aziz Acharki
Roberto Nickson
Neil Rosenstech
Miroslava
Taylor Kiser
Simon Matzinger
Daiga Ellaby
Pablo Lancaster Jones
Rawpixel
Element5 Digital
Juliane Liebermann
Andrew Neel
Alex Geerts
Attentie Attentie
Edward Boulton
Artem Bali
Andrés Medina
Alexandra Golovac
Dan Gold
James Sutton
Mike Kenneally
Tracey Hocking

Bin Thiều
Georgia de Lotz
Kyle Loftus
Alex Blăjan
Christin Hume
Kelly Sikkema
Rose Elena
Rhand McCoy
Ryan Christodoulou
Alexandre Croussette
Becca Tapert
Icons8 team
Benjamin Voros
Zuza Reinhard
Aiony Haust
Daryn Stumbaugh
Anthony Tran
Yuvraj Singh
Cristian Palmer
Matheus Frade
Joanna Kosinska
Max Bender
Marvin Meyer
Anna Sullivan
Roberto Salinas
Laura Marques
Chris Jarvis
Julie Johnson
Dan Gold
Les Anderson
Edward Virvel
Clem Onojeghuo
Geert Pieters
Nathan Peterson
Mi Pham

Matthew LeJune
Severin Höin
Joseph Barrientos
Faye Cornish
Lyndon Li
Paulius Dragunas
Toa Heftiba
Thomas Heintz
Lera Freeland
Alexander Michl
Kirill Zakharov
Easton Oliver
Willian Justen de Vasconcellos
Kyle Loftus
Dominik Jirovský
Shari Sirotnak
Sebastien Gabriel
Huan Minh
Jason Briscoe
Giulia Bertelli
Charlotte Karlsen
Eric Nopanen
Joseph Pearson
Daniel Silva Gaxiola
Kinga Cichewicz
Yoann Boyer
Danielle MacInnes

OIL BLENDS

Olivia Bauso
Marvin Meyer
Daiga Ellaby

Alora Griffiths
Kevin Grieve
Atikh Bana
Jason Leung
Victor Vorontsov
Jon Moore
Annie Spratt
Kelly Sikkema
Caroline Hernandez
Ben White
Michael Podger
Kiana Bosman
Blake Meyer
Robert Collins
Justin Young
Thao Le Hoang
Naomi Koelemans
Ricardo Resende
Sharon McCutcheon
Charles Deluvio
Hilary Hahn
Sarah Shaffer
Raul Petri
Heather Schwartz
Nick West
Rodion Kutsaev
Ksenya von Shlezinger
Loverna Journey
Andy HYD
Tomas Sobek
Oleg Ivanov
Thomas Rey
Alan Caishan
Dominik Jirovsky

SUPPLEMENTS

Ben White
Jared Erondu
Jenn Evelyn-Ann
Rawpixel
Tim Tiedemann
Brooke Lark
Vincent Foret
Jay Wennington
Shangyou Shi
Clique Images
Tomas Anton Escobar
Ja Ma
Albert Melu
Joshua Yu
Taylor Kiser
Brooke Lark
Erwan Hesry
Annie Spratt
Ivan Jevtic
Kinga Cichewicz
Alexandr Podvalny
Lon Christensen
Gesing Kunkel

AILMENT PROTOCOLS

Qingbao Meng

EMOTIONS & ENERGY

Anders Jildén
Geetanjal Khanna
Feliphe Schiarolli
Simon Migaj
Savs
Dev
Jason Rosewell

Bruce Mars
Fotografia.ges
Vitaliy Paykov
Annie Spratt
Hutomo Abrianto
Sharon Garcia
Warren Wong
JC Gellidon
Ian Espinosa
Ian Dooley
Pawel Janiak
Tim Mossholder
Andy Omvik
Marek Mucha

LIFESTYLE PROTOCOLS

Julia Caesar
Austin Neill
Brandon Bynum
Darius Bashar
Alexander Redl
Laura Marques
Julie Johnson
Myung-Won Seo
Janko Ferlič
Paola Aguilar
Hannah Grace
Aziz Acharki
Karl Fredrickson
Chad Madden
Matheus Ferrero
Manuel Meurisse
Jorge Barahona
Brook Anderson
Sebastián León Prado
Sai De Silva
Toa Heftiba
Mari Lezhava
Ben White
Lopez Robin

Brooke Cagle
Kevin Ku
Calum MacAulay
Caleb Jones

Protocol Tracker

Name of Protocol Used — Page #

Start Date

Who is it for?

End Date

Severity of Condition Prior *(circle one)*

0 1 2 3 4 5 6 7 8 9 10

Severity of Condition After *(circle one)*

0 1 2 3 4 5 6 7 8 9 10

Products Used *(highlight favorites)*

#1

#2

#3

#4

#5

#6

#7

Goals for the Protocol *(fill out before)*

What Went Well *(fill out after)*

Products to Continue and New Products to Try for Support *(fill out after)*

Protocol Tracker

Name of Protocol Used — Page #

Start Date

Who is it for?

End Date

Severity of Condition Prior *(circle one)*

0 1 2 3 4 5 6 7 8 9 10

Severity of Condition After *(circle one)*

0 1 2 3 4 5 6 7 8 9 10

Products Used *(highlight favorites)*

#1

#2

#3

#4

#5

#6

#7

Goals for the Protocol *(fill out before)*

What Went Well *(fill out after)*

Products to Continue and New Products to Try for Support *(fill out after)*

Protocol Tracker

Start Date

Who is it for?

End Date

Severity of Condition Prior *(circle one)*

0   1   2   3   4   5   6   7   8   9   10

Severity of Condition After *(circle one)*

0   1   2   3   4   5   6   7   8   9   10

Products Used *(highlight favorites)*

#1

#2

#3

#4

#5

#6

#7

Goals for the Protocol *(fill out before)*

What Went Well *(fill out after)*

Products to Continue and New Products to Try for Support
(fill out after)

Protocol Tracker

Name of Protocol Used — Page #

Start Date

Who is it for?

End Date

Severity of Condition Prior *(circle one)*

0 1 2 3 4 5 6 7 8 9 10

Severity of Condition After *(circle one)*

0 1 2 3 4 5 6 7 8 9 10

Products Used *(highlight favorites)*

#1

#2

#3

#4

#5

#6

#7

Goals for the Protocol *(fill out before)*

What Went Well *(fill out after)*

Products to Continue and New Products to Try for Support *(fill out after)*

References

Protocol Tracker

Name of Protocol Used *Page #*

Start Date

Who is it for?

End Date

Severity of Condition Prior *(circle one)*

0 1 2 3 4 5 6 7 8 9 10

Severity of Condition After *(circle one)*

0 1 2 3 4 5 6 7 8 9 10

Products Used *(highlight favorites)*

#1

#2

#3

#4

#5

#6

#7

Goals for the Protocol *(fill out before)*

What Went Well *(fill out after)*

Products to Continue and New Products to Try for Support *(fill out after)*

Protocol Tracker

Start Date

Who is it for?

End Date

Severity of Condition Prior *(circle one)*

0   1   2   3   4   5   6   7   8   9   10

Severity of Condition After *(circle one)*

0   1   2   3   4   5   6   7   8   9   10

Products Used *(highlight favorites)*

#1

#2

#3

#4

#5

#6

#7

Goals for the Protocol *(fill out before)*

What Went Well *(fill out after)*

Products to Continue and New Products to Try for Support *(fill out after)*

References

Protocol Tracker

Name of Protocol Used *Page #*

Start Date

Who is it for?

End Date

Severity of Condition Prior *(circle one)*

0 1 2 3 4 5 6 7 8 9 10

Severity of Condition After *(circle one)*

0 1 2 3 4 5 6 7 8 9 10

Products Used *(highlight favorites)*

#1

#2

#3

#4

#5

#6

#7

Goals for the Protocol *(fill out before)*

What Went Well *(fill out after)*

Products to Continue and New Products to Try for Support *(fill out after)*

Protocol Tracker

Start Date

Who is it for?

End Date

Severity of Condition Prior *(circle one)*

0   1   2   3   4   5   6   7   8   9   10

Severity of Condition After *(circle one)*

0   1   2   3   4   5   6   7   8   9   10

Products Used *(highlight favorites)*

#1

#2

#3

#4

#5

#6

#7

Goals for the Protocol *(fill out before)*

What Went Well *(fill out after)*

Products to Continue and New Products to Try for Support *(fill out after)*

References

335

"Magic is believing in yourself. If you can do that,
you can make anything happen."

-Johann Wolfgang von Goethe